Atlas of
Liver Pathology

Current Histopathology

Consultant Editor
Professor G. Austin Gresham, TD, ScD, MD, FRCPath.
Emeritus Professor of Morbid Anatomy and Histopathology,
University of Cambridge

Volume Twenty-three

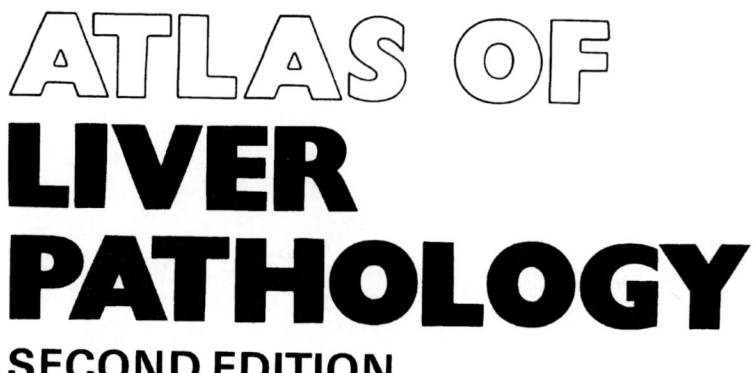

ATLAS OF
LIVER
PATHOLOGY
SECOND EDITION

By
D. G. D. WIGHT
Department of Histopathology
University of Cambridge
Addenbrooke's Hospital
Cambridge, UK

 Springer-Science+Business Media, B.V.

Library of Congress Cataloging-in-Publication Data

Wight, D. G. D.
  Atlas of liver pathology / by D.G.D. Wight.—2nd ed.
    p.   cm. — (Current histopathology ; v. 23)
  Includes bibliographical references and index.
  ISBN 978-0-7923-8819-7 (casebound)
  1. Liver—Diseases—Diagnosis—Atlases.
  I. Title. II. Series.
  [DNLM: 1. Liver Diseases—pathology—atlases.
  2. Liver—pathology—atlases. W1 CU788JBA v.23
1993 / WI 17 W657a 1993]
RC847.W48 1993
616.3'6207583—dc20
DNLM/DLC
for Library of Congress   93-17187
                                                   CIP

Contents

Current Histopathology Series

Other volumes currently scheduled in this series include the following titles

Atlas of AIDS Pathology

Atlas of Bone Tumours

Atlas of Correlative Surgical Neuropathology and Imaging

Atlas of Endocrine Pathology

Atlas of Ocular Pathology

Atlas of Renal Transplantation Pathology

Atlas of Soft Tissue Pathology

Consultant Editor's Note

At the present time books on morbid anatomy and histopathology can be divided into two broad groups: extensive textbooks often written primarily for students and monographs on research topics.

This takes no account of the fact that the vast majority of pathologists are involved in an essentially practical field of general diagnostic pathology providing an important service to their clinical colleagues. Many of these pathologists are expected to cover a broad range of disciplines and even those who remain solely within the field of histopathology usually have single and sole responsibility within the hospital for all this work. They may often have no colleagues in the same department. In the field of histopathology, no less than in other medical fields, there have been extensive and recent advances, not only in new histochemical techniques but also in the type of specimen provided by new surgical procedures.

There is a great need for the provision of appropriate information for this group. This need has been defined in the following terms:

1. It should be aimed at the general clinical pathologist or histopathologist with existing practical training, but should have value for the trainee pathologist.

2. It should concentrate on the practical aspects of histopathology taking account of the new techniques which should be within the compass of the worker in a unit with reasonable facilities.

3. New types of material, e.g. those derived from endoscopic biopsy should be covered fully.

4. There should be an adequate number of illustrations on each subject to demonstrate the variation in appearance that is encountered.

5. Colour illustrations should be used wherever they aid recognition.

Consultant histopathologists, pathologists in training, clinicians and medical students will find the second edition of this popular atlas to be a useful addition to their learning and practice. Expanding knowledge about infective liver disease, disorders associated with new therapeutic agents, autoimmune hepatitis and other topics are dealt with in this new addition. Pictures have been added and changed but the basic principles enunciated by the author remain. He emphasizes the increasing importance of clinico-pathological correlation and the need to try to understand the pathogenetic mechanisms of liver disorders. Medical students and pathologists in training will find this approach of great value.

It is a special pleasure to introduce a second edition in this series of Atlases by a colleague of long standing. The original aim of the series to produce up-to-date bench manuals for those at the sharp end of histopathology is an achievement that is being maintained.

G. A. Gresham

Foreword

Although the technique of needle biopsy of the liver was introduced as long ago as 1883 by Paul Ehrlich, it has only come into general use in the last 10–20 years. It is now an accepted procedure in most large general hospitals. Concurrently with new advances and interest in liver disease, there have been considerable advances in the design of biopsy needles. Moreover, surgeons and laparoscopists are more likely to biopsy the liver under direct vision than in the past. The consequence of these changes has been that increasing demands are being made upon pathologists.

This book is intended for the practising pathologist, the trainee pathologist and for the clinician who performs biopsies of the liver. It is designed to provide, with the help of many colour illustrations, a practical guide to histopathological diagnosis of liver disorders. Particular emphasis is placed upon clinicopathological correlation and the need for the pathologist to be in full possession of all the available clinical information for his opinion to be of value.

Whilst it is in no way attempting to compete with larger texts, the book is intended to be more than just an atlas and thus each section includes a brief description of the main clinical and pathological features of the subject under discussion. Pathogenetic mechanisms are discussed where these are known and where morphology can contribute to their understanding. Similarly, although the majority of the illustrations are of histological preparations, macro-photographs are included where these are helpful. It has not been thought necessary to state magnification factors for the micrographs. H&E stain has been used unless specified otherwise.

Where appropriate, attention will also be drawn to the limitations of biopsy. A biopsy represents only a tiny fraction of the liver as a whole and although many diseases are diffuse, the biopsy may not be entirely representative. Amongst our own material, approximately 25% of biopsies provide no positive diagnosis, despite the fact that a proportion of these patients are subsequently shown to be suffering from primary liver disease.

Because of the emphasis on clinicopathological correlations and pathogenetic mechanisms, I believe the book will also be of use to postgraduates and residents in other branches of medicine, especially those studying for higher examinations, and to senior medical students.

In this new edition, the basic philosophy remains the same, but many advances, for example in viral hepatitis, have required that many chapters have had to be rewritten or extensively revised, and many new illustrations have been added.

All illustrations are of sections stained with haematoxylin and eosin unless otherwise stated. Magnifications are no longer included since they are now widely recognized as having little or no value.

ACKNOWLEDGEMENTS

I am deeply indebted to many people without whose help this book would never have been written. In particular, I am grateful to Dr Janice Anderson for much help and encouragement; to Chris Burton and the late Peter Haslam for the macroscopic photography; to the technical staff of the Department of Histopathology, Addenbrooke's Hospital, for invaluable technical help; to the members of my slide club for sending me numerous sections over many years; to Dr David Ansell, Professor M S R Hutt, Dr Fernando Paradinas, Dr Bernard Portmann and Prof Michel Reynès for letting me have specific sections to photograph (indicated in the relevant sections); to Miss Susen Green for help with typing the manuscript; and finally to my colleagues in Histopathology and to my family for their tolerance during another long period of gestation.

Liver Biopsy

1

Pathological examination of the liver is essential for the understanding and classification of liver disease. Furthermore, liver biopsy is now an essential step in the management of patients with a wide range of different diseases affecting or apparently affecting the liver. It is thus vital, following a procedure which carries a small but definite risk to the patient[1], that the pathologist extracts the maximum possible information from the specimen that is available.

In contrast to disease in other parts of the body, the whole organ is usually only available for study at autopsy, or, in the increasing number of centres where it is practised, following liver transplantation. Many benign and non-progressive diseases never reach that stage and thus it is the correct interpretation of biopsies that is the principal concern of practising pathologists.

Liver disease may be either focal or diffuse. Unfortunately it is not always possible to know as a result of clinical examination and investigation from which of these types the patient suffers. However, modern diagnostic procedures such as radioisotope and ultrasonic scans, computerized tomography (CT) and magnetic resonance imaging (MRI), have greatly increased the chances of detecting and localizing focal disease. When disease is shown to be localized the yield of positive biopsies is vastly increased if the lesion is biopsied directly. At its simplest, this may be under direct vision at laparotomy or laparoscopy[2], or it may be possible to aim a percutaneous needle directly at the lesion. If malignant disease is suspected, fine needle aspiration biopsy has been shown to produce excellent results, at minimal risk to the patient[3].

In the majority of cases, however, biopsy is blind and the disease, presumptively at least, diffuse. There are two main types of biopsy needle/the Menghini or aspiration type[4,5], and the cutting type exemplified by the Trucut® needle[6]. The choice of needle is largely determined by factors such as personal preference and economics, but each tends to have its advantages and disadvantages[7]. With aspiration needles the sample can be quite large, which is particularly desirable if the biopsy has to be divided for chemical analysis or electron microscopy as well as histological examination. The principal disadvantage of this needle is its tendency to cause fragmentation in the presence of fibrous tissue, much of which can be left behind (although this is much less of a problem with modern ultra-sharp disposable needles). Conversely this is precisely the type of case in which the cutting type of needle is so effective. If there are contraindications to percutaneous biopsies, such as a haemorrhagic tendency or biliary obstruction, transvenous biopsy may be a satisfactory alternative[8].

HANDLING THE BIOPSY

Once obtained, the biopsy must be properly handled if maximum information is to be obtained. Inspection, although not always helpful, may occasionally be useful and thus the appearance should always be recorded. For example, tumour appears pale and may involve only part of the biopsy; or the colour may provide a pointer towards the disease, e.g. in biliary obstruction it will be dark green, in haemochromatosis brown, in Dubin Johnson syndrome black, or in congestive states, dark red. If chemical analysis or electron microscopy are required, part must be set aside at this stage. For best results, needle biopsies should be fixed flat–for example on a small piece of wooden spatula. Fixation, ideally in 10% buffered formal saline, should not be rushed, a minimum of 6 hours being necessary for best results, although with modern vacuum-assisted tissue-processing machines, this can be greatly reduced. If very long, the biopsy probably should be cut into 1.0–1.5 cm lengths. Wedge biopsies should be cut into 1.0 mm slices at right angles to the capsule, with a portion being set aside as a reserve in case, for example, frozen section should subsequently prove necessary.

The sample is then ready for processing through to paraffin wax in the usual way. The number of sections cut and stains performed is a matter for individual choice, but in this laboratory it is the practice to cut a serial ribbon and mount ten consecutive slides, each with about four to six sections. The first and last sections are then stained with haematoxylin and eosin (H & E) and the remainder retained for special stains. In the vast majority of cases, these provide a representative view of the biopsy and further sections or serialization of the whole biopsy are quite unnecessary. With the relatively greater amount of tissue available in a wedge biopsy, it is our practice to cut two or three step sections with several sections mounted at each level.

SPECIAL STAINS

The choice of stains is also a matter for preference, but we have found considerable advantages in performing four or five stains as a matter of routine. One of the most valuable of these is the *reticulin* stain with which one can appreciate architectural changes so much more readily than in H & E (Figure 1.1). This is especially true of thin bands of collagen which may be completely inapparent in the H & E. Recently orcein as well as being required to demonstrate both copper associated protein and HBsAg (Figure 1.2), has acquired a new role in the differentiation of collapse (which is unstained) from fibrosis, both of which may appear very similar in reticulin preparations[9]. The *Perl's* stain with a counterstain such as neutral red, as well as demonstrating iron in iron overload states, is particularly valuable for assessing the distribution of other pigments, such as bile and lipofuscin (Figure 1.3). *Periodic acid–Schiff* (PAS) after diastase digestion demonstrates basement membranes, bile and lipofuscin, as well as ceroid in active Kupffer cells (Figure 1.4). The globules of α_1-anti-trypsin in α_1-anti-trypsin deficiency may be completely missed without it. A connective tissue stain such as *trichrome* or *elastic van Gieson* (EVG) is used for the detection and assessment of collagen in conditions such as cirrhosis and alcoholic liver disease (Figure 1.5). Other stains can be used as necessary (Figure 1.6). The remaining unused spare sections are stored, along with the block, for possible use at a later date.

OTHER TECHNIQUES

Occasionally other techniques are required. From time to time it may be necessary to perform a rapid frozen section,

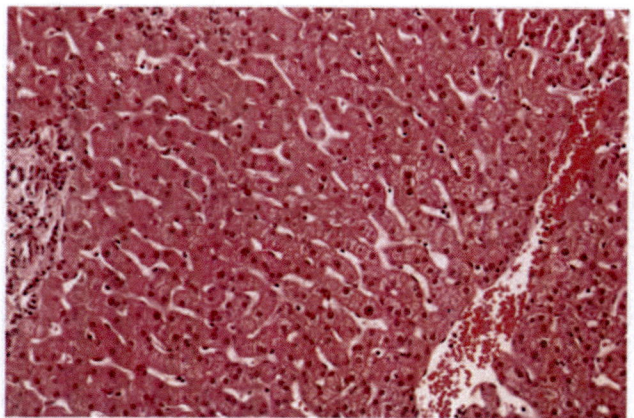

Figure 1.7 Normal liver. A portal tract is seen to the left and central vein to the right. Note the one-cell-thick liver cell plates radiating from the central vein. Kupffer cells are inconspicuous but can be seen as flattened nuclei on the sinusoidal aspect of some hepatocytes.

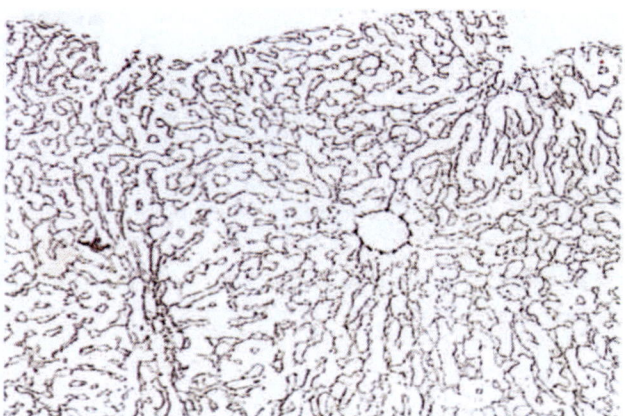

Figure 1.8 Normal liver. Normal reticulin framework. Reticulin.

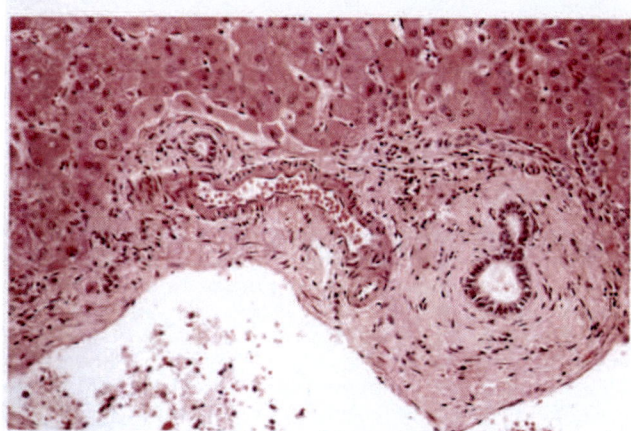

Figure 1.9 Normal liver. This section shows a large portal tract showing a branch of the portal vein inferiorly. hepatic artery and two bile ducts. The bile duct on the right shows an interlobular branch entering a septal duct. Note the ductules (or canals of Hering) leaving the liver (top right). Note also the normal concentric arrangement of collagen fibres around the septal duct. This should not be over-interpreted when associated with disease (see Chapter 20).

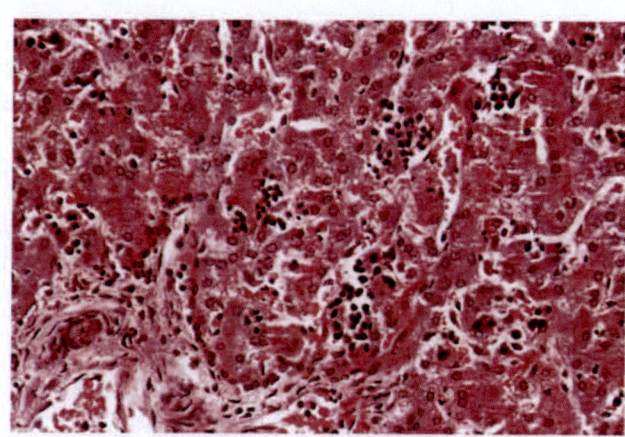

Figure 1.10 Neonatal liver. Note the broad liver cell plates and abundant sinusoidal erythropoiesis.

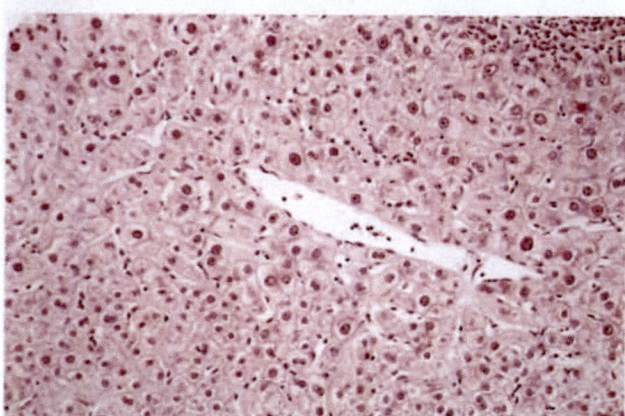

Figure 1.11 Senile liver. Note the increased size of many of the hepatocyte nuclei (due to polyploidy) around the central vein, in this biopsy from an elderly man.

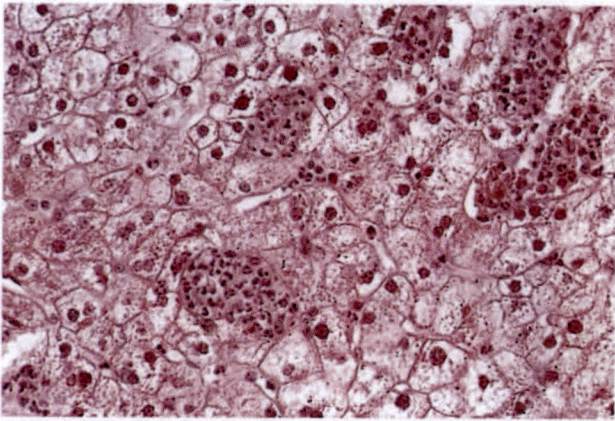

Figure 1.12 Operation artefact. Note the replacement of several hepatocytes by aggregates of neutrophils, whilst the remaining liver cells are entirely normal. The biopsy was taken at the end of a cholecystectomy operation.

for example in tumour diagnosis. On the whole this, wherever possible, is to be avoided, much better results being obtained by rapid processing which can now be achieved in some 3 hours. Water-soluble plastic embedding media are being increasingly used in histopathology. In the liver they are very useful for studying cytological features, since 1 μm sections can be cut quite easily and, with practice, most routine stains give satisfactory results[10]. Ultrastructure and chemical or enzyme analyses also both have a role to play, particularly in metabolic diseases, but play little part in day-to-day practice.

Increasingly immunoperoxidase techniques are being applied to the study of antigens such as HBsAg and α_1-anti-trypsin, and applications of the techniques are almost certain to increase in the next few years.

INTERPRETATION

A liver biopsy may represent only one fifty-thousandth part of the organ and thus it is important to know how representative and reproducible the results can be. A number of studies have confirmed that truly diffuse conditions, such as alcoholic and viral hepatitis, leukaemic infiltration and non-specific inflammation, show a high degree of correlation on multiple biopsies[11]. As perhaps would be expected, focal conditions, such as metastases, and diseases of variable intensity, such as chronic active hepatitis, show a much lower correlation[11,12], but clearly, the larger the biopsy the more likely it is to be diagnostic in this type of condition[13]. Inevitably there may also be significant variation between different observers[14], although this is much less between specialists in the field.

NORMAL FINDINGS

Normal lobular anatomy is illustrated in Figures 1.7–1.9. In functional terms it would be more proper to consider the liver in terms of Rappaport's acinus[15], a concept which has been readily grasped by histopathologists. However, old habits die hard and the terms centrilobular and periportal remain in common usage because application of acinar terminology is somewhat cumbersome in practice. Furthermore, even if not a functional reality, the lobule certainly exists as an anatomical entity, and no one seems to have created a term for the smallest bile ducts and portal venules other than 'interlobular'. Thus in this volume both terms tend to be used interchangeably, with the acinus especially mentioned when necessary to help in the understanding of a particular condition.

For the correct interpretation of the abnormal, it is necessary to be aware of the normal variation that exists in the liver. Portal tracts just beneath the capsule, especially at the anterior edge of the liver which is the main source of wedge biopsies, are frequently more fibrotic and have an abnormal inter-relationship which may simulate cirrhosis. However, these changes rarely extend deeper than 2 mm and thus, provided the biopsy is sectioned at right angles to the capsule, should not cause real difficulty. In infancy, twinning of liver cell plates, indicating active growth of liver cells in an adult, is a normal feature lasting for several years (Figure 1.10). Foci of extramedullary haemopoiesis and an excess of stainable iron may both persist for several weeks after birth. Hepatocyte nuclear vacuolation is regularly seen throughout childhood and has no significance. At the other extreme of life, the ageing liver commonly shows an increase of lipofuscin and increased ploidy of hepatocyte nuclei giving them a pleomorphic appearance (Figure 1.11). The latter should not be interpreted as evidence of regeneration. Increasing quantities of fat too are seen with increasing age[16].

ARTEFACTS

Artefacts are quite common and must be recognized for what they are. Processing and staining artefacts can be avoided by proper technique, but occasionally they may cause confusion. They should be suspected if any change such as cell swelling or shrinkage, or differential staining, is related to the edges of the biopsy, rather than to the micro-anatomy of the liver. Surgical biopsies, especially if taken at the end of the operation rather than the beginning, may show a very characteristic focal neutrophilic infiltration of hepatocytes within the liver cell plates (Figure 1.12). This can usually be readily distinguished from alcoholic hepatitis or other inflammatory disease by the complete absence of any other abnormality.

SECONDARY CHANGES

From time to time, although the liver appears to be affected by primary disease, the biochemical and histological changes may merely be a response to disease elsewhere in the body (Chapter 21). The liver changes are usually relatively non-specific, but when severe can be confused with viral hepatitis or other primary disease. Similarly, the biopsy needle may sample the vicinity of a focal lesion, such as tumour or an abscess, rather than the lesion itself. Changes such as sinusoidal dilatation, cholestasis in a non-jaundiced patient or granulation tissue should all alert one to the possibility of nearby focal disease.

SYSTEMATIC EVALUATION

Having considered all these other factors, the biopsy should then be examined in a systematic way. As with all small biopsies, it is most important that every part of every available slide is examined. In every case, the overall *architecture* should be assessed and the presence of collapse or fibrosis noted. *Hepatocytes* should be examined both for the integrity of liver cell plates and for degenerative changes, nuclear vacuolation, cholestasis and pigmentation amongst other features. Kupffer cells respond to injury mainly by increasing in activity, but the number and distribution of *Kupffer cells* should be noted and related to other changes, such as cholestasis or hepatocyte necrosis. *Adventitious cells* such as inflammatory cells, should be sought and their distribution, whether focal or uniform, portal tract or sinusoidal; and nature, whether lymphocytes, plasma cells or neoplastic, for example, should all be carefully noted. *Portal tracts* should be assessed, bearing in mind factors such as their size, presence or absence of fibrosis, the state of the *bile ducts* and vessels.

It is often a good idea to make a preliminary assessment in this way, before being made aware of the clinical data, thus avoiding bias. However, it cannot be emphasized too strongly that it is vital for the pathologist to have available to him all the clinical and investigational results before attempting a final diagnosis. In the absence of proper clinico-pathological correlations, not only will mistakes be made, but, more importantly, much valuable information to the benefit of the patient which could have been obtained from the biopsy is liable to be lost.

REFERENCES

1. Perrault, J., McGill, D. B., Ott, B. J. and Taylor, W. F. (1978). Liver biopsy complications in 1,000 in-patients and outpatients. Gastroenterology, 74, 103–106
2. Balfour, T. W. (1976). Laparoscopy in liver disease. Lancet, 1, 612–613
3. Ho, C. S., McLoughlin, M. J., Tao, L. C., Blendis, L. and K, E. W. (1981). Guided percutaneous fine needle aspiration biopsy of the liver. Cancer, 47, 1781–1785

4. Menghini, G., Lauro, G. and Caraceni, M. (1975). Some innovations in the technique of the one second needle biopsy of the liver. Am J Gastroenterol, 64, 175–180

5. Greenwald, R., Chiprut, R. O. and Schiff, E. R. (1977). Percutaneous aspiration liver biopsy using a large calibre disposable needle preliminary report. Am J Dig Dis, 22, 1109–1114

6. Rake, M. O., Murray-Lyon, I. M., Ansell, I. D. and Williams, R. (1969). Improved liver-biopsy needle. Lancet, 2, 1283

7. Bateson, M. C., Hopwood, D., Duguid, H. L. D. and Bouchier, I. A. D. (1980). Comparative trial of liver biopsy needles. J Clin Pathol, 33, 131–133

8. Lebrec, D., Degott, C., Rueff, B. and Benhamou, J.-P. (1978). Transvenous (transjugular) liver biopsy. An experience based on 100 biopsies. Am J Dig Dis, 23, 302–304

9. Scheuer, P. J. and Maggi, G. (1980). Hepatic fibrosis and collapse. Histopathology, 4, 487–490

10. Zerpa, H., Malik, N. J., Arborgh, B. A. M. and Scheuer, P. J. (1981). Application of routine and immunohistochemical staining methods to liver tissue embedded in water soluble resin. Liver, 1, 62–66

11. Abdi, W., Millan, J. C. and Mezey, E. (1979). Sampling variability on percutaneous liver biopsy. Arch Intern Med, 139, 667–669

12. Soloway, R. D., Baggenstoss, A. H., Schoenfield, L. J. and Summerskill, W. H. J. (1971). Observer error and sampling variability tested in evaluation of hepatitis and cirrhosis by liver biopsy. Am J Dig Dis, 16, 1082–1086

13. Hølund, B., Poulsen, H. and Schlichting, P. (1980). Reproducibility of liver biopsy diagnosis in relationship to size of specimen. Scand J Gastroenterol, 15, 329–335

14. Theodossi, A., Skene, A. M., Portmann, B., Knill-Jones, R. P., Patrick, R. S., Tate, R. A., Kealey, W., Jarvis, K. J., O'Brian, D. J. and Williams, R. (1980). Observer variation in assessment of liver biopsies including analysis by Kappa statistics. Gastroenterology, 29, 232–241

15. Rappaport, A. M. (1976). The microcirculation, acinar concept of normal and pathological hepatic structure. Beitr Pathol, 157, 215–243

16. Hilden, M., Christoffersen, P., Suhl, E. and Dalgaard, J. B. (1977). Liver histology in a normal population examination of 503 consecutive fatal traffic casualties. Scand J Gastroenterol, 12, 593–597

Viral Hepatitis

2

Although a number of different viruses may affect the liver the unqualified term viral (or virus) hepatitis usually implies infection by one of the hepatotrophic viruses, defined as infections in which the liver is the prime target and thus producing hepatitis as the major clinical manifestation. Although technically this definition might encompass some of the exotic viruses described in Chapter 3, such as yellow fever, by convention the term is restricted to those viruses now designated by letters of the alphabet. Five are well-characterized and called hepatitis A (or infectious hepatitis), hepatitis B (serum hepatitis) hepatitis C (parenteral non-A, non-B), hepatitis D (delta agent) and hepatitis E (epidemic non-A, non-B). Progress into our understanding of the organisms and the diseases that they cause has been spectacular in recent years.

Hepatitis A and hepatitis E are both self-limiting infections without chronic sequelae, whilst both hepatitis B and hepatitis C, although producing a similar acute illness, have a high rate of progression to chronic disease. Hepatitis D is a unique organism which forms a hybrid between its own viral core and surface components supplied by hepatitis B acting as a helper virus.

HEPATITIS A (HA)

Hepatitis A virus (HAV) is a highly contagious and ubiquitous virus, transmitted by the faecal–oral route. The virus has a 27 nm single stranded RNA genome without an envelope and is closely related to the picorna viruses; to date only one serotype has been recognized. HAV is shed in the stools for up to 2 weeks before the onset of acute hepatitis[1] and then disappears within a day or two of clinical illness. Virus multiplication takes place exclusively in the cytoplasm of hepatocytes and the organism returns to the gut after being shed in membrane-bound vesicles into the bile canaliculi and thence the biliary tree[2]. The infection has a relatively short incubation period of 15–40 days, tends to be seasonal and is maximal in children and young adults. Anicteric infection is common, particularly in children, and acute cases form the main reservoir. Serological evidence of past infection is present in from 29% of urban adults in Switzerland to 97% in former Yugoslavia[3]. Chronic liver disease and the carrier state are not seen, although, in common with the other hepatitis viruses, it can rarely cause fulminant disease which is often fatal (about 0.1% of all infections). Diagnosis is confirmed by finding IgM antibody to HAV, which indicates recent infection.

Pathogenesis of HA

It is not clear whether the organism has a primary replication phase in the intestine[4], but it is not known to be associated with any extrahepatic pathology. HAV grows only slowly in cells in culture without causing cytopathic effect, and hepatitis only occurs in vivo after the appearance of antibody, suggesting that the liver cell damage has a immunopathological basis[5].

HEPATITIS E (HE)

HE is an epidemiologically distinct form of non-A, non-B (NANB) hepatitis, principally transmitted by the faecal-oral route and found especially in poorer parts of the world where it is often water-borne[6]. The virus (HEV) is a non-enveloped 32–34 nm single positive strand RNA virus related to the caliciviruses[7,8]. Infection is often epidemic and the incubation period averages 6 weeks. Most patients develop a self-limited acute hepatitis, without chronic sequelae. Fulminant disease occurs overall in about 1%, but in as many as 20% or more of those infected during the third trimester of pregnancy[9]. There are currently no serological markers for HE, diagnosis being based on epidemiological evidence combined with absence of other markers. Close contact between damaged hepatocytes and lymphoid cells in experimental HE in cynomolgous monkeys suggests an immunological pathogenesis in this model[10], although nothing is known of the mechanism in humans.

HEPATITIS B (HB)

The Dane particle or complete virus (HBV) measures 42 nm in diameter and is composed of a central 27 nm core (HBcAg) containing a circular double stranded DNA nucleocapsid, surrounded by an envelope of surface antigen (HBsAg). Uniquely, HBV utilizes a linear RNA intermediate during replication, which is converted back to DNA by reverse transcriptase[11]. HBV also has the smallest genome of any DNA virus known to infect animals. The incubation period is relatively long ranging from 50 to 180 days and infection can occur in any age group. Transmission is usually by blood or blood products, for example following transfusion or drug addiction, or by intimate sexual or family contact. Perinatal spread from mother to infant is also important in many parts of the world. Slight or inapparent infection (about 70% of all infections), the carrier state and chronic liver disease are all commonly encountered and are seen most often amongst young males, homosexuals and drug addicts. Chronic carriers form the principal reservoir of infection and their incidence varies greatly amongst different populations, ranging from 0.1% in Britain and the USA to 15% or more in parts of Africa and the Far East. Fatal fulminant disease occurs in less than 1% of acute infections[4]. Diagnosis is based upon finding markers of HB in the serum, particularly HBsAg and HBeAg, the latter being a useful marker of active virus replication[12].

Pathogenesis of HB

There is little correlation between the severity of the illness and the amount of virus in the liver, chronic carriers often having large amounts of HBsAg and HBcAg but little inflammation or necrosis. This suggests that the virus is not itself cytopathic, and that failure to clear the virus in the carrier state is due to a failure of an adequate immune response. The acute hepatocellular necrosis during acute infection is thus thought to result not from the direct action of virus-mediated cytolysis but from the recognition of viral antigens upon the surface of infected liver cells by the T lymphocytes of an intact immune system. The resulting cell destruction liberates virus which may then be destroyed by T cells or neutralized by antibody. This explains why in acute disease immunological methods detect viral antigens only in small quantities in Kupffer cells but rarely or not at all in hepatocytes. The major target of the immune response is thought to be membrane-bound HBcAg[13]. Antibodies to the preS components appear early in the course of infection and are thought to be important in the clearance of HBV.

HEPATITIS D (HD)

HD (also known as the delta agent)[14] was first discovered amongst drug abusers in Northern Italy who were already infected with HBV. The virus (HDV), the smallest known human virus, consists of a circular single-stranded RNA genome within an envelope of HBsAg. Coincident or pre-existing HB infection is essential for replication of the virus which thus tends to have a similar geographic distribution to HBV. Infection is endemic in the tropics and the prevalence falls off towards temperate zones, where it tends to be restricted to high risk groups such as drug addicts. The outcome of infection depends upon the HBV status of the patient. Infection by HDV acquired at the same time as HBV may run a biphasic course with two peaks of liver cell necrosis a few weeks apart[15], and is more often complicated by fulminant disease than HBV infection alone[16]. When chronic carriers of HBV are superinfected by HDV, the disease often becomes progressive, particularly when replication of HBV is active[17]. The virus is thus thought to be directly cytopathic. Diagnosis is based upon finding IgM antibody to HDV in the serum.

HEPATITIS C (HC)

Until recent recognition of the hepatitis C virus (HCV)[18] and of the hepatitis E virus[7], these organisms were considered together as *non-A, non-B (NANB) viruses*, diagnosis being mainly by exclusion (although it was clear quite early on that there was more than one virus concerned[19]). HCV has now been fully sequenced[18] and shown to be a single-stranded positive sense RNA virus with a lipid envelope. Its nearest relatives are flaviviruses (which include yellow fever and Dengue viruses) and the pestiviruses (which cause diseases in a number of animals).

Now that a scrum marker for HCV is available, it has been shown that this virus is responsible for most post-transfusion NANB hepatitis, and also for most community acquired NANB hepatitis in the developed world. As with HB, other forms of parenteral transmission such as parenteral drug abuse, and sexual and perinatal transmission may also be important[16,20]. Up to 40% of infections within families and within the community have no known parenteral explanation[21] and thus, in these cases, transmission may be by non-percutaneous routes. Although many related viruses are insect-transmitted, there is not yet any evidence of insect involvement in the spread of HCV. The incubation period is usually between 6 and 12 weeks and clinically HC is indistinguishable from other forms of hepatitis, although about 75% of cases are subclinical. Conversely, fulminant disease also occurs, often with late onset weeks or months after first symptoms[22], and has a high fatality rate. The risk of progression to chronic disease may be as high as 50%[20].

Little is known of pathogenic mechanisms in HC infection, but the presence of degenerative changes in hepatocytes in association with little inflammation might suggest a direct cytopathic effect of the virus[23].

OTHER VIRUSES

The possibility that there are other NANB viruses remains since a proportion of patients with acute hepatitis remain negative to all known markers[24]. One such agent may be

related to measles virus and has been associated with syncytial giant-cell formation[25].

HISTOPATHOLOGY

All the agents of viral hepatitis cause an essentially similar picture, and cannot be reliably distinguished other than with techniques for demonstrating the virus[16]. In the acute stage there are basically three morphological components each of which is independently variable[26]. These are (a) acute hepatocyte damage; (b) inflammation; and (c) regeneration.

(a) *Acute Hepatocyte Damage*. Liver cell changes develop throughout the acinus but vary in intensity and are most severe in perivenular (centrilobular) regions. One of the most striking histological features of the liver in acute viral hepatitis is the lobular disarray (Figure 2.1). This is due to the great variation in size and staining quality of liver cells, representing both degeneration and regeneration. Enlarged cells tend to encroach upon sinusoids and may give a false impression of twinning as well as leading to obliteration of the normal radial arrangement of liver cell plates. Some of the larger cells, up to twice normal size, may have empty non-staining cytoplasm apart from a little perinuclear condensation and occasional granules of bile. This appearance is often called ballooning degeneration (Figure 2.2). Spotty necrosis may be both cytolytic and coagulative. Lytic lesions are poorly defined but cause defects in the liver cell plates which are more or less filled with proliferating Kupffer cells and lymphocytes. Necrosis affects single cells which become shrunken, rounded and heavily eosinophilic with a pyknotic or absent nucleus (Figure 2.3). These acidophil (Councilman, apoptotic) bodies are extruded from the plate into the perisinusoidal space and tend to persist longer than the other liver cell changes. In most cases, small bile pigment precipitates are seen within a few canaliculi. Fatty change is most unusual in viral hepatitis, although it may be observed after corticosteroid therapy[27], and is also seen particularly in HD and HC (see below).

(b) *Inflammation*. Inflammatory cell infiltration occurs nearly simultaneously with the liver cell changes (Figure 2.4). There is proliferation of existing portal tract lymphoid tissue ranging from minimal to marked and this may spill out into the parenchyma, blurring the outline of limiting plates. This should not be confused with piecemeal necrosis, in that although periportal liver cells may be separated and surrounded by mononuclear cells, they remain healthy and do not show degenerative changes (see Chapter 7). Although lymphocytes predominate, there may also be a few macrophages, neutrophils and even plasma cells, although the last are rarely numerous. Bile ductular proliferation may be quite marked in a few cases, but it is not usually a prominent feature.

Within the parenchyma, in addition to variable numbers of sinusoidal lymphocytes (Figure 2.5), there is hypertrophy and hyperplasia of Kupffer cells. Ceroid pigment, recognizable by staining with PAS after diastase digestion, is present in many of these cells which are often found in small clusters (Figure 2.6). They may also contain a diffuse hazy deposit of iron (Figure 2.7), presumably like the ceroid released from hepatocytes[28]. Later, similar ceroid and iron containing macrophages accumulate in portal tracts where they may persist for some months after the acute episode has subsided (Figure 2.8). Collapse and condensation of the centrilobular reticulin framework may be seen at this stage (Figure 2.9).

(c) *Regeneration*. Regeneration is always recognizable by the time of the onset of symptoms and tends to be

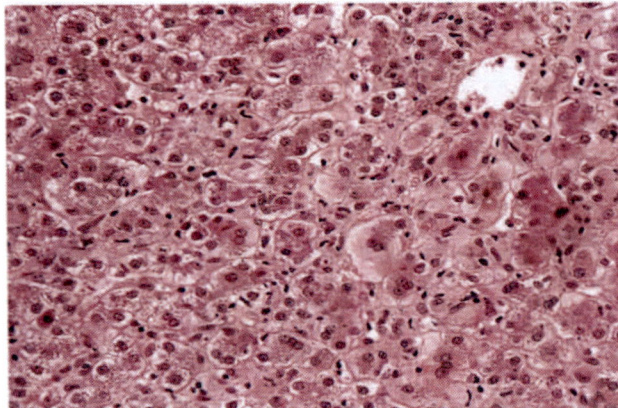

Figure 2.1 Acute viral hepatitis showing lobular disarray with irregular swelling of cells around the central vein (top right), regenerative changes and an acidophil body (bottom left).

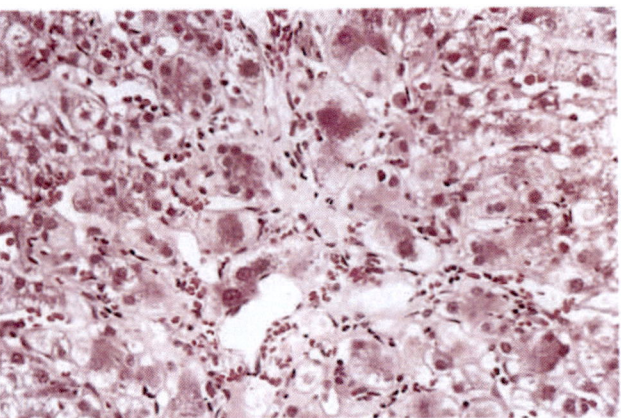

Figure 2.2 Acute viral hepatitis showing ballooning degeneration of centrilobular hepatocytes.

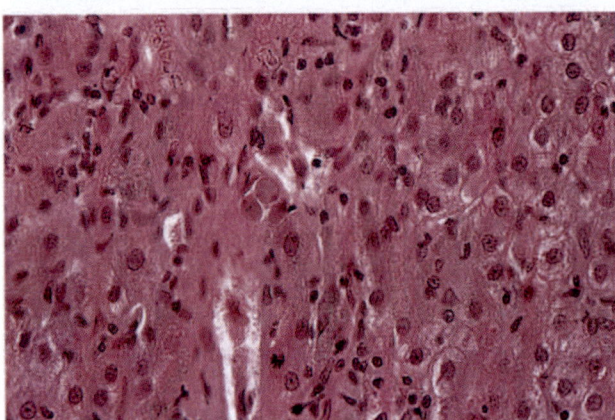

Figure 2.3 Acute viral hepatitis showing several foci of Kupffer cells filled with yellow-brown ceroid pigment and a group of three acidophil bodies (left to centre), all grouped around a central vein.

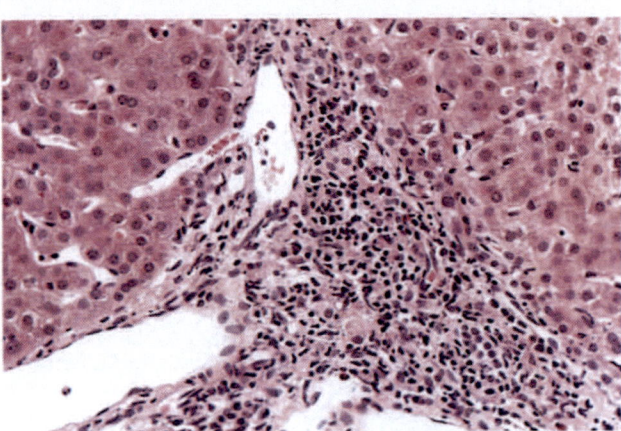

Figure 2.4 Acute viral hepatitis. The portal tract is expanded and contains a light lymphocytic infiltrate associated with slight bile ductular proliferation. Note the lobular disarray in the surrounding parenchyma.

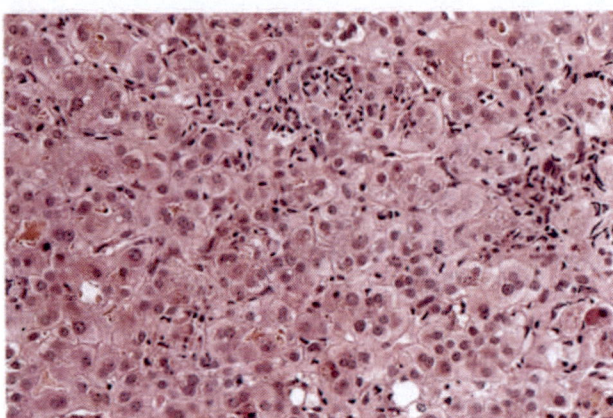

Figure 2.5 Acute viral hepatitis. Same case as Figure 2.4. The parenchyma shows lobular disarray with scattered sinusoidal lymphocytes. Note also the acidophil body (lower right) and cholestasis (left border).

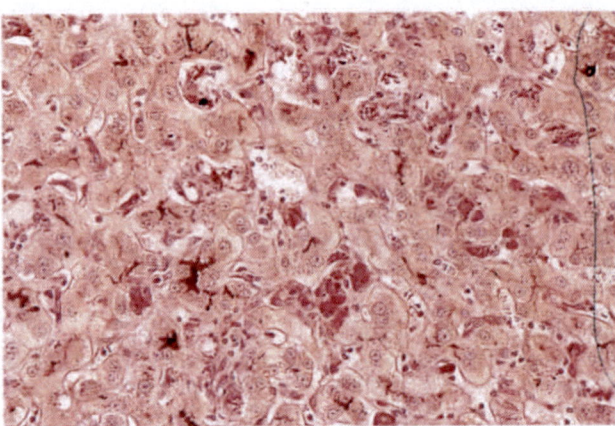

Figure 2.6 Acute viral hepatitis. Lobular disarray with clumps of ceroid-filled Kupffer cells between liver cell plates. Note also the many distended bile canaliculi filled with faintly PAS-positive bile thrombi in this cholestatic case. PAS diastase.

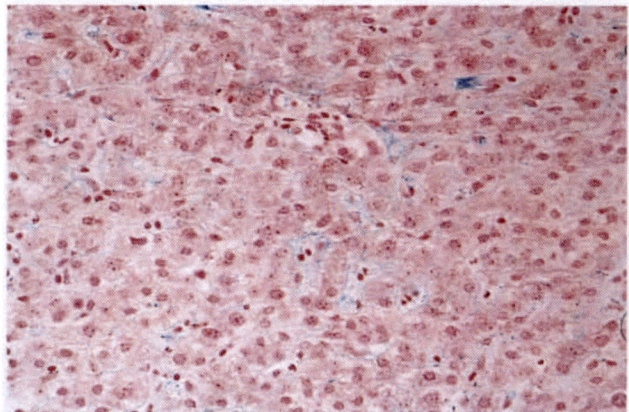

Figure 2.7 Acute viral hepatitis. Diffuse hazy deposition of iron in Kupffer cells. Perl's Prussian blue.

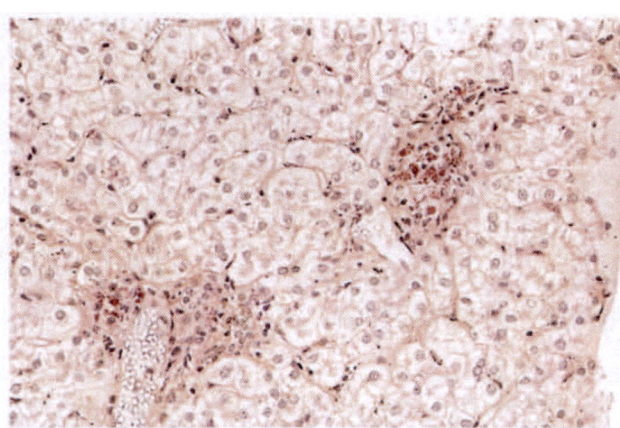

Figure 2.8 Post-viral hepatitis. Typical acute viral hepatitis 9 months prior to liver biopsy. Residual ceroid-filled macrophages are now confined to portal tracts. PAS diastase.

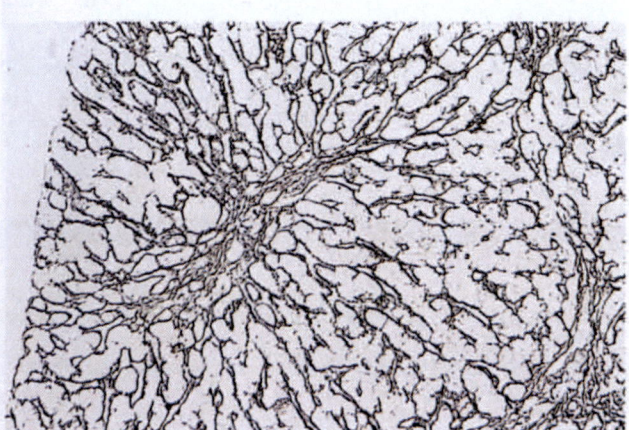

Figure 2.9 Acute viral hepatitis. Condensation of the reticulin framework adjacent to a terminal venule. Reticulin.

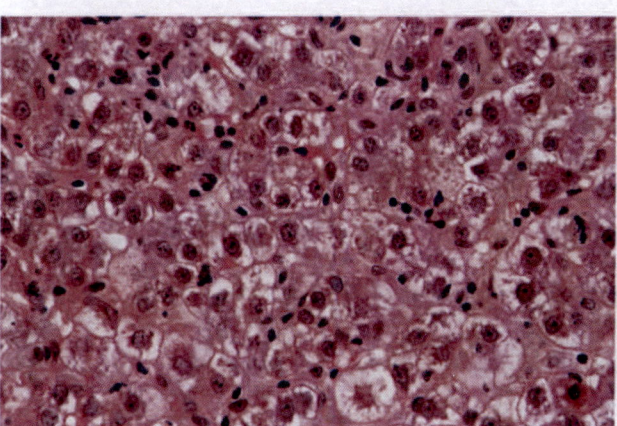

Figure 2.10 Acute viral hepatitis. Regenerative activity in the form of twin liver cell plates with marked regularity of the nuclei dominating the periportal region in this biopsy. Note also scanty sinusoidal lymphocytes.

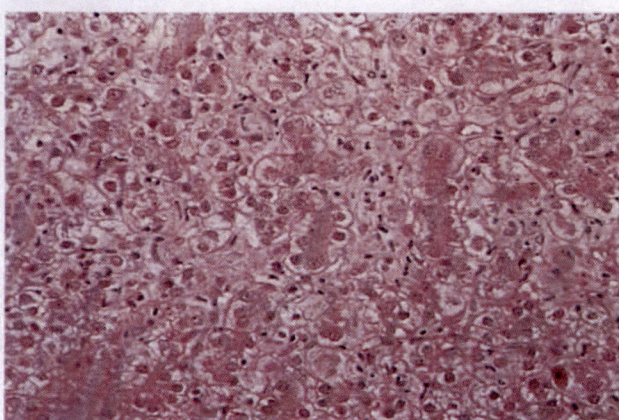

Figure 2.11 Acute viral hepatitis. Regenerative activity. Twinning of liver cell plates is more striking in this biopsy. Note the position of the hepatocyte nuclei on the sinusoidal aspect of the liver cells.

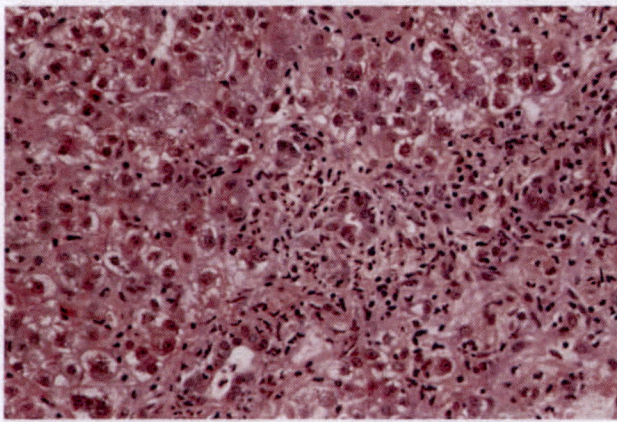

Figure 2.12 Cholestatic viral hepatitis. An expanded portal tract showing bile duct proliferation and cellular infiltration, in this case dominated by neutrophils.

more prominent in the periportal regions. As the disease progresses, it is this emphasis on regeneration which further effaces the liver cell plate–sinusoid arrangement. Twin cell plates, mitotic figures and binucleate and multinucleate cells may all be seen. Although there may be considerable cytoplasmic pleomorphism, often with reduced amounts of lipofuscin, nuclei tend to be more uniform with much less polyploidy than in normal liver (Figures 2.10 and 2.11). Thin residual fibrous septa radiating from a few portal tracts may also be seen at this stage.

There are no qualitative histological differences between icteric and non-icteric hepatitis.

Late stages

The parenchymal changes gradually subside whilst the mesenchymal changes persist. Liver cell pleomorphism is now confined to the perivenular region, where there may also be some canalicular cholestasis and hydropic swelling. Inflammation, too, tends to be mainly centrilobular or in portal tracts which are now much more clearly demarcated from the parenchyma. As stated above, acidophil bodies and ceroid-filled Kupffer cells may persist for long periods. There are varying degrees of collapse and condensation of reticulin and delicate collagenous extensions from portal tracts may also be present, but neither has prognostic significance.

VARIANTS OF ACUTE VIRAL HEPATITIS (AVH)

Cholestasis

Occasionally viral hepatitis may mimic obstructive jaundice. Histologically, the changes are basically those of viral hepatitis with cholestasis, which may be impressive, superimposed (Figure 2.6). The changes are maximal around terminal venules and take the form of coarse granules of bile pigment in liver cells and in Kupffer cells and bile thrombi in dilated canaliculi between liver cells. Occasionally bile thrombi may be surrounded by a tubular arrangement of liver cells (see cholestasis, Chapter 16). Polymorphonuclear leukocytes are also liable to be more numerous (Figure 2.12) and in the late stage some ducts may contain inspissated bile. All these portal changes increase the resemblance to large duct obstruction (Chapter 16), but in the latter, in contrast to the lobular disarray seen in hepatitis, the radial pattern of liver cell plates is not only preserved but may even be accentuated.

The prognosis of cholestatic hepatitis is no worse than uncomplicated virus hepatitis and, although the jaundice may persist for 6 months or more, recovery is usually complete.

Fulminant hepatitis (hepatitis with massive necrosis)

The overall mortality from acute viral hepatitis is probably about 1–2 per 1000. Any patient passing into hepatic coma as a result of viral hepatitis is regarded as having fulminant hepatic failure (FHF). FHF may be caused by any of the hepatotrophic viruses, but also by any of the other viruses described in Chapter 3, and, quite commonly, by paracetamol overdose[29]. Survival appears to be to some extent dependent on the aetiological agent[30], survival rates being lowest in FHF due to NANB hepatitis. Severity is mainly a reflection of the quantity of liver cell necrosis. At its most extreme, liver cells may be almost totally eliminated[31]. In such a case, the liver is greatly shrunken with a wrinkled capsule and a reddish cut surface showing a nutmeg pattern and crowding of major ducts and vessels. Other livers contain nodules of surviving and regenerating parenchyma often pale yellow or green in colour (Figure 2.13).

Microscopically, liver acini may be entirely devoid of liver cells (so-called multiacinar or multilobular necrosis) with merely a little cellular debris and a few inflammatory cells all that remain (Figure 2.14), yet there is little or no collapse of the reticulin framework at this early stage. Inflammatory changes are rarely conspicuous[32,33]. Inflammatory cells may, however, be quite numerous in portal tracts where proliferating bile ductules are often very conspicuous, especially if the patient survives for more than 10 days. Changes mimicking large duct obstruction, namely dilated ducts containing inspissated bile, microcalculi with focal necrosis, neutrophil infiltration and even occasional bile extravasates are not rare in fulminant disease[34]. Survival for weeks and months (submassive necrosis) may lead to the appearance of bulging nodules of regenerating liver in some places and parenchyma totally devoid of hepatocytes in others.

Histological recovery from fulminant and subacute hepatitis can be complete[33], although subsequent scarring may be followed by the development of portal hypertension[35]. Subsequent chronic hepatitis is most unusual.

Hepatitis with confluent necrosis (subacute hepatic necrosis)

The significance of different types of confluent necrosis has been greatly clarified by an understanding of the acinar structure of the liver[36]. Portal to portal links occur merely by expansion of portal tracts which may be due to extension of periportal piecemeal necrosis (Chapter 7) or to scarring, and have no additional significance. True confluent necrosis takes place at the periphery of Rappaport's complex acinus and is usefully considered as having three degrees of severity.

Minor necrosis is seen as classic centrilobular necrosis alone (Figure 2.15), and is quite common in acute viral hepatitis (as well as following exposure to certain drugs and toxins, Chapter 10). Liver cell regeneration normally replaces the lost cells and there are no lasting consequences. When the necrosis is slightly more extensive, affecting most of zone 3 of the complex acinus, there will be central to central links through the nodal point of Mall, so called bridging hepatic necrosis (BHN). These are typically bent or vaulted, as would be expected on anatomical grounds, and they, too, heal readily by regenerative activity. If the necrosis is even more extensive, it will involve the whole of zone 3 causing now, for the first time, portal to hepatic venule (central) bridges (Figures 2.16 and 2.17), as well as the hepatic venule (central) to hepatic venule (central) links which will always be present at this stage. This, too, is perfectly capable of healing unless the liver cells at the margins of the bridge are affected by piecemeal necrosis (Chapter 7). The key to the significance of BHN thus seems to be whether or not piecemeal necrosis spreads from the portal tracts to the surviving cells lining the portal to central bridge. When this occurs, the chances of subsequent chronic hepatitis and cirrhosis developing are significantly increased, but taken alone its prognostic value in predicting subsequent chronic hepatitis[37] has probably been overemphasized[38–41]. In contrast BHN is associated with a high mortality in the acute phase, especially in patients over 40[26] in whom the regenerative capacity is more likely to be impaired.

Periportal necrosis

In this form of acute hepatitis there may be dramatic portal inflammation with spillover into the zone 1 parenchyma (Figure 2.18), and a high proportion of plasma cells in the infiltrate. True piecemeal necrosis, with irregular

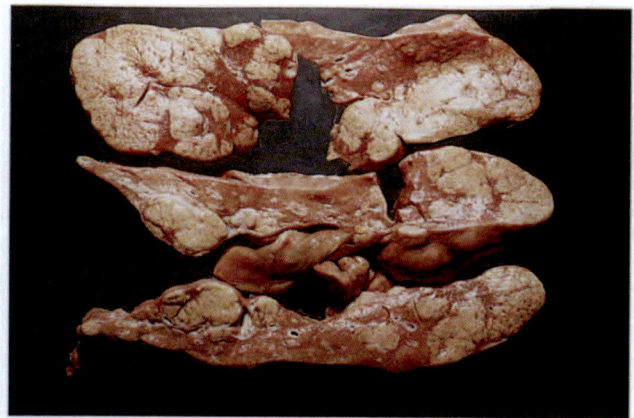

Figure 2.13 Fulminant viral hepatitis. A 52-year-old female patient with acute viral hepatitis who became increasingly jaundiced and died in coma two months after onset. Note the extensive reddish-brown multilobular necrosis and the yellowish foci of regeneration.

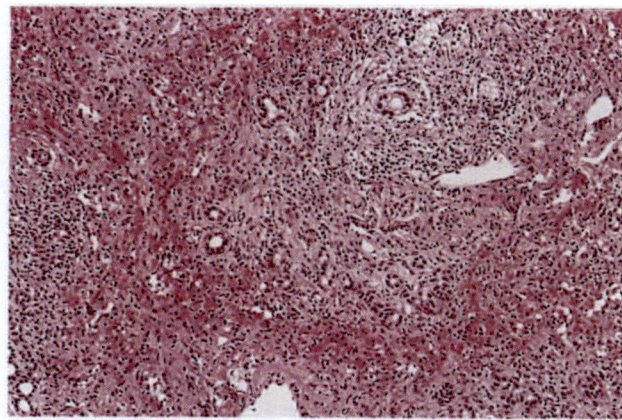

Figure 2.14 Fulminant viral hepatitis. Multilobular necrosis with total absence of liver cells. A terminal venule (bottom left of centre) is surrounded by a light infiltrate of lymphocytes and macrophages, but no surviving hepatocytes. Similar cells are present in the expanded portal tracts which also show some bile duct proliferation.

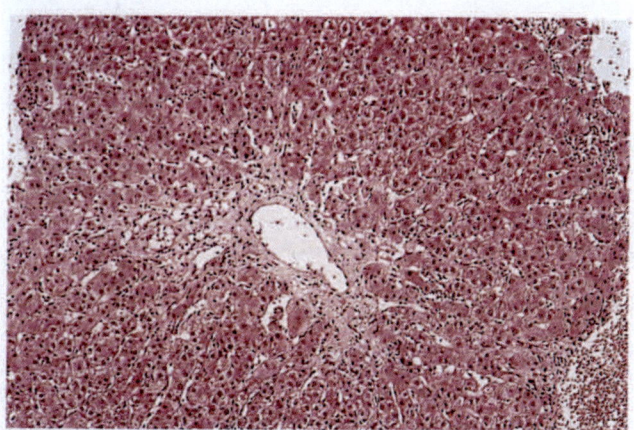

Figure 2.15 Acute viral hepatitis. Centrilobular liver cell loss, which was followed by an uneventful recovery in this patient (same biopsy as Figure 1.1).

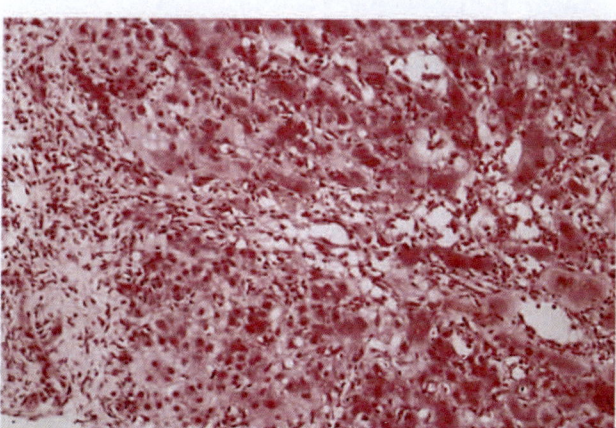

Figure 2.16 Acute viral hepatitis. Bridging hepatic necrosis which is creating a bridge between the terminal venule (right) and portal tract (left).

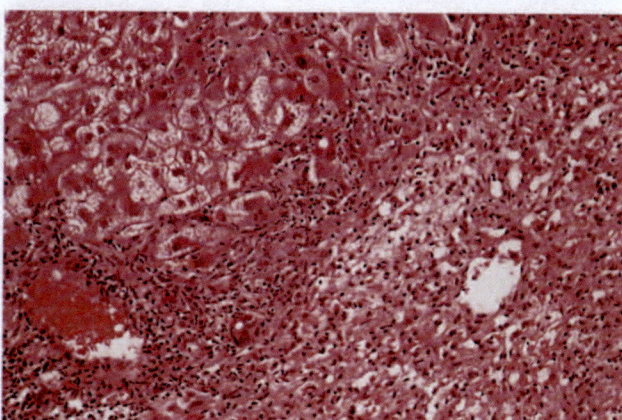

Figure 2.17 Acute viral hepatitis. Bridging hepatic necrosis, still more severe, now involving most of Rappaport's zones 3 and 2. Marked perivenular liver cell loss with broad bridge linking the terminal hepatic venule (right) with portal tract (left). Note the surviving hepatocytes in zone 1 (above the portal tract).

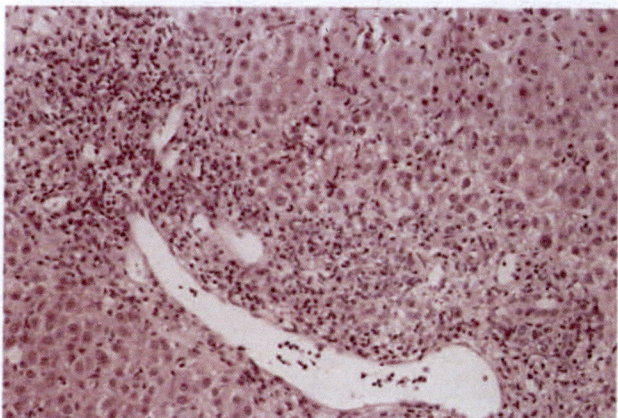

Figure 2.18 Acute hepatitis A. Note the expanded portal tract filled with mononuclear cells, predominantly lymphocytes, which are spilling out into the adjacent periportal parenchyma in a manner very similar to that seen in chronic active hepatitis (Chapter 7). The patient made an uneventful recovery.

destruction of the limiting plate, may, however, occasionally be seen in patients with acute viral hepatitis who subsequently recover completely[40]. Many of these cases may actually be due to infection by hepatitis A virus (see below). Differentiation from hitherto silent chronic active hepatitis (CAH) in an acute exacerbation may be difficult or impossible, with serial biopsies and the passage of time being necessary to establish the correct diagnosis[42]. However points in favour of CAH include variation in intensity from one lobule to another and no particular tendency to involve the centrilobular region.

Persistence of acute viral hepatitis

In a few patients, AVH is persistent or recurrent. The histological appearances are usually identical to those seen in the original acute phase. Similarly, there is a group of patients in whom the typical biopsy changes of AVH persist for as long as 2 years (chronic lobular hepatitis, Chapter 7) yet also recover fully eventually. Many of these cases probably represent chronic hepatitis C[43].

HISTOLOGICAL CHANGES RELATED TO PARTICULAR VIRUSES

There are more similarities than differences between the various aetiological categories of acute hepatitis[42], but certain patterns are more commonly seen in association with certain viruses:

In *hepatitis A* infection, hepatitis is more likely to be cholestatic and associated with periportal hepatitis (Figure 2.18)[44,45]. Severe forms with bridging or multiacinar necrosis are probably less common in hepatitis A than hepatitis B. The histological picture in infection with *hepatitis E* is said to be very similar to that of HA[46], with a mainly periportal cholestatic hepatitis.

Acute *hepatitis B* is often characterized by severe hepatocellular necrosis, but all degrees of severity of necrosis may be seen (Figure 2.19). Lymphocytes may sometimes be seen in close proximity to hepatocytes (Figure 2.20) and even appear within them[47]. Lymphoid aggregates or follicles are sometimes seen in HB as in HC. Ground-glass cells containing HBsAg (Chapter 7) are not seen in acute infection—indeed even sensitive techniques generally reveal very little evidence of HB antigens in acute hepatitis because they are cleared from the liver early in infection. Coinfection with *hepatitis D* may increase the severity of the hepatitis but is not associated with specific histological features. Although microvesicular fatty change has been recorded in a number of outbreaks[48], this is not a specific finding.

Hepatitis C: Various histological patterns have been described in the parenteral form of NANB hepatitis[47,49,50], but were hampered by the lack of specific markers of infection. Recent studies have, however, generally confirmed the earlier observations[43]. Cytopathic changes in the form of prominent acidophil bodies showing intense granular eosinophilia are well described (Figures 2.21 and 2.22), as is the presence of lipid in hepatocytes (Figures 2.21 and 2.23), but probably the most distinctive appearance is the presence of lymphoid aggregates in portal tracts, often surrounding damaged bile ducts (Figures 2.23 and 2.24)[43,49,51]. The high risk of transition to chronicity in HC has already been noted (see also Chapter 7).

DIFFERENTIAL DIAGNOSIS

Classical acute viral hepatitis can usually be diagnosed confidently by clinical and biochemical parameters combined with recognition of serum markers specific to the individual viruses. Thus the indications for biopsy in such a case are limited and so the classical biopsy appearances are relatively uncommonly seen in routine practice. Biopsy then tends to be reserved for cases with unusual clinical features which may also be atypical histologically.

Apart from AVH, recurrent AVH and chronic lobular hepatitis (or unresolved AVH), the classic lobular changes may also be seen in hepatitis due to drugs and toxins (Chapter 10), as well as in chronic hepatitis as mentioned above. Frequently the diagnosis depends more on the history than the biopsy findings, but additional features such as fatty change, periportal bile stasis or numerous eosinophils might suggest drug idiosyncrasy (Chapter 10).

Autoimmune chronic hepatitis. This form of hepatitis, discussed in Chapter 7, has no specific histological features and may be difficult to distinguish from AVH at the start of the illness before chronic features have appeared.

Infectious mononucleosis. This condition may sometimes clinically and biochemically mimic AVH. Morphologically, parenchymal changes are usually greatly overshadowed by inflammatory changes (Chapter 3). There is usually intense portal infiltration by mononuclear cells, with similar cells in strings in sinusoids. The diagnosis is confirmed by detection of heterophile antibody in the blood.

Heat stroke. This can also resemble AVH clinically and biochemically, but here the history is clearly the most important diagnostic pointer. Microscopically the necrosis is strictly centrilobular and there is little parenchymal or portal inflammation[52].

Non-specific reactive hepatitis (Chapter 21). Although portal inflammation may be quite intense it is usually not uniform, whereas lobular inflammation is more likely to be diffuse than focal.

Biliary obstruction. As mentioned above, portal tract changes may resemble those seen in biliary obstruction and may cause especial confusion during the phase of resolution. Although by now they may be much less conspicuous, lobular changes such as centrilobular liver cell swelling, and parenchymal inflammation should all help to establish the diagnosis of AVH. Prominent Kupffer cells filled with ceroid pigment are present in both conditions but their distribution tends to differ. In hepatitis they tend to occur in clusters, whilst in cholestasis they are much more evenly spread, and are closely related to the cholestasis.

PROGNOSIS OF AVH

The mortality of hepatitis with acute liver failure is high probably in excess of 80% and correlates quite well with the presence of multiacinar and BHN. It does, however, remain extremely difficult to predict accurately the likely development of chronic hepatitis in any individual during the acute illness, whether by biopsy or other parameters[53]. However, it is clear that the identity of the virus is at least as important as any morphological features: hepatitis A and hepatitis E do not go on to chronic disease, whilst hepatitis B has a small risk, and hepatitis D and hepatitis C have a high risk of chronicity. In chronic disease, HB and HD can be readily identified immunologically in histological sections (Chapter 7).

REFERENCES

1. Dienstag, J. L., Feinstone, S. M., Kapikian, R. Z., Purcell, R. H., Boggs, J. D. and Conrad, M. E. (1975). Faecal shedding of hepatitis A antigen. Lancet, 1, 765–767
2. Cohen, J. I. (1989). Hepatitis A: insights from molecular biology. Hepatology, 9, 889–895
3. Szmuness, W., Dienstag, J. L., and Purcell, R. H. (1977). The prevalence of antibody to hepatitis A antigen in various parts of the world. A pilot study. Am. J. Epidemiol., 5, 392–398

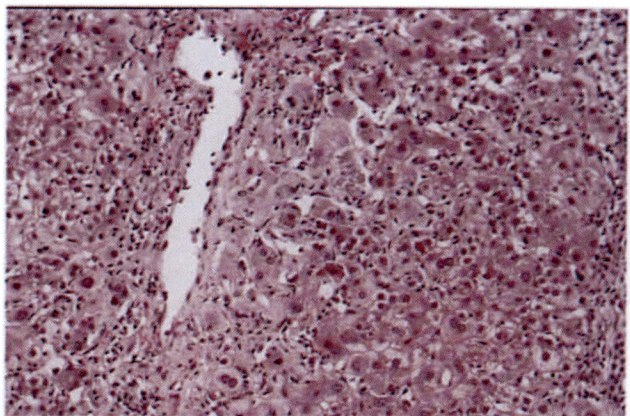

Figure 2.19 Acute hepatitis B. Note the dropout around the terminal hepatic venule (left of centre) and the lobular disarray with an occasional acidophil body. There are scattered lymphocytes in sinusoids and in the portal tract (right). These appearances are in no way diagnostic of hepatitis B.
The author is deeply indebted to Dr B C Portmann who kindly supplied the slide from which Figure 2.19 was prepared.

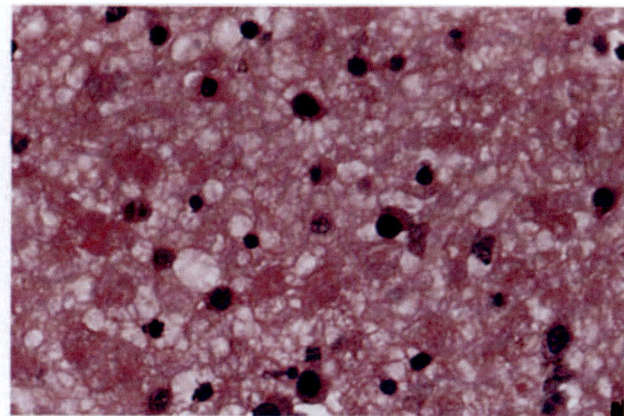

Figure 2.20 Fulminant hepatitis B. This 28-year-old man developed fulminant hepatic failure and died within five days of onset of his first symptom. The autopsy was performed within three hours of death and thus the extensive autolysis of hepatocytes seen in this field is at least partly the consequence of the hepatitis. Note the well-preserved lymphocytes, some activated, in contact with the hepatocytes.

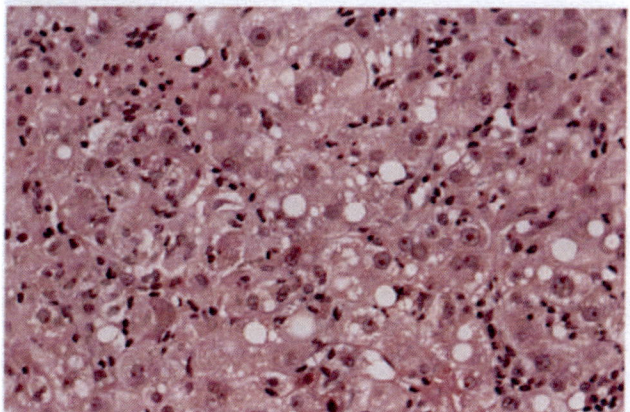

Figure 2.21 Acute hepatitis C. Acute lobular disarray with scattered acidophil bodies and sinusoidal lymphocytes. Note also the parenchymal fat droplets.

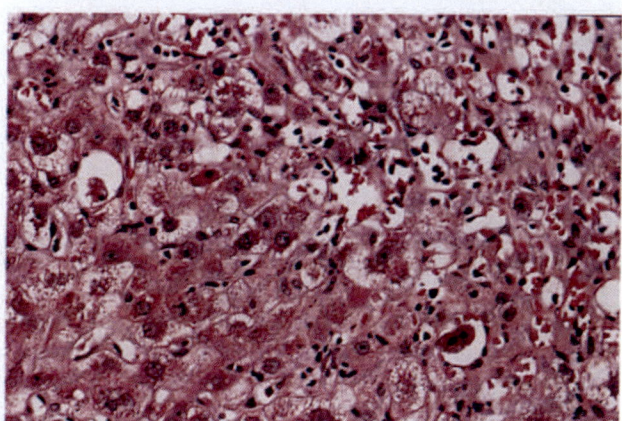

Figure 2.22 Acute hepatitis C. A very similar case to that shown in Figure 2.21, again with quite prominent angular acidophil bodies. Nevertheless, the changes are in no way diagnostic of HC (cf. Figure 2.19).

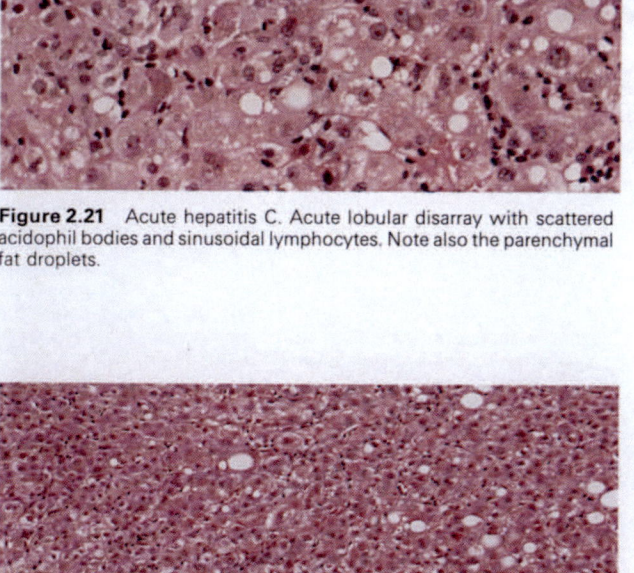

Figure 2.23 Acute hepatitis C. Note the lymphoid aggregate in a portal tract and the scattered parenchymal fat droplets.

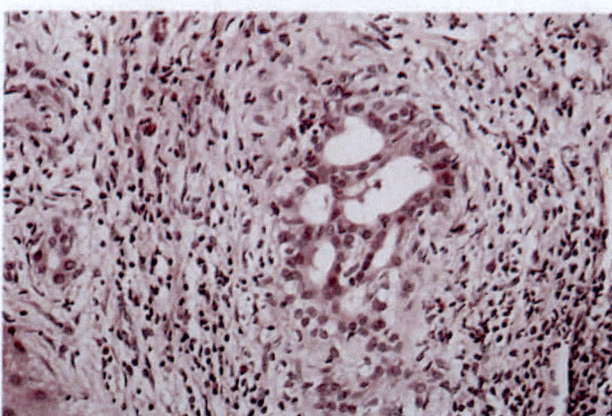

Figure 2.24 Acute NANB viral hepatitis, probably hepatitis C. The portal tract contains a bile duct showing epithelial proliferation with multilayering leading to a cribriform appearance (quite different from the bile duct damage in primary biliary cirrhosis (Chapter 17).

4. Feinstone, S. M. and Gust, I. D. (1991). Hepatitis A. In McIntyre, N., Benhamou, J.-P., Bircher, J., Rizetto, M. and Rodes, J. (eds). Oxford Textbook of Clinical Hepatology. pp. 565–571. Oxford: Oxford University Press

5. Vallbracht, A., Gabriel, P., Maier, K., Hartmann, F., Steinhardt, H. J., Müller, C., Wolf, A., Manncke, K. H. and Fleming, B. (1986). Cell–mediated cytotoxicity in hepatitis A virus infection. Hepatology, 6, 1308–1314

6. Krawczynski, K. (1991). Hepatitis type E–enterically transmitted (epidemic) non-A, non-B hepatitis. In McIntyre, N., Benhamou, J.-P., Bircher, J., Rizetto, M. and Rodes, J. (eds). Oxford Textbook of Clinical Hepatology. pp. 617–620. Oxford: Oxford University Press

7. Tam, A. W., Smith, M. M., and Guerra, M. E. (1991). Hepatitis E virus: molecular cloning and sequencing of the full-length viral genome. Virology, 185, 120–131

8. Reyes, G. R., Bradley, D. W. and Lovett, M. (1992). New strategies for isolation of low abundance viral and host cDNAs: application to cloning of the hepatitis E virus and analysis of tissue-specific transcription. Semin. Liver Dis. 12, 289–300

9. Ramalingaswami, V. and Purcell, R. H. (1988). Waterborne non-A, non-B hepatitis. Lancet, 1, 571–573

10. Soe, S., Uchita, T., Suzuki, K., Komatsu, K., Azumi, J., Okuda, Y., Iida, F., Shikata, T., Rikihisa, T. and Mizuno, K. (1989). Enterically transmitted non-A, non-B hepatitis in cynomolgous monkeys: morphology and probable mechanism of hepatocellular necrosis. Liver, 9, 135–145

11. Miller, R. H. (1991). Comparative molecular biology of the hepatitis viruses. Semin. Liver Dis., 11, 113–120

12. Hoofnagle, J. H. and Di Bisceglie, A. M. (1991). Serologic diagnosis of acute and chronic viral hepatitis. Hepatology, 11, 758–763

13. Mondelli, M. and Eddleston, A. L. W. F. (1984). Mechanisms of liver cell injury in acute and chronic hepatitis B. Semin. Liver Dis., 4, 47–58

14. Bonino, F., Brunetto, M. R., Negro, F., Smedile, A. and Ponzetto, A. (1991). Hepatitis D, a model of liver cell pathology. J. Hepatol., 13, 260–266

15. Govindarajan, S., Kaliniuck, B. and Peters, L. (1986). Relapse of B viral hepatitis–role of delta agent. Gut, 27, 19–22

16. Lavine, J. E., Bull, F. G., Millward-Sadler, G. H. and Arthur, M. J. P. (1992). Acute viral hepatitis. In Millward-Sadler, G. H., Wright, R. and Arthur, M. J. P. (eds). Wright's Liver and Biliary Disease. 3rd edn. pp. 679–786. London: W B Saunders

17. Smedile, A., Rosina, F., Saracco, G., Chiaberge, E., Lattore, V., Fabiano, A., Brunetto, M. R., Verme, G., Rizetto, M. and Bonino, F. (1991). Hepatitis B replication modulates pathogenesis of hepatitis D virus in chronic hepatitis D. Hepatology, 13, 413–416

18. Houghton, M., Weiner, A., Kuo, G. and Choo, Q.-L. (1991). Molecular biology of the hepatitis C viruses: implications for diagnosis, development and control of viral disease. Hepatology, 14, 381–388

19. Tsiquaye, K. N., Bird, R. E., Tovey, G., Wyke, R. J., Williams, R. and Zuckerman, A. J. (1980). Further evidence of cellular changes associated with non-A, non-B hepatitis. J. Med. Virol. 5, 63–71

20. Genseca, P., Esteban, J. I. and Alter, H. J. (1991). Blood–borne non-A, non-B hepatitis: hepatitis C. Semin. Liver Dis., 11, 147–164

21. Alter, H. J., Hadler, S. C., Judson, F. N., Mares, A., Alexander, W. J., Hu, P. Y., Miller, J. K., Moyer, L. A., Fields, H. A. and Bradley, D. W. (1990). Risk factors for acute non-A, non-B hepatitis in the United States and association with hepatitis C virus infection. JAMA, 264, 2231–2235

22. Williams, R. and Wendon, J. (1991). Clinical syndrome and aetiology of fulminant hepatic failure. In Williams, R. and Hughes, R. D. (eds). Acute Liver Failure. pp. 1–5. London: Mitre Press

23. Alberti, A. and Realdi, G. (1991). Parenterally-acquired non-A, non-B (type C) hepatitis. In McIntyre, N., Benhamou, J.-P., Bircher, J., Rizetto, M. and Rodes, J. (eds). Oxford Textbook of Clinical Hepatology. pp. 605–617. Oxford: Oxford University Press

24. Article, L. (1990). The A to F of viral hepatitis. Lancet, 336, 1158–1160

25. Phillips, M. J., Blendis, L. M., Poucell, S., Patterson, J., Petric, M., Roberts, E., Levy, G. A., Superina, R. A., Greig, P. D., Cameron, R., Langer, B. and Purcell, R. H. (1991). Syncytial giant-cell hepatitis. Sporadic hepatitis with distinctive pathological features, a severe clinical course, and paramyxoviral features. N. Engl. J. Med., 324, 455–460

26. Peters, R. L. (1975). Viral hepatitis; a pathologic spectrum. Am. J. Med. Sci. 270, 17–31

27. Bianchi, L., DeGroote, J., Desmet, V., Gedigk, P., Korb, G., Popper, H., Poulsen, H., Scheuer, P. J., Schmid, M., Thaler, H. and Wepler, W. (1971). Morphological criteria in viral hepatitis. Lancet, 1,

333–337

28. Petersen, P., Christoffersen, P., Elling, P., Juhl, E., Dietrichson, O., Faber, V., Iversen, K., Nielsen, J. O. and Poulsen, H. (1974). Acute viral hepatitis; a survey of 500 patients. Scand. J. Gastroenterol. 9, 607–613

29. Bernuau, J. and Benhamou, J.-P. (1992). Fulminant and subfulminant liver failure. In Millward-Sadler, G. H., Wright, R. and Arthur, M. J. P. (eds). Wright's Liver and Biliary Disease. 3rd edn. pp. 923–942. London: W B Saunders

30. O'Grady, J., Alexander, G. J. M., Hayllar, K. M. and Williams, R. (1989). Early indicators of prognosis in fulminant hepatic failure. Gastroenterology, 97, 439–445

31. Trey, C. and Galdabini, J. J. (1973). Case 46–1973. Case records of Massachusetts General Hospital. N. Engl. J. Med. 280, 1082–1088

32. Horney, J. T. and Galambos, J. T. (1977). The liver during and after fulminant hepatitis. Gastroenterology, 73, 639–645

33. Karvountzis, G. G., Redeker, A. G. and Peters, R. L. (1974). Long-term follow-up studies of patients surviving fulminant viral hepatitis. Gastroenterol. 67, 870–877

34. Schmid, M. and Cueni, B. (1972). Portal lesions in viral hepatitis with submassive hepatic necrosis. Hum. Pathol. 3, 209–216

35. Popper, H. (1979). Pathology of viral hepatitis. Isr. J. Med Sci. 15, 240–247

36. Rappaport, A. M. (1976). The microcirculation, acinar concept of normal and pathological hepatic structure. Beitr. Pathol. 157, 215–243

37. Boyer, J. L. and Klatskin, G. (1970). Pattern of necrosis in acute viral hepatitis. Prognostic value of bridging (subacute hepatic necrosis). N. Engl. J. Med. 283, 1063–1071

38. Busher, G. L., Skidmore, S. J., McKendrick, M. W. and Geddes, A. M. (1981). Sporadic non-A non-B hepatitis in Birmingham. J. Infect. 3, 45–49

39. Ware, A. J., Cuthbert, J. A., Shorey, J., Gurian, L. E., Eigenbrodt, E. H. and Canbes, B. (1981). A prospective trial of steroid therapy in severe viral hepatitis. The prognostic significance of bridging necrosis. Gastroenterology, 80, 219–224

40. Houthoff, H. J., Niermeijer, P., Gips, C. H., Arends, A., Hofstee, N. and van Guldener, M. (1980). Hepatic morphological findings and viral antigens in acute hepatitis B. A longitudinal study. Virchow's Arch. A Pathol. Anat. Histol., 380, 153–166

41. Combes, B. (1986). The initial morphological lesion in chronic hepatitis, important or unimportant. Hepatology, 6, 518–522

42. Scheuer, P. J. (1993). Acute hepatitis. In Wight, D. G. D. (ed). Liver, Biliary Tract and Exocrine Pancreas. Vol. 11. Systemic Pathology. Symmers, W. S. C. Series ed. 3rd edn. Edinburgh: Churchill Livingstone

43. Scheuer, P. J., Ashrafzadeh, P., Sherlock, S., Brown, D. and Dusheiko, G. (1992). The pathology of hepatitis C. Hepatology, 15, 567–571

44. Teixera, M. R., Weller, I. V. D., Murray, A., Bamber, M., Thomas, H. C., Sherlock, S. and Scheuer, P. (1982). The pathology of hepatitis A in man. Liver, 2, 53–60

45. Okuno, T., Sano, A., Deguchi, T., Katsuma, Y., Ogasawara, T., Okanoue, T. and Takina, T. (1984). Pathology of acute hepatitis A in humans; comparison with acute hepatitis B. Am. J. Clin. Pathol., 81, 162–169

46. Dienes, H. P., Hütteroth, T., Bianchi, L., Grün, M. and Thoenes, W. (1986). Hepatitis A-like non-A, non-B hepatitis: light and electron microscopic observations of three cases. Virchows Arch. [A], 409, 657–667

47. Dienes, H. P., Popper, H., Arnold, W. and Lobeck, H. (1982). Histologic observations in human hepatitis non-A, non-B. Hepatology, 2, 562–571

48. Lefkowitch, J. H., Goldstein, H., Yatto, R. and Gerber, M. A. (1987). Cytopathic injury in acute delta virus hepatitis. Gastroenterology, 92, 1262–1266

49. Schmid, M., Pirovino, M., Altorfer, J., Gudat, F. and Bianchi, L. (1982). Acute hepatitis non-A, non-B, are there any specific light microscopic features? Liver, 2, 61–67

50. Lefkowitch, J. H. and Apfelbaum, T. F. (1989). Non-A, non-B hepatitis: Characterisation of liver biopsy pathology. J. Clin. Gastroenterol., 11, 225–232

51. Poulsen, H. and Christoffersen, P. (1969). Abnormal bile-duct epithelium in liver biopsies with histological signs of viral hepatitis. Acta Pathol. Microbiol. Scand. 76, 383–390

52. Bianchi, L., Ohnacker, H., Beck, K. and Zimmerli-Ning, M. (1972). Liver damage in heatstroke and its regression. Hum. Pathol., 3, 237–248

53. Tygstrup, N. and Nielsen, J. O. (1979). Prognosis of viral hepatitis. Isr. J. Med. Sci. 15, 257–260

Non-Hepatotrophic Viruses including HIV and AIDS

3

NON-HEPATOTROPHIC VIRUS INFECTIONS

A great number of viruses may infect the liver. Those which were discussed in Chapter 2 are called hepatitis or hepatotrophic viruses, because they primarily or exclusively infect the liver. Apart from the hepatotrophic viruses, there is a number of others which may also involve the liver (Table 3.1). Many of these, particularly in the developed West, are opportunistic, but there are also several tropical viral haemorrhagic fevers which have a high mortality and show regular involvement of the liver.

Herpes viruses

Infectious mononucleosis

This is caused by the Epstein-Barr (EB) virus. Most primary infection is acquired in childhood and is entirely asymptomatic, whilst that acquired in adolescence or adult life is usually associated with fever, pharyngitis, malaise and lymphadenopathy, the clinical syndrome of glandular fever. Following entry through the epithelial cells of the pharynx, B lymphocytes are infected through binding of the virus with the complement receptor 2^1, new viral antigens are then expressed on the B cell surface. T lymphocytes react against these neoantigens and become transformed into the characteristic 'atypical mononuclear cells' in the peripheral blood.

Clinical hepatitis, with jaundice and elevated serum transaminases, occurs in about 15% of cases but is rarely serious and thus biopsy is seldom indicated and the histological changes rarely seen[2]. Microscopically the most characteristic finding is a heavy mononuclear cell infiltrate, which includes mature lymphocytes, large lymphoblastoid cells and also a few plasma cells in portal tracts (Figure 3.1)[3]. They may also be found in sinusoids (Figure 3.2), either diffusely distributed or in the form of small aggregates. Liver cells are usually unaffected or may show regenerative changes, but fatal hepatic necrosis with herpes-like intranuclear inclusions has been described[4].

The main histological differential diagnosis is from leukaemia or lymphoma which it may closely resemble (Chapter 25). The presence of heterophile antibodies and atypical mononuclear cells in the blood should help to confirm the diagnosis in the majority of cases.

In common with all the herpes viruses, EBV establishes latency and may reactivate into saliva and cervical secretions, such patients forming the main reservoir of infection. Immunocompromised individuals are at risk of subsequent development of B-cell lymphoproliferative disease (see below, and Chapter 26).

Cytomegalovirus infection

Cytomegalovirus, another member of the herpes virus group, is, like EB virus, very widely disseminated and in some population groups up to 100% of adults have antibodies[5], silent infection most often having been acquired in childhood. Primary infection *in utero* or in the neonatal period can result in multisystem disease with anaemia, thrombocytopenia, hepatosplenomegaly and hepatitis, pneumonitis and central nervous system damage, although even in this age group the majority of infections are probably inapparent[6].

Overt clinical infection in normal adults is most unusual but may present as a glandular fever-like syndrome (without heterophile antibody)[7], unexplained pyrexia, a respiratory infection or as liver disease. Even in the presence of liver involvement, it is usually obvious that

Table 3.1 Non-hepatotrophic viruses that may infect the liver*

Family	Genus	Virus
Herpesviridae	Lymphocryptovirus	Epstein-Barr virus (EBV)
	Cytomegalovirus	Cytomegalovirus (CMV)
	Simplexvirus	Herpes simplex virus (HSV) Type 1
		HSV Type 2
	Varicellavirus	Varicella-Zoster virus (VZV)
Adenoviridae	Mastadenovirus	Adenovirus
Paramyxoviridae	Paramyxovirus	Mumps
	Morbillivirus	Measles
Togaviridae	Rubivirus	Rubella
Picornaviridae	Enterovirus	Coxsackie
		ECHO
Exotic viruses		
Flaviviridae	Flavivirus	Yellow fever
Arenaviridae	Arenavirus	Lassa virus
		Junin
		Machupo
Filoviridae	Filovirus	Marburg virus
		Ebola virus
Bunyaviridae	Nairovirus	Congo-Crimean haemorrhagic fever
	Phlebovirus	Rift valley fever
Retroviridae	Lentivirus	Human immunodeficiency virus

* based on Foster, C. S. (1993). Infections and infestations of the liver. In Wight, D. G. D. (ed). *Liver, Biliary Tract and Exocrine Pancreas*, vol. 11, Systemic Pathology, 3rd edn. Edinburgh: Churchill Livingstone

the patient is suffering from a systemic infection rather than a viral hepatitis[8], although CMV is occasionally responsible for neonatal hepatitis[9]. Some cases occur in pregnancy or following multiple blood transfusions, but the majority are seen in debilitated or immunocompromised patients. CMV infection is one of the commonest opportunist organisms in transplant patients (Chapter 26), and in patients with acquired immunodeficiency syndrome (AIDS) (see below). Infection is confirmed by culture of the organism, detection of inclusion-containing cells in the urine or by demonstrating a rising titre of specific antibodies in the blood.

The histological findings in the liver are characteristic in only about 20% of cases[10], when typical cytomegalic cells are found. These measure 40 μm or more in diameter with a large nucleus containing a central eosinophilic inclusion body surrounded by a clear halo, the so-called 'owl's eye' cell (Figure 3.3). The same cells may also contain smaller and more basophilic cytoplasmic inclusions. They are found both in liver cells and in portal tracts. In liver cells they occur in any part of the acinus and may be in intact liver cell plates or partly or wholly extruded into sinusoids. The latter are usually surrounded by a cuff of inflammatory cells which include both neutrophil polymorphs and mononuclear cells (Figures 3.4 and 3.5). In portal tracts, cytomegalic cells may be seen in vascular endothelium and especially in the biliary epithelium. Non-parenchymal cell involvement appears more common in patients with significant degrees of immunosuppression and thus are rarely seen in those who appear to be otherwise fit.

In the absence of cytomegalic cells, non-specific changes may closely resemble viral hepatitis (Figures 3.6 and 3.7)[10]. The mixed inflammatory cell infiltrate, which although based on portal tracts may also extend into the parenchyma, can include large immature appearing lymphocytes as well as other acute and chronic inflammatory cells. Kupffer cells are often prominent and may show erythrophagocytosis and siderosis. A granulomatous response has also been described[11]. Widespread necrosis[12] or cholestasis are most unusual and complete recovery of the liver is the rule if the patient survives the systemic infection. Changes in the neonatal period are essentially similar, although cytomegalovirus is well recognized as one cause of a giant cell hepatitis (Chapter 8). Diagnosis can now be confirmed by use of monoclonal antibodies to the early proteins[13], which have a reported sensitivity of 70 to 80%, or by in situ hybridization[14]. Such techniques demonstrate that CMV is present in many normal–appearing cells in a great variety of tissues around the body[15].

Herpes simplex

This is the third virus of the herpes virus group and like the others is ubiquitous. Population studies show antibodies to herpes simplex virus (HSV) I and/or 2 in 50–100% of those adults screened. Typically the primary infection is inapparent or consists of a vesicular eruption at a mucocutaneous border on the lips (HSV I) or cervix uteri (HSV 2).

In most patients the virus will become latent, only to become reactivated as the typical 'cold sore' or genital sore at times of stress. Generalized infection is most unusual and as a rule only occurs in the neonatal period or in an immunocompromised older child or adult. Neonatal infection is usually acquired directly from the mother, during passage through the birth canal rather than transplacentally, and is usually HSV Type 2. It causes a severe generalized disease associated with fever, vesicular skin eruption, encephalitis, keratitis and haematological disorders as well as hepatitis[16]. In the older subject there is

usually evidence of debility, malnutrition or immunosuppression due to conditions such as Hodgkin's disease[17], following transplantation or in AIDS, but very occasionally there may be no obvious predisposing cause[18].

The pathological findings are very similar at all ages. Macroscopically the liver contains numerous yellowish foci of necrosis 1–2 mm in diameter often surrounded by a haemorrhagic halo. Histologically these represent foci of coagulative necrosis (Figure 3.8), often with associated haemorrhage. There may be a mononuclear cell reaction at the periphery of the necrosis, but this is often inconspicuous. Surviving liver cells in this region, however, do show conspicuous eosinophilic intranuclear inclusion bodies (Figure 3.9). Diagnosis can be confirmed by application of labelled antibodies[19]. In the neonatal cases giant cell transformation is unusual. In disseminated disease the changes observed in other organs are closely similar.

Varicella zoster

This is the fourth of the herpes virus group, and is normally a benign, almost universal, disease of childhood associated with a vesicular rash. Disseminated infection by this virus is very uncommon and more or less confined to immunodeficient patients, especially transplant recipients. Hepatic involvement is then usually part of fatal systemic disease[20], although in recent years treatment with the drug acyclovir has been successful.

The liver, in common with other organs such as the lung, is the site of multiple miliary foci of necrosis (Figure 3.10) not unlike those associated with herpes simplex infection. Adjacent liver cells contain Cowdry type A intranuclear inclusions, as may Kupffer cells and bile duct cells (Figure 3.11). Distinction from herpes simplex is mainly determined by clinical, virological and serological parameters.

Adenoviruses

Adenoviruses are ubiquitous and commonly infect children, causing subclinical or mild and self-limited disease with symptoms such as rhinitis and keratoconjunctivitis. Immunocompromised patients, however, may develop severe generalized disease with hepatic involvement, which is often fatal[21,22]. The liver shows extensive haemorrhagic necrosis, with distinctive 'smudgy' basophilic intranuclear inclusions in surviving hepatocytes bordering the necrotic zones (Figure 3.12). Distinctive crystalline arrays of virions are easily found by electron microscopy. Similar inclusions may be found in other affected organs, particularly the lungs.

Exotic virus infections

Yellow fever

Yellow fever is caused by a group B arbovirus which is transmitted to man by infected mosquitoes. Whilst there has been great success in the control of yellow fever, especially by control of the vector, it remains endemic in certain parts of South America and equatorial Africa, where the prevalence may even be on the increase[23].

Infection is probably often silent, but when severe it causes a systemic disease with fever, prostration, haemorrhage and jaundice. Microscopically, in the classical case there is a mid-zonal eosinophilic necrosis of hepatocytes, giving rise to the so-called Councilman or acidophil bodies. Many of these are vacuolated and the necrosis tends to be bordered by liver cells showing large and small droplet fatty change. Spotty necrosis may be seen in other parts of the lobule where there may also be ballooning degeneration of liver cells. The cellular

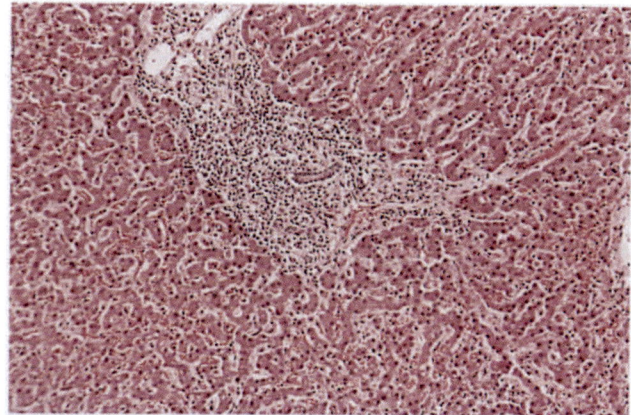

Figure 3.1 Infectious mononucleosis. There is a moderately dense mononuclear cell infiltration of portal tracts and sinusoids. The limiting plate is intact and liver cells are healthy.

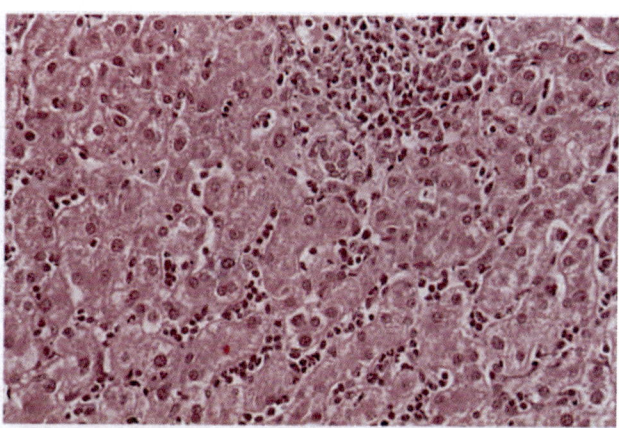

Figure 3.2 Infectious mononucleosis. A different patient, showing similar infiltration of portal tracts and sinusoids, resembling leukaemia. Most of the cells can be seen to be lymphocytes. Note the complete lack of hepatocellular damage.

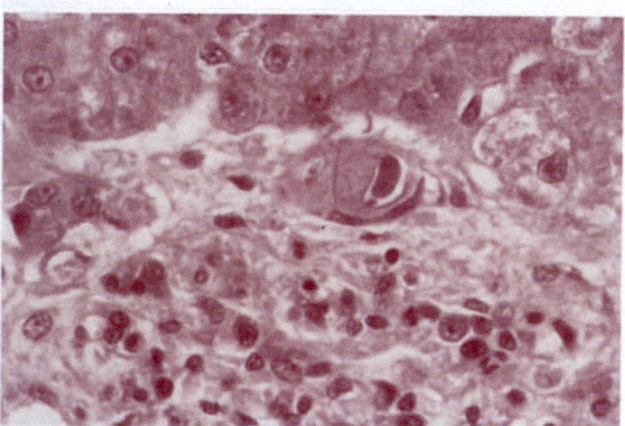

Figure 3.3 Cytomegalovirus hepatitis. A portal cell, possibly endothelial, is transformed into a typical cytomegalocyte or 'owl's eye' cell. In this instance, there is little or no cellular reaction.

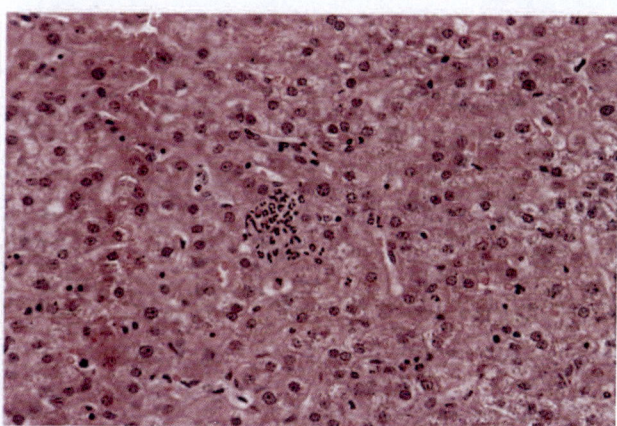

Figure 3.4 Cytomegalovirus hepatitis. Focal collection of inflammatory cells almost totally composed of neutrophils.

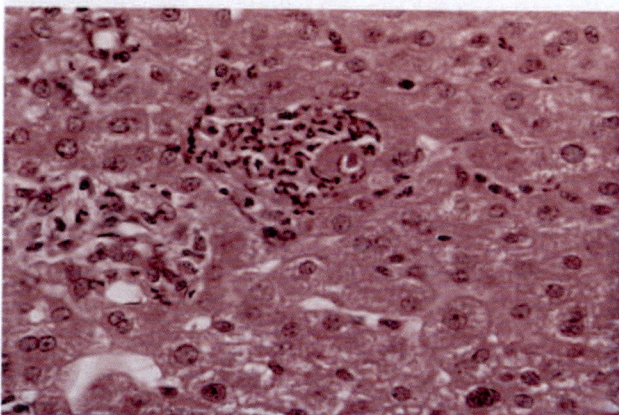

Figure 3.5 Cytomegalovirus hepatitis. Sections of Figure 3.4 cut at deeper levels revealed that the inflammatory cells were related to a typical cytomegalocyte.

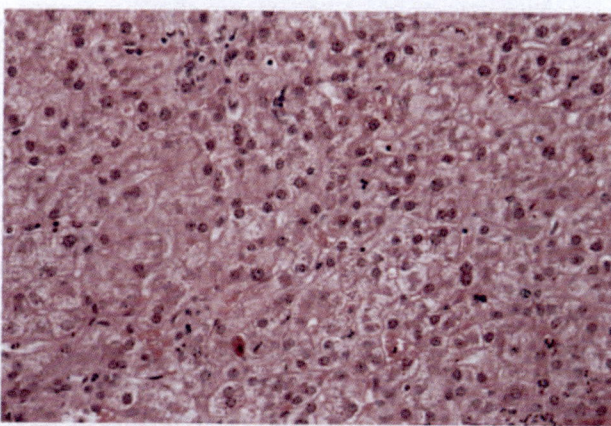

Figure 3.6 Cytomegalovirus hepatitis. Renal transplant recipient, with a hepatitic clinical picture, from whom CMV was cultured. The histological picture was non-specific and closely resembled acute viral hepatitis. Note an acidophil body (below centre), minor inflammatory activity and regenerative changes.

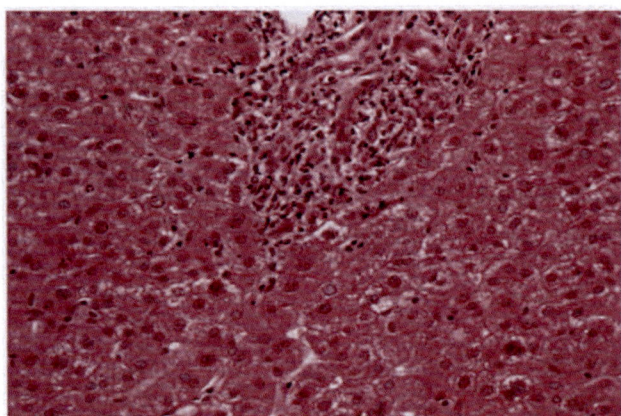

Figure 3.7 Cytomegalovirus hepatitis. Same patient as Figure 3.6. Portal tract showing entirely non-specific inflammatory changes.

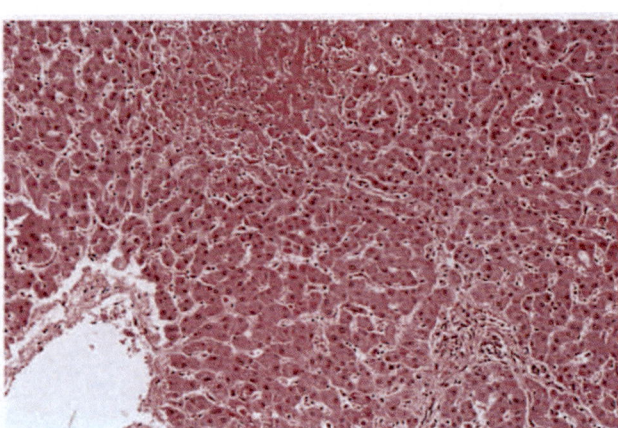

Figure 3.8 Herpes simplex virus hepatitis. A 23-year-old male treated with chemotherapy for lymphoma. Died with terminal vesiculopapular rash from which virus was cultured. There is a small focus of coagulative necrosis in the section which is exciting a negligible cellular reaction.

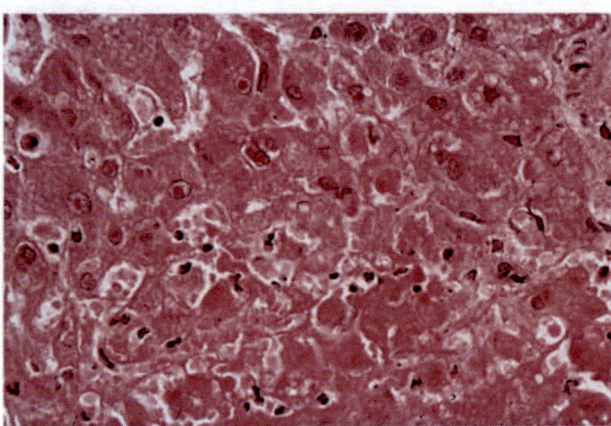

Figure 3.9 Herpes simplex virus hepatitis. Same case as Figure 3.8, showing intranuclear inclusion bodies in the hepatocyte nuclei at the margin of the necrotic zone.

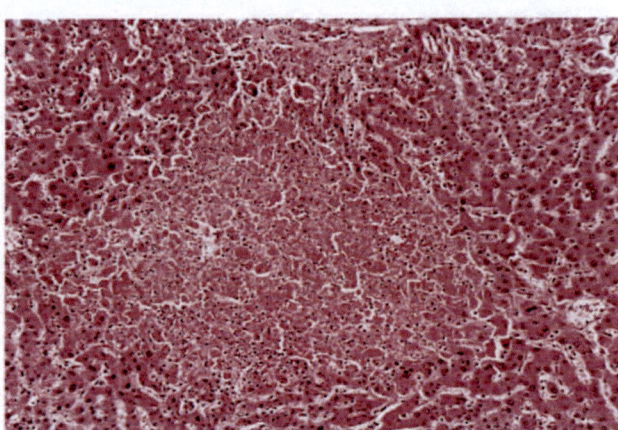

Figure 3.10 Herpes zoster hepatitis. Adult patient treated with chemotherapy for Hodgkin's disease. Rapid deterioration with generalized bullous eruption from which zoster virus was harvested. All organs, including the liver, contained focal necroses very similar to those in Figures 3.8 and 3.9 due to HSV.

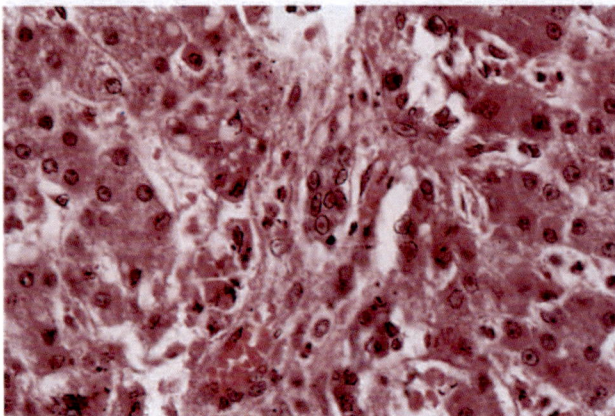

Figure 3.11 Herpes zoster hepatitis. Eosinophilic inclusion bodies in both hepatocytes and biliary epithelium.

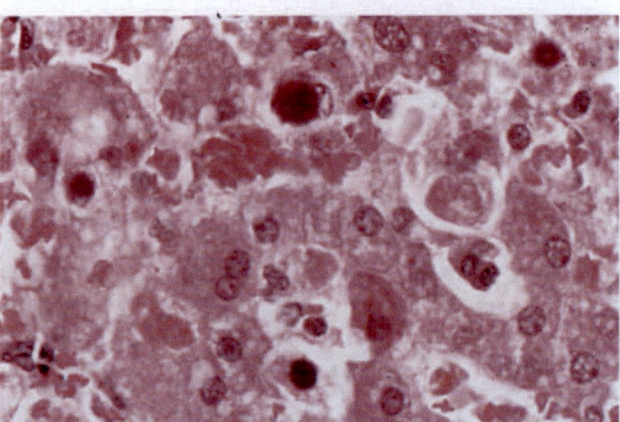

Figure 3.12 Adenovirus hepatitis. Adult transplant patient who developed a systemic haemorrhagic illness and died within a few days. At autopsy, irregular foci of hepatic necrosis were seen with these characteristic smudgy basophilic intranuclear inclusions in adjacent viable hepatocytes.

response is rather slight, is composed of mononuclear cells and tends to be related to the Councilman bodies. The reticulin framework remains intact and cholestasis is not seen. Kupffer cells may be prominent and contain iron and ceroid pigment. Lipofuscin is sometimes prominent in liver cells.

These classical changes are only seen in the first week of illness[24]. Thereafter the appearances become non-specific and indistinguishable from viral hepatitis. This can cause some diagnostic problems in the sporadic case, since complement fixation tests do not become positive until about 20 days after onset of disease.

Other exotic viruses

There was considerable interest in three 'new' viral diseases, all described for the first time about ten years ago, mainly because of their very high case fatality rate. These are *Marburg virus disease*, *Lassa fever* and *Ebola virus* infection, all of which may involve the liver[25].

All three infections probably involve an animal reservoir and despite the high case fatality ratio amongst patients admitted to hospital, the relatively frequent finding of specific antibodies in patients from endemic areas suggests the existence of unrecognized or mild infections. The clinical illness tends to be non-specific with fever and prostration and the differential diagnosis includes such diverse conditions as malaria, typhoid, yellow fever and even influenza and measles. Histologically the liver is the principal target in Lassa infection[26], and is involved as part of more generalized disease in Marburg[27] and Ebola virus infections. All three are associated with eosinophilic necrosis of hepatocytes, singly or in small groups and without a zonal distribution, with little accompanying inflammation. The causative virus may be visible on electron microscopy. Diagnostic procedures must be carried out in maximum security laboratories by virus isolation and specific antibody assays[28]. Other exotic viruses are discussed by Howard and colleagues[29].

Other viruses

Rubella virus may involve the liver, amongst other organs in the congenital rubella syndrome[30], and very occasionally in adults[31]. Abnormalities of liver biochemistry may be seen in up to 80% of adults admitted to hospital with *measles*[32], but they are usually subclinical and self-limited. Occasionally, hepatitis may be clinically significant, although rarely seen histologically. Liver dysfunction may follow infection with both *Coxsackie viruses* (groups A and B) and *ECHO viruses*[33], but are generally only significant in the neonatal period.

HUMAN IMMUNODEFICIENCY VIRUS (HIV) AND THE LIVER

During the 1980s, a hitherto unrecognized disease, acquired immunodeficiency syndrome, reached epidemic proportions in all countries of the world[34]. The discovery in 1981 of the causative RNA retrovirus, HIV, led to considerable understanding of its epidemiology and pathogenic mechanisms. HIV infection of helper/inducer (T4) lymphocytes by binding to their CD4 receptor is the fundamental biological event whereby the immune system becomes crippled[35], rendering the host susceptible to a wide variety of opportunistic infections[36] and neoplasms, including malignant lymphoma and Kaposi's sarcoma[37,38].

The multisystem pathological effects of HIV infection in AIDS have been described in a number of autopsy studies[39]. Although there is as yet no evidence that HIV directly infects any of the cells of the liver[40], liver disease nevertheless contributes substantially to morbidity and mortality in AIDS[41,42,43]. Lesions fall into three categories[42]: 1. complications of immune paresis, 2. infection by the hepatitis viruses, 3. changes secondary to multisystem disease[44]—there are no changes specific to HIV infection. Liver biopsy produces a high yield of positive diagnoses[41], but, as yet, the information provided by biopsy rarely leads to improved survival of the patient[45].

Infections

Many different infectious agents, including bacteria, viruses, fungi and protozoa, have been found in the liver in HIV infection (Table 3.2), and, in as many as 25% of cases, liver biopsy will yield an infectious diagnosis[43,46]. Opportunist infections usually reflect a disseminated process. Mycobacteria have been the most frequent bacteria to infect the liver, and they include atypical organisms such as *Mycobacterium avium-intracellulare* and *M. kansasii* as well as *M. tuberculosis*[45,46] (see also Chapter 19). In the immunodeficient patient, granulomas form poorly or not at all—raising comparisons with lepromatous leprosy—and the bacteria are found in dense clusters within foamy macrophages or even within single sinusoidal Kupffer cells. It is therefore important to use an acid-fast Ziel-Nielsen stain in all biopsies from AIDS patients. *Mycobacterium avium-intracellulare* also stains with silver stains which also demonstrate fungi (Table 3.2) and the rare instances of disseminated *Pneumocystis carinii*[47]. The latter organisms are found in nodules of pale-staining amorphous exudate, not unlike that seen more frequently in the alveolar spaces of the lung.

Infection with or reactivation of viruses of the herpes family can cause serious problems in patients with AIDS. Herpes simplex and varicella-zoster both cause a similar picture, although in AIDS patients the histological features may be less distinctive, with more widespread and less discrete areas of necrosis[41]. Persons at risk of infection by HIV are also at risk from infection by the various hepatitis viruses[48], particularly hepatitis B. Some 10–20% of AIDS patients have chronic hepatitis B infection. Coexistent infection with the delta virus or hepatitis D is extremely common in some patients with AIDS, and, as in immunocompetent individuals (Chapter 2), is associated with progressive disease. Patients at risk of HIV are similarly exposed to risk of HCV infection.

Table 3.2 Infections associated with AIDS*

Bacteria	*Mycobacterium avium-intracellulare*
	Mycobacterium kansasii
	Mycobacterium tuberculosis
	Klebsiella pneumoniae
	Staphylococcus aureus
Fungi	*Candida albicans*
	Coccidioides
	Cryptococcus
	Histoplasma
Viruses	Herpes viruses
	Herpes simplex (Types 1 & 2)
	Cytomegalovirus
	Varicella-Zoster
	Epstein-Barr virus
	Hepatitis viruses
	Hepatitis B
	Hepatitis C
	Hepatitis D
Protozoa	Cryptosporidium
	Pneumocystis carinii
	Toxoplasma

* based upon Foster, C. S. (1993). Infections and infestations of the liver. In Wight, D. G. D. (ed). *Liver, Biliary Tract and Exocrine Pancreas.* vol 11, Systemic Pathology. Edinburgh: Churchill Livingstone

Neoplasms

Kaposi's sarcoma may involve the liver as part of general dissemination[46], and can be recognized by proliferating spindle cells with extravasated red cells and hyaline globules, as at other sites. The link between Kaposi's sarcoma and HIV infection, or with other viruses such as CMV, remains unclear, although recent molecular genetic evidence suggests that it may be due directly to HIV itself[49]. Malignant lymphomas in AIDS are usually high grade B-cell neoplasms[50], and may apparently arise in the liver. As in patients immunosuppressed for transplantation, the tumour has been linked with EBV infection.

Other complications

Non-specific changes may be attributable to such factors as malnutrition, hypotension, various drugs, including zidovudine, sepsis or other conditions[44], but do not differ from those seen in patients similarly ill without HIV infection.

REFERENCES

1. Fingeroth, J. D., Weiss, J., Tedder, T. F., Strominger, J. L., Biro, P. A. and Fearon, D. T. (1984). Epstein-Barr virus receptor of human B lymphocytes is the C3d receptor CR2. Proc. Natl Acad. Sci., 81, 4510–4514
2. White, N. J. and Juel-Jensen, B. E. (1984). Infectious mononucleosis hepatitis. Semin. Liver Dis., 4, 301–306
3. Gowing, N. F. C. (1975). Infectious mononucleosis, histopathologic aspects. Pathol. Ann., 10, 1–20
4. Chang, M. Y. and Campbell, W. G. (1975). Fatal infectious mononucleosis associated with liver necrosis and herpes-like virus particles. Arch. Pathol., 99, 185–191
5. Krech, V. (1973). Complement fixing antibodies against CMV in different parts of the world. Bull. WHO, 40, 103–106
6. Griffiths, P. D. (1984). Cytomegalovirus and the liver. Semin. Liver Dis., 4, 307–313
7. Snover, D. C. and Horwitz, C. A. (1984). Liver disease in cytomegalovirus mononucleosis: a light microscopical and immunoperoxidase study of six cases. Hepatology, 4, 408–412
8. Toghill, P. J., Bailey, M. E., Williams, R., Zeegen, R. and Brown, R. (1967). Cytomegalovirus hepatitis in the adult. Lancet, i, 1351–1354
9. Watkins, J. B., Katz, A. J. and Grand, R. J. (1977). Neonatal hepatitis. A diagnostic approach. Adv. Pediatr., 24, 399–454
10. Henson, D. E., Grimley, P. M. and Strano, A. J. (1974). Postnatal cytomegalovirus hepatitis. Hum. Pathol., 5, 93–103
11. Clarke, J., Craig, R. M., Saffro, R., Murphy, P. and Yokoo, H. (1979). Cytomegalovirus granulomatous hepatitis. Am. J. Med., 66, 264–269
12. Schusterman, N. H., Frauenhoffer, C. and Kinsey, M. D. (1978). Fatal massive hepatic necrosis in cytomegalovirus mononucleosis. Ann. Intern. Med., 88, 810–812
13. Stirk, P. R. and Griffiths, P. D. (1987). Use of monoclonal antibodies. J. Med. Virol., 21, 329–337
14. Naoumov, N. V., Alexander, G. J., O'Grady, J. G., Aldio, P., Portmann, B. C. and Williams, R. (1988). Rapid diagnosis of cytomegalovirus infection by in situ hybridization in liver grafts. Lancet, 1, 1361–1364
15. Myerson, D., Hackman, R. C., Nelson, J. A., Ward, D. C. and McDougall, J. K. (1984). Widespread presence of histologically occult cytomegalovirus. Hum. Pathol., 15, 430–439
16. White, J. G. (1963). Fulminant infection with herpes simplex virus in premature and newborn infants. N. Engl. J. Med., 269, 455–460
17. Lee, J. C. and Fortuny, I. E. (1972). Adult herpes simplex hepatitis. Hum Pathol., 3, 277–281
18. Connor, R. W., Lorts, G. and Gilbert, D. N. (1979). Lethal herpes simplex virus type 1 hepatitis in a normal adult. Gastroenterology, 76, 590–594
19. Marrie, T. J., McDonald, A. R., Conen, P. E. and Boubrean, S. F. J. (1982). Herpes simplex hepatitis. Use of immunoperoxidase to demonstrate the viral antigen in hepatocytes. Gastroenterology, 82, 71–76
20. Morishita, K., Kodo, M., Asano, S., Fuji, H. and Miwa, S. (1985). Fulminant varicella hepatitis following bone marrow transplantation. JAM., 253, 511
21. Carmichael, G. P., Zahradnik, J. M., Moyer, G. H. and Porter, D. D. (1979). Adenovirus hepatitis in an immunosuppressed adult patient. Am. J. Clin. Pathol., 71, 352–355
22. Zahradnik, J. M., Spencer, M. J. and Porter, D. D. (1980). Adenovirus infection in the immunocompromised patient. Am. J. Med., 68, 725–732
23. Leading article. (1981). Yellow fever cause for concern? Br. Med. J., 282, 1735–1736
24. Francis, T. I., Moore, D. L., Edington, G. M. and Smith, J. A. (1972). A clinico-pathological study of human yellow fever. Bull. WHO, 46, 659–667
25. Zuckerman, A. J. and Simpson, D. H. (1979). Exotic virus infections of the liver. In Popper, H. and Schaffner, F. (eds). Progress in Liver Diseases. V. pp. 425–438. New York: Grune and Stratton
26. Winn, W. C. and Walker, D. H. (1975). The pathology of human Lassa fever. Bull. WHO, 52, 535–545
27. Bechtelsheimer, H., Korb, G. and Gedigk, P. (1972). The morphology and pathogenesis of 'Marburg virus' hepatitis. Hum. Pathol., 3, 255–264
28. Zuckerman, A. J. and Ellis, D. S. (1991). Exotic virus infections of the liver. In McIntyre, N., Benhamou, J.-P., Bircher, J., Rizzetto, M. and Rodes, J. (eds). Oxford textbook of clinical hepatology. pp. 638–646. Oxford: Oxford University Press
29. Howard, C. R., Ellis, D. S. and Simpson, D. I. H. (1984). Exotic viruses and the liver. Semin. Liver Dis., 4, 361–374
30. Esterly, J. R. and Oppenheimer, E. H. (1973). Intrauterine rubella infection. In Rosenberg, H. S. and Bolande, R. P. (eds). Perspectives in Pediatric Pathology. 1. pp. 313–338. Chicago: Year Book Medical Publishers
31. Onji, M., Kumon, I., Kanaoka, M., Miyaoka, H. and Ohta, Y. (1988). Intrahepatic lymphocyte subpopulations in acute hepatitis in an adult with rubella. Am. J. Gastroenterol., 83, 320–322
32. Shalev Zimels, H., Weizman, Z., Lotan, C., Gavish, D., Ackerman, Z. and Morag, A. (1988). Extent of measles hepatitis in various ages. Hepatology, 8, 1138–1139
33. Modlin, J. F. (1985). Coxsackievirus and echovirus. In Mandell, G. L., Douglas, R. G. and Bennett, J. E. (eds). Principles and practice in infectious disease. pp. 814–825. New York: Wiley and Sons
34. Friedman, S. L. (1992). AIDS: a review for the hepatologist. Semin. Liver Dis., 12, No 2 (whole issue)
35. Edelman, A. S. and Zoller-Pasner, S. (1989). AIDS: a syndrome of immune dysregulation, dysfunction and deficiency. FASEB J., 3, 22–30
36. Glatt, A. E., Chirgivin, K. and Landesman, S. H. (1988). Treatment of infections associated with human immunodeficiency virus. N. Engl. J. Med., 318, 1439–1448
37. Biggar, R. J., Horm, J., Goedert, J. J. and Melbye, M. (1987). Cancer in a group at risk of acquired immunodeficiency syndrome (AIDS) through 1984. Am. J. Epidemiol., 126, 578–586
38. Kaplan, M. H., Susin, M., Pahwa, S. G. and et al. (1987). Neoplastic complications of HTLV-III infection. Lymphomas and solid tumours. Am. J. Med., 82, 389–396
39. Wilkes, M. S., Felix, J. C., Fortin, A. H., Godwin, T. A. and Thompson, W. G. (1988). Value of necropsy in acquired immunodeficiency syndrome. Lancet, 2, 85–88
40. Lafon, M.-E. and Kirn, A. (1992). Human immunodeficiency virus infection of the liver. Semin. Liver Dis., 12, 197–204
41. Schaffner, F. (1990). The liver in HIV infection. Progr. Liver Dis., 9, 505–522
42. Lefkowitch, J. H. (1991). Pathologic aspects of the liver in human immunodeficiency virus (HIV) infection. In McIntyre, N., Benhamou, J.-P., Bircher, J., Rizzetto, M. and Rodes, J. (eds). Oxford textbook of hepatology. pp. 630–635. Oxford: Oxford University Press
43. Bach, N., Theise, N. D. and Schaffner, F. (1992). Hepatic histopathology in the acquired immunodeficiency syndrome. Semin. Liver Dis., 12, 205–212
44. Cappell, M. S. (1991). Hepatobiliary manifestations of the acquired immune deficiency syndrome. Am. J. Gastroenterol., 86, 1–15
45. Schneiderman, D. J., Arenson, D. M., Cello, J. P. et al. (1987). Hepatic disease in patients with the acquired immunodeficiency syndrome. Hepatology, 7, 925–930
46. Lebovics, E., Dworkin, B. M., Heier, S. K. and Rosenthal, W. S. (1988). The hepato-biliary manifestations of immunodeficiency virus infection. Am. J. Gastroenterol.
47. Poblete, R. B., Rodriguez, K., Foust, R. T., Reddy, K. R. and Suldana, M. J. (1989). Pneumocystis carinii hepatitis in the acquired immunodeficiency syndrome (AIDS). Ann. Intern. Med., 110, 737–738
48. Foster, C. S. (1993). Infections and infestations of the liver. In Wight, D. G. D. (ed). Liver, Biliary Tract and Exocrine Pancreas. 11 pp. Edinburgh: Churchill Livingstone
49. Sinkovics, J. G. (1991). Kaposi's sarcoma: its 'oncogenes' and growth factors. Crit. Rev. Oncol. Hematol., 11, 87–107
50. Herndier, B. G. and Friedman, S. L. (1992). Neoplasms of the gastrointestinal tract and hepatobiliary system in acquired immunodeficiency syndrome. Semin. Liver Dis., 12, 128–141

Bacterial and Fungal Infections

4

Bacteria may affect the liver either as a result of parenchymal or biliary invasion, or as a systemic manifestation of bacteraemia or toxaemia. Any serious bacterial infections by, for example, pyogenic cocci, enterobacteria, or the Legionnaire's organism, may be complicated by jaundice[1]. Jaundice occurs in over 40% of young children with bacteraemia[2]. The mechanism in these cases is not always clear but is usually only partly attributable to haemolysis. Microscopically, in the absence of abscess formation (Chapter 5), the changes in the liver are rarely distinctive, with non-specific reactive hepatitis (Chapter 21) being the most common finding. However, focal necroses of hepatocytes may also occasionally be seen, especially in young children, when infection is an important cause of hepatic necrosis. Intrahepatic cholestasis, particularly ductular cholestasis, may be found in any severe bacterial infections (Figure 4.1)[3].

Staphylococcus aureus and *Clostridium perfringens* may both cause hepatic dysfunction as a consequence of toxin production. In the *toxic shock syndrome* complicating *Staph. aureus* infection there may be evidence of cholestasis and cholangitis[4].

Characteristically bacteria and other micro-organisms may be associated with granuloma formation (further discussed in Chapter 19) or with abscess formation (further discussed in Chapter 5). Space only permits a discussion of selected organisms in this chapter–an extended account of bacterial infections of the liver is given by Kibbler[5] and of infections and infestations by Foster[6].

SPECIFIC BACTERIAL INFECTIONS
Listerosis

Listeria monocytogenes is a Gram-positive bacillus which causes infection with increasing frequency in humans. It is usually asymptomatic in adults, and is probably mainly food-borne[5]. It is rarely clinically significant outside the neonatal period[7], when it is generally acquired transplacentally from the mother, and may lead to fatal disseminated disease. Histologically, it is characterized by rounded granuloma-like foci of macrophages[8], often undergoing necrosis, in many other organs as well as the liver (Figure 4.2).

Typhoid fever

Abnormalities of liver function are common in typhoid fever but hepatomegaly and jaundice are only encountered in a minority of patients in most[9] but not all series[10]. Nevertheless morphological changes are almost invariably present. The most constant are non-specific and consist of mononuclear cell infiltration of portal tracts with focal ballooning degeneration and necrosis of liver cells[11]. Small droplet fatty change is common. There may be some sinusoidal dilation and congestion with scattered lymphocytes and proliferation of Kupffer cells. The most distinctive lesion, seen less often but not apparently related to severity or duration of disease[9] is the 'typhoid nodule' (Figure 4.3). This is found most often in the periportal region and is composed of a nodular aggregate of lymphocytes and macrophages. Central necrosis may

or may not be present but is much more likely to be seen post-mortem.

This spectrum of histological changes is very similar to those seen in other bacterial septicaemias[12] and in primary malaria[13] and can only be distinguished with confidence if organisms are demonstrated in the typhoid nodules.

Tuberculosis

This is discussed in Chapters 5 and 19.

Leprosy

Mycobacterium leprae affects the liver in most cases of lepromatous leprosy, but is usually entirely asymptomatic[6]. Histologically, miliary collections of foamy macrophages are seen scattered throughout both portal tracts and parenchyma[14], sometimes forming ill-defined granulomas. Large numbers of organisms can readily be demonstrated in the cytoplasm of these cells with the appropriate stain. In tuberculoid leprosy, granulomata are rare but indistinguishable from those in tuberculosis.

Syphilis

This may involve the liver in congenital infection, or as part of secondary or tertiary disease.

In congenital syphilis the liver commonly appears morphologically entirely normal[15], although in virtually every case numerous organisms can easily be demonstrated with silver stains. In a small proportion of cases, the well-known pericellular fibrosis is seen. Here there is widespread portal tract fibrosis as well as diffuse intercellular fibrosis separating and surrounding single and small groups of liver cells (Figure 4.4). Rarely, gummas (see below) may be seen in the neonatal period.

In early (secondary) syphilis some 10% of cases show evidence of liver damage[16], and in some parts of the world the incidence is increasing[17]. A recent report suggests that in early disease the changes may be indistinguishable from those of viral hepatitis[18]. More typically there is widespread infiltration of portal tracts and sinusoids by neutrophil and eosinophil polymorphs and lymphocytes. Vessels in portal tracts may show thickening of their walls with fibrin deposition and infiltration with both neutrophils and mononuclear cells. Focal parenchymal necroses occur in periportal and central locations, the latter being fairly characteristic and associated with the same mix of acute and chronic inflammatory cells. Silver stains demonstrate organisms in about half of these foci. Healing may be followed by some pericellular fibrosis.

The characteristic hepatic lesion of *late* syphilis is the gumma (Figure 4.5). These are almost always asymptomatic and may be single or multiple. Although they are now quite rare in the developed world, their importance lies in the fact that they may be confused with metastases or other space occupying lesions in the liver[19]. Macroscopically and microscopically they are indistinguishable from gummata in other organs. There is central necrosis surrounded by vascular granulation tissue containing numerous plasma cells and lymphocytes and occasional giant cells. Obliterative endarteritis of the adjacent small vessels is one of the most characteristic features of a

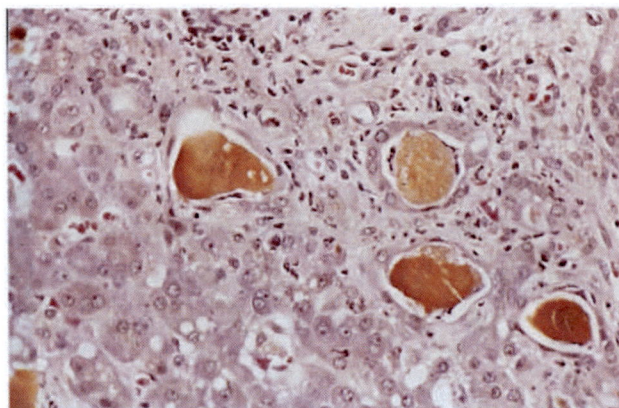

Figure 4.1 Ductular cholestasis in systemic sepsis, showing distended bile ductules filled with inspissated bile.

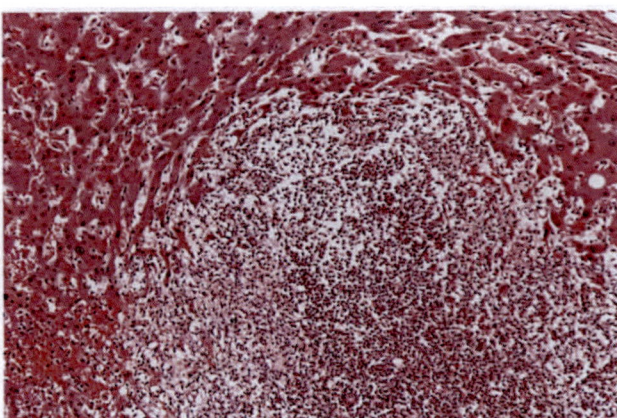

Figure 4.2 Disseminated infection with Listeria monocytogenes. Terminal septicaemic illness in a 70-year-old patient with disseminated malignancy. Microabscesses were visible in many organs. In the liver there is a central core containing neutrophils, surrounded by macrophages.

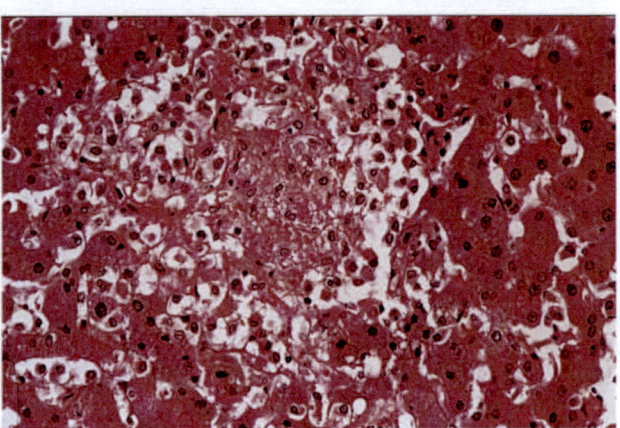

Figure 4.3 Typhoid fever. Post-mortem liver 'biopsy' shows a typical typhoid nodule, composed of macrophages and lymphocytes and undergoing central necrosis. The adjacent liver is unremarkable.

The author is deeply indebted to Professor MSR Hutt who kindly provided the slides from which Figure 4.3 was prepared.

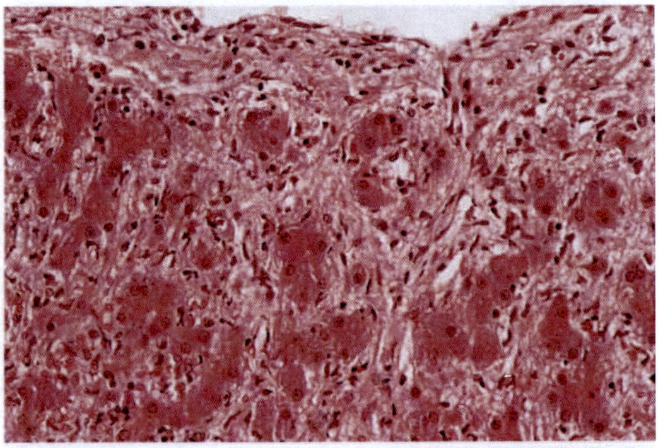

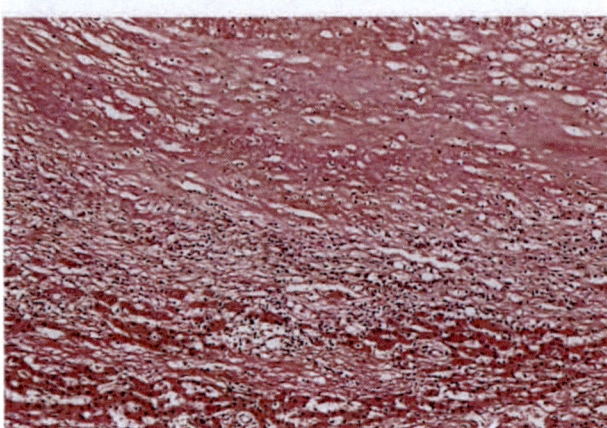

Figure 4.4 Congenital syphilis. Classic pericellular fibrosis with individual hepatocytes and small groups of cells separated and surrounded by fibrous tissue.

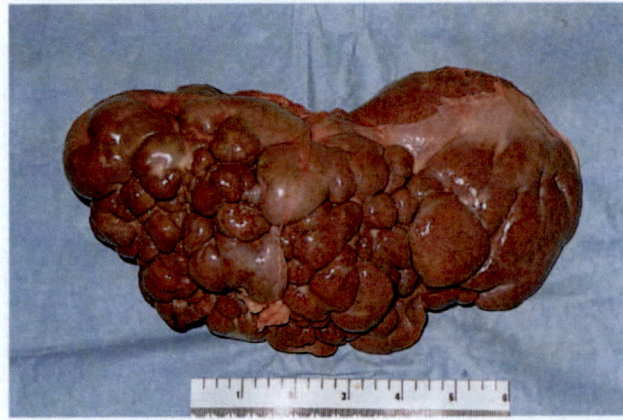

Figure 4.5 Gumma. There is central avascular necrosis surrounded by a poorly developed inflammatory response composed mainly of lymphocytes and plasma cells.

Figure 4.6 Hepar lobatum, not in this instance due to syphilis, but a modern equivalent which is the result of shrinkage of liver metastases by chemotherapy. Each of the deep furrows in the capsule is caused by contraction of underlying tumour.

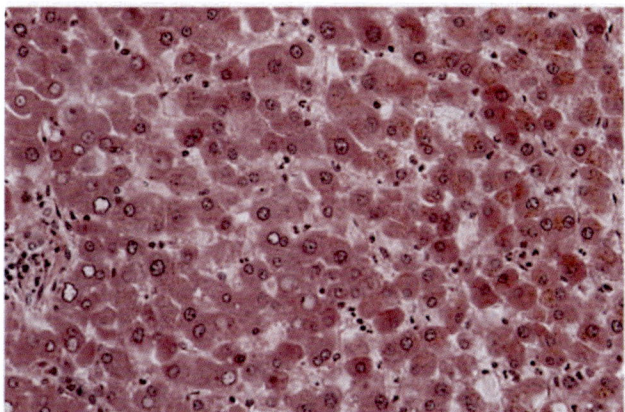

Figure 4.7 Weil's disease. Post-mortem section of liver from a fatal case in a 61-year-old coal miner. Note the striking rounding-off and lipofuscin pigmentation of the centrilobular liver cells (right). There is also periportal glycogen vacuolation of nuclei.

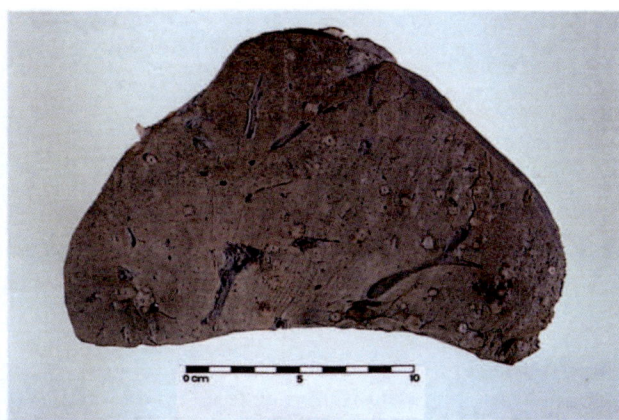

Figure 4.8 Disseminated candidiasis. A 41-year-old patient with non-Hodgkin's lymphoma treated with chemotherapy. Rapid deterioration and death, no symptoms referable to the liver. At post-mortem there was mucormycosis of lungs and candidal abscesses in liver, kidneys and oesophagus.

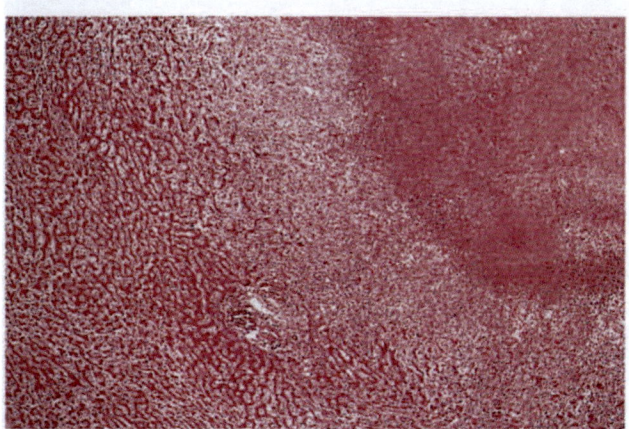

Figure 4.9 Candidiasis. Same patient as Figure 4.8. This abscess has a necrotic centre surrounded by mononuclear cells. No organisms are visible.

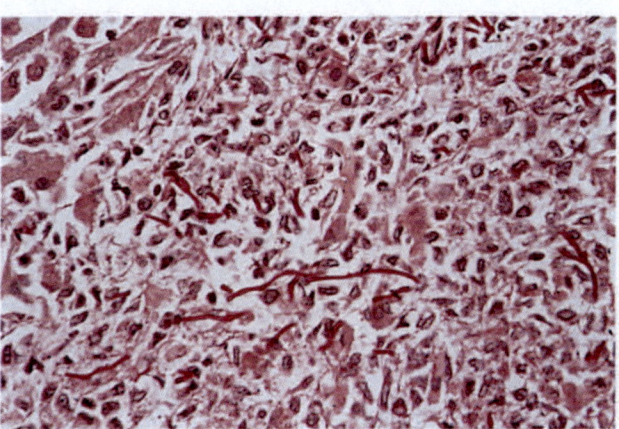

Figure 4.10 Candidiasis. Same patient as Figures 4.8 and 4.9. The pseudohyphae are readily seen, surrounded by mononuclear cells, with PAS diastase.

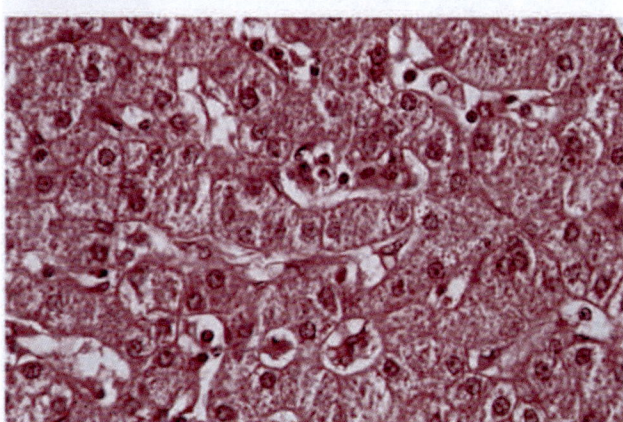

Figure 4.11 Disseminated infection with Histoplasma capsulatum. In this case the organisms, which measure only 2–3 mm in diameter, are confined to Kupffer cells (a good example just below centre) where they have excited no cellular response. PAS staining would easily distinguish the fungi from leishmania which are PAS-negative.

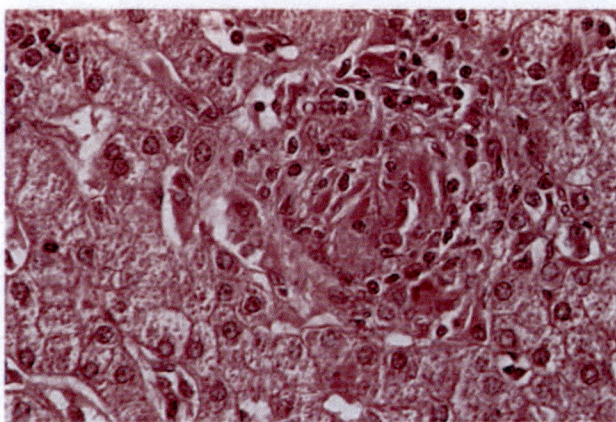

Figure 4.12 Histoplasmosis. Same patient as Figure 4.11. An ill-defined granuloma composed of macrophages and lymphocytes. A few organisms can just be discerned, but they were readily demonstrated with PAS stain.

gumma. Healing may lead to the deeply furrowed 'hepar lobatum' of the older literature (Figure 4.6). Late syphilis does not progress to cirrhosis, the concomitant cirrhosis in some of the older reports almost certainly would today be attributed to hepatitis B or alcohol.

Lyme disease

Lyme disease is a zoonosis caused by the Gram–negative spirochaete, *Borrelia burgdorferi*. It is transmitted by ticks and is a chronic multisystem disorder in which diagnosis is often delayed. Hepatitis may be a significant clinical feature[5] and may also be observed histologically[20].

Leptospirosis

Infection by the leptospire *Leptospira interrogans* is usually acquired by contact with rat urine (subtype *icterohaemorrhagiae*) or, less frequently, infected dogs (subtype *canicola*), and thus certain professions such as farm workers and refuse collectors have the greatest risk. Serious infection is uncommon–there being only about 50 cases per annum in the United Kingdom.

Weil's disease is the name given to any leptospiral illness. Infection is systemic and is typically characterized by fever, jaundice, renal and hepatic failure and has a high mortality[1]. However, it is probable that many infections are much less severe and in the absence of jaundice may go unrecognized. The pathogenesis of the jaundice is not clear although assumed to be due to a hepatotoxic reaction.

Histologically, the liver lesions may be unexpectedly trivial in view of the severity of the jaundice, although ultrastructural damage may be much more dramatic. Most descriptions are based upon autopsy material where disruption of liver cell plates with rounding and separation of liver cells is the most striking feature (Figure 4.7). In biopsies this is usually absent[21] the appearances being rather non-specific with some liver cell swelling, occasional acidophil bodies and frequent hepatocyte mitosis. Focal necroses are seen in less than 10%. Cholestasis is common. Leptospirae are only detectable in the liver in about 25% of cases by means of silver stains such as the Warthin-Starry technique[21]. If the patient survives, the liver returns to normal without any adverse sequelae.

RICKETTSIAE

The Rickettsiae basically cause two types of disease, typhus and haemorrhagic fever. Of the typhus group, only Q fever, caused by *Coxiella burnetii*, is associated with a hepatitis[22]. Although typically an influenza-like pulmonary infection, hepatomegaly and minor disturbances of liver function are common and jaundice occurs in about 5%. Biopsy changes may be present even in the absence of biochemical abnormality. Granulomas are almost always present. These are mostly lobular but also occur in portal tracts. Many of these have a very distinctive and pathognomonic appearance characterized by a central clear space, resembling a fat vacuole, surrounded by a halo of fibrinoid material which stains positively with Masson and Mallory's PTAH[23] at the centre of an otherwise ordinary epithelioid and giant cell granuloma. Serial sections may be necessary to demonstrate this pattern, which is also occasionally encountered in other conditions which include toxoplasmosis, leishmaniasis and drug sensitivity[24]. Apart from the granulomas, fatty change, of variable degree, minor focal necroses and inflammatory changes are common.

In contrast, in the haemorrhagic fevers liver involvement is part of systemic infection. In Rocky Mountain spotted fever there is portal tract infiltration by both mononuclear cells and neutrophil polymorphs and this may be accompanied by a striking vasculitis[25]. *Rickettsia prowazeki* can be demonstrated by immunofluorescence in the majority of cases, but liver biopsy is not a practicable diagnostic procedure because these patients invariably suffer from a severe haemorrhagic diathesis.

FUNGAL INFECTIONS

Systemic mycoses broadly fall into two groups. There are those ubiquitous and generally harmless fungi which only cause disease in patients with defective defences. The main offenders in this opportunistic group are Candida, Aspergillus and Mucor, and infection by them has become increasingly common in recent years with increased use of steroids and other immunosuppressive drugs, and as part of the acquired immunodeficiency syndrome (AIDS) (Chapter 3). In contrast, there is a number of other fungi, many with a relatively restricted geographic distribution, which regularly cause infection in apparently normal individuals. These include Histoplasma (which has infected more than 30×10^6 people in the USA), Coccidioides and the organisms responsible for North and South American blastomycosis. The latter two may affect patients with AIDS in the areas where they are prevalent. Both groups may from time to time affect the liver but, in general, liver involvement is asymptomatic and only recognized at autopsy in fatal cases of generalized disease (Figures 4.8–4.10).

The most characteristic tissue response to fungal infection is a suppurative granuloma in which a central neutrophil abscess is surrounded by epithelioid and giant cells. Occasionally, particularly in histoplasmosis, there may be caseous necrosis so that the lesions are almost indistinguishable from tuberculosis[26], or the granulomas may be sarcoid-like. Granulomas, however, are by no means invariable, and there may merely be non-specific chronic inflammation or, especially in disseminated disease, there may be a relatively inconspicuous cellular response (Figures 4.11 and 4.12).

The key to the diagnosis of fungal infection, therefore, lies in the detection and subsequent identification of the organism. Ideally, culture methods should be employed, but where fresh tissue is not available it is possible to identify most organisms with morphological methods[27]. Many organisms are at best only poorly visualized by haematoxylin and eosin stains, but PAS and Grocott's modification of the methenamine silver stain both demonstrate fungi well. More recently, plant lectins have been used with considerable success in the identification of specific fungi[28].

REFERENCES

1. Holdstock, G., Blanchard, T., Robertson, D. A. F. and Millward-Sadler, G. H. (1992). The liver in infection. In Millward-Sadler, G. H., Wright, R. and Arthur, M. J. P. (eds). Wright's Liver and Biliary Disease. pp. 1039–1078. London: W B Saunders
2. Franson, T. R., Hierholzer, W. J. and LaBreque, D. R. (1985). Frequency and characteristics of hyperbilirubinaemia associated with bacteraemia. Rev. Infect. Dis., 7, 1–9
3. Lefkowitch, J. H. (1982). Bile ductular cholestasis: an ominous histopathological sign related to sepsis and 'cholangitis lenta'. Hum. Pathol., 13, 13–24
4. Ishak, K. G. and Rogers, W. A. (1981). Cryptogenic acute cholangitis–association with toxic shock syndrome. Am. J. Clin. Pathol., 76, 619–626
5. Kibbler, C. C. (1991). Bacterial infections and the liver. In McIntyre, N., Benhamou, J.-P., Bircher, J., Rizetto, M. and Rodes, J. (eds). Oxford Textbook of Clinical Hepatology, pp. 656-682. Oxford: Oxford University Press
6. Foster, C. S. (1993). Infections and infestations of the liver. In Wight, D. G. D. (ed). Liver, Biliary Tract and Exocrine Pancreas. 11 pp. Edinburgh: Churchill Livingstone

7. Yu, V. L., Miller, W. P., Wing, E. J., Romano, J. M., Ruiz, C. A. and Bruns, F. J. (1982). Disseminated listeriosis presenting as acute hepatitis. Am. J. Med., 73, 773–777

8. Gebauer, K., Hall, J. C., Donlon, J. B., Herrman, R., Rofe, S. and Platell, C. (1989). Hepatic involvement in listeriosis. Aust. NZ. J. Med., 19, 486–487

9. Bernard, P., Imbert, J. C. and Elkabbaj, M. (1980). L'atteinte hepatique au cours de la fievre typhoide. Nouv. Presse Med., 9, 256–257

10. De Brito, T., Vieira, W. T. and Dias, M. D. (1977). Jaundice in typhoid hepatitis: a light and EM study based on liver biopsies. Acta Hepatogastroenterol., 24, 426–433

11. Khosla, S. N. (1990). Typhoid hepatitis. Postgrad. Med. J., 66, 923–925

12. El Kabbaj, M., Bernard, P., El Hachimi, A. and Imbert, J. C. (1979). Atteinte hépatique au cours de la fièvre typhoide. Gastroenterol. Clin. Biol., 3, 651–656

13. Ramchandran, S. and Perera, M. V. F. (1976). Jaundice and hepatomegaly in primary malaria. J. Trop. Med. Hyg., 79, 207–210

14. Karat, A. B. A., Job, C. K. and Rao, P. S. S. (1971). Liver in leprosy: histological and biochemical findings. Br. Med. J., 1, 307–310

15. Wright, D. J. M. and Berry, C. L. (1974). Liver involvement in congenital syphilis. Br. J. Vener. Dis., 50, 241

16. Fehér, J., Somogyi, T., Timmer, M. and Jósza, L. (1975). Early syphilitic hepatitis. Lancet, 2, 896–899

17. Greenspon, J. S. (1991). Syphilitic hepatitis. Mayo Clin. Proc., 66, 114

18. Bukharovich, A. M., Sokol, A. N., Knigovskii, A. M. and Khilko, I. N. (1989). Liver involvement in secondary new syphilis. Vestn. Dermatol. Venerol., 9, 58–61

19. Parnis, R. (1975). Gumma of the liver. Br. J. Surg., 62, 236

20. Steere, A. C., Hutchinson, G. J., Rahn, D. W. et al. (1983). Treatment of the early mainfestations of Lyme disease. Ann. Intern. Med., 99, 22–26

21. De Brito, T., Machado, M. M., Monstans, S. D., Hoshino, S. and Freymüller, E. (1967). Liver biopsy in human leptospirosis: a light and electron microscopic study. Virch. Arch. [A]., 342, 61–69

22. Hofmann, C. E. and Heaton, J. W. (1982). Q fever hepatitis. Clinical manifestations and pathologic findings. Gastroenterology, 83, 474–479

23. Pellegrin, M., Delsol, G., Auvergnat, J. C., Familiades, J., Faure, H., Guin, M. and Voigt, J. J. (1980). Granulomatous hepatitis in Q fever. Hum. Pathol., 11, 51–57

24. Marazuela, M., Moreno, A., Yebra, M., Cerezo, E., Gomez, G. C. and Vargas, J. A. (1991). Hepatic fibrin-ring granulomas: a clinicopathologic study of 23 patients. Hum Pathol., 22, 607–13

25. Adams, J. S. and Walker, D. H. (1981). The liver in Rocky mountain spotted fever. Am. J. Clin. Pathol., 75, 156–161

26. Smith, J. W. and Utz, J. P. (1972). Progressive disseminated histoplasmosis. Ann. Intern. Med., 76, 557–565

27. Anthony, P. P. (1973). A guide to the histological identification of fungi. J. Clin. Pathol., 26, 828–831

28. Stoddart, R. W. and Herbertson, B. M. (1978). The use of fluorescein labelled lectins in the detection and identification of fungi pathogenic for man: a preliminary study. J. Med. Microbiol., 11, 315–324

5

Liver Abscess

In developed countries pyogenic infection accounts for the large majority of cases of liver abscess, whilst in the rest of the world amoebic abscess is the more common. Both may present in a non-specific way with vague symptoms of ill health and fever and not necessarily showing any localizing features referable to the liver: thus nothing can replace clinical awareness and suspicion. Both continue to have a high mortality if untreated[1]. Fortunately, when they are considered, investigations such as isotope scanning, ultrasound, and CT have greatly increased diagnostic accuracy.

PYOGENIC ABSCESS

Infection may spread to the liver directly, from the biliary tree, or in portal or hepatic artery blood. Direct extension is most often from an infected gallbladder, but may also be from any other adjacent infection, such as a subphrenic abscess. Trauma, either penetrating or closed, is becoming increasingly frequent, but biliary tract disease is now the commonest cause of abscess and is usually associated with obstruction, often intermittent, by stones, stricture or tumours. It may be a sequel of suppurative cholangitis and the abscesses are then centred upon portal tracts and are small and multiple. Extension of infection from a source of intra-abdominal sepsis, such as a perforated appendix or diverticular disease, used to be the most common mechanism before the antibiotic era but now accounts for only a small proportion[2]. Bacteraemia or septicaemia from any cause may be followed by liver abscess. In the neonatal period, infection may spread from the umbilical region, especially if a catheter is used. There remains a significant proportion without obvious aetiological factors amounting to 10–15% of all cases.

Almost any organism may be associated with liver abscess[3,4]. Most of the early reports emphasize the importance of Gram-negative aerobes, such as *E. coli* and *Klebsiella pneumoniae*, but they all include a significant number paradoxically labelled as 'sterile'. The probable explanation is that a significant proportion of liver abscesses are caused by, or have a major contribution from, microaerophilic organisms, such as *Streptococcus milleri* (Figure 5.2)[5], or anaerobes, such as *Bacteroides spp* [6], which will not have been detected by inadequate culture techniques.

The diagnosis of abscess is rarely made solely by biopsy, indeed the role of biopsy is somewhat controversial[7], but fine-needle aspiration should improve the chances of obtaining a satisfactory specimen for culture in most cases, especially when guided by ultrasound or CT scanning[1,4]. However, abscesses are not uncommonly seen in wedge biopsies or resection specimens, since surgical drainage or resection remain the treatment of choice.

Abscesses may be single or multiple (Figures 5.1–5.4). Those associated with biliary tract disease are nearly always multiple and accompanied by obstructive jaundice[3]. Cholestasis is not invariable however, since, as explained in Chapter 15, infection is more common when obstruction is intermittent or incomplete. Some portal tracts may only show the changes of cholangitis with oedema, bile duct proliferation and neutrophilic infiltration (Figure 5.5), whilst others contain abscesses of varying sizes. These are usually obviously located within portal tracts and may contain biliary debris (Figure 5.6).

Solitary abscesses vary greatly in size but are rarely more than a few centimetres in diameter and are filled with greenish pus, often foul-smelling if due to anaerobic organisms. If relatively acute they may have very little in the way of a capsule. More chronic lesions have a thick capsule composed of hyaline collagen resembling the wall of an empyema (Figure 5.1). Exuberant fibrosis like this has few other causes and thus an abscess should always be suspected when it is encountered in biopsy material, particularly if associated with a few tell-tale polymorphs. A Gram stain occasionally will be positive in such circumstances (Figure 5.2).

AMOEBIC ABSCESS

Although much more common in tropical than temperate climates[1], amoebic abscess, caused by Entamoeba histolytica, is occasionally seen in the latter. It is important to appreciate that abscess may occur many years after the primary gut infection and well over half of all patients have no evidence of large bowel disease at the time of presentation. Presentation is usually with pyrexia and right upper quadrant pain and tenderness[8], and affects men far more often than women[1], for reasons which are not clear.

Abscesses are usually single but may be multiple and typically are found in the posterior aspect of the dome of the right lobe. They can be very large, sometimes occupying the whole lobe. Characteristically the cavity contains reddish-brown pus resembling anchovy sauce and aspiration is regarded as a safe diagnostic procedure. Organisms are seen in the aspirated fluid only in a minority of cases, but modern immunological techniques will detect amoebic antigen in over 90%[9].

Histologically there are three distinct layers around an abscess (Figure 5.7). The innermost layer is composed of liver showing coagulative necrosis and occasional amoebae may be visible in this zone. They measure about 60 μm in diameter and have a spherical nucleus. Ingested red blood cells may or may not be present (Figure 5.8). Viable trophozoites are surrounded by a clear halo (Figure 5.9). Although fairly readily seen in routine preparations, they are best demonstrated by PAS or Heidenhein's iron haematoxylin[4]. The next layer contains a few inflammatory cells, mostly mononuclear, together with rather variable quantities of granulation tissue and fibrosis—often very little. This is then surrounded by compressed but otherwise normal liver.

Complications of amoebic abscess include rupture into adjacent structures and secondary pyogenic infection following aspiration. The prognosis with appropriate drug treatment is excellent[1,9].

ACTINOMYCOSIS

Actinomycosis is another rare cause of liver abscess. *Actinomyces israelii, A. bovis* and *A. naeslundii* are common inhabitants of the normal mouth, but only rarely are pathogenic, possibly because they require the co-operation of another organism before they become established. Traditionally the facial and ileocaecal regions are regarded as the main primary sites of infection, but

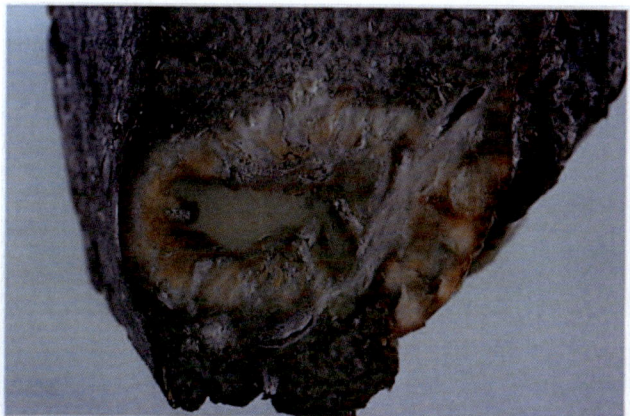

Figure 5.1 Pyogenic liver abscess. The patient had acute appendicitis 3 months previously, recurring pyrexia ever since. Liver abscess treated by surgical excision. The photograph shows a central cavity filled with pus surrounded by a thick fibrous wall.

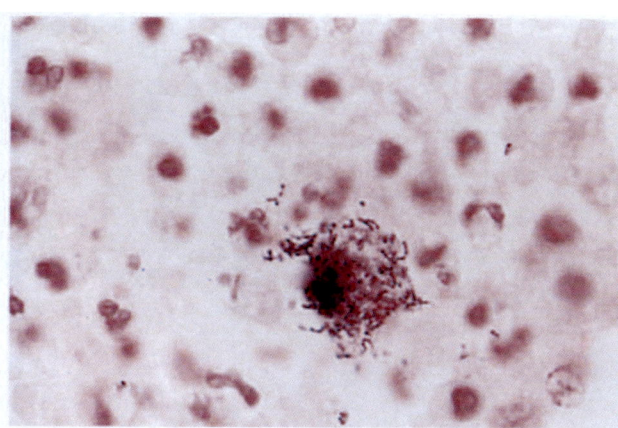

Figure 5.2 Pyogenic liver abscess. Same case as Figure 5.1. *Streptococcus milleri* was cultured and a Gram stain shows clumps of positive cocci.

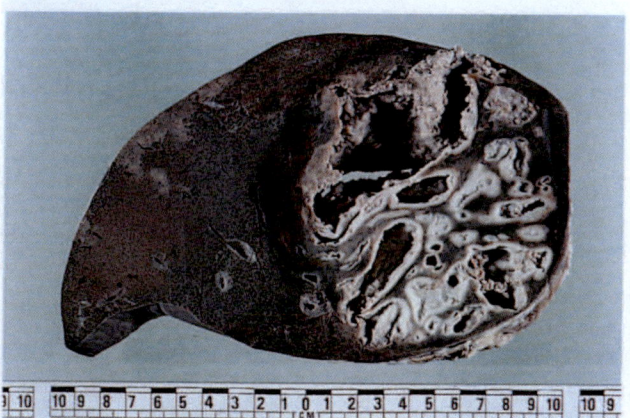

Figure 5.3 Pyogenic liver abscess. A 75-year-old man had recurrent pyrexia for one week and died before a diagnosis was made. At postmortem no cause was found for this large multilocular abscess, from which Strep. milleri was cultured.

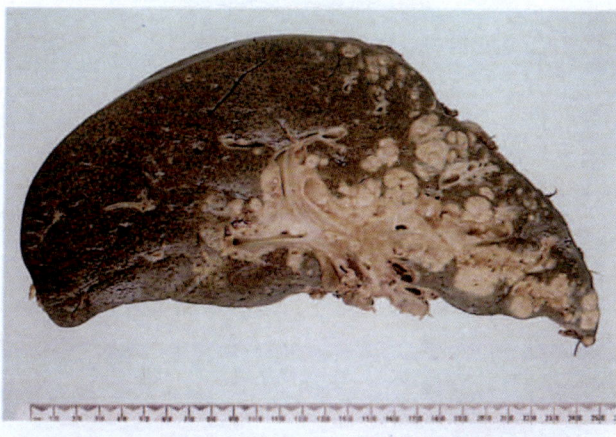

Figure 5.4 Ascending cholangitis in a patient undergoing transplantation for primary sclerosing cholangitis. Multiple small abscesses are confined to the left lobe of the liver. A carcinoma, not apparent macroscopically, was found to be obstructing the left hepatic duct at the hilum.

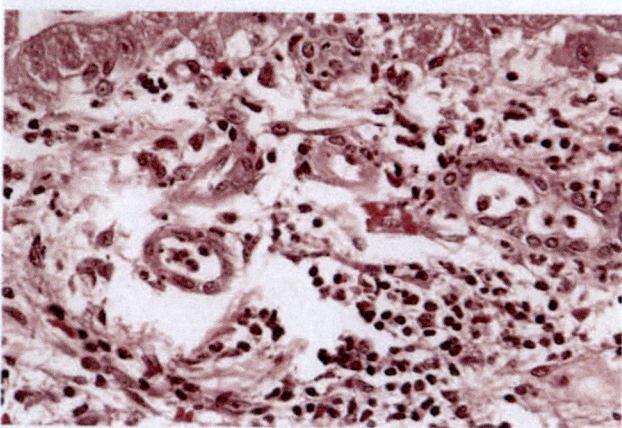

Figure 5.5 Ascending cholangitis without abscess formation. This patient presented with recurrent pyrexia and subsequently was shown to have sclerosing cholangitis. Biopsy shows expanded oedematous portal tracts with neutrophils both within and between bile ducts.

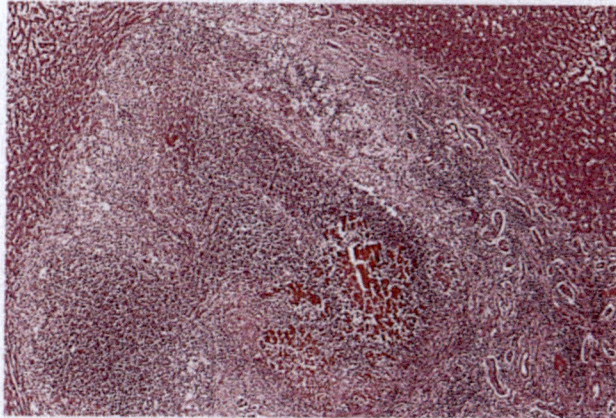

Figure 5.6 Ascending cholangitis. An elderly patient with multiple gall-stones and a duodeno-colic fistula had numerous abscesses centred upon portal tracts. Yellow-brown debris is surrounded by neutrophil polymorphs and a zone of foamy macrophages.

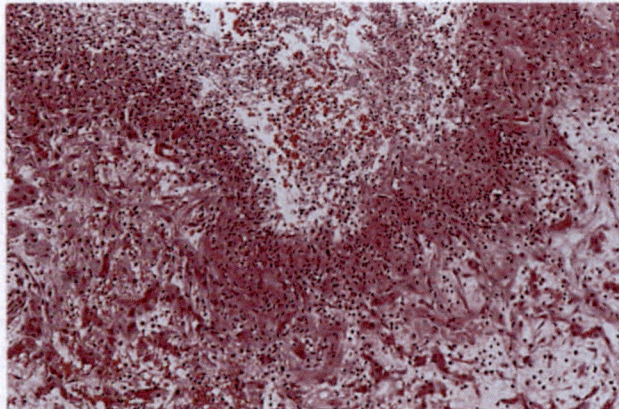

Figure 5.7 Amoebic liver abscess. This patient presented with abdominal pain and fever after return from the tropics. There was no history of amoebic dysentery. Laparotomy was performed and the wedge biopsy shows a characteristic abscess wall composed of a zone of coagulative necrosis and pus cells, surrounded by oedematous liver. The lumen contains necrotic debris and occasional amoebae. See Figure 5.8.

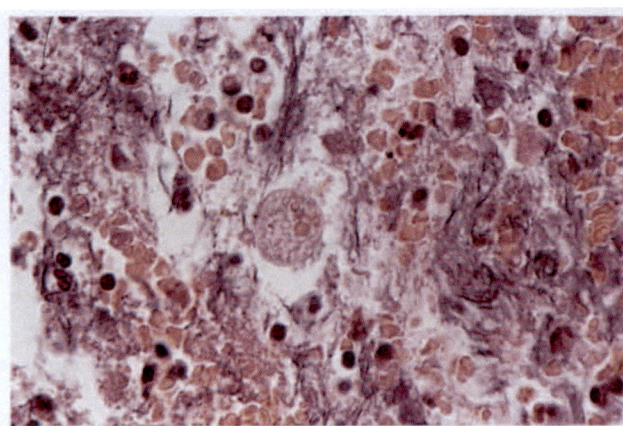

Figure 5.8 Amoebic liver abscess. Same case as Figure 5.7. Necrotic debris, inflammatory cells and red blood cells from the lumen of the abscess. At the centre there is a circular amoeba containing two ingested red cells adjacent to, and the same size as, the nucleus.

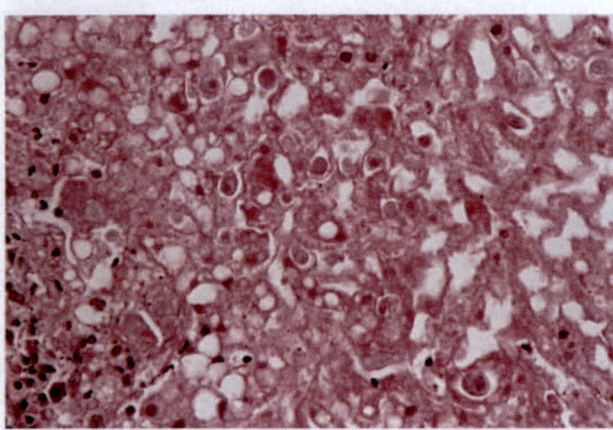

Figure 5.9 Amoebic liver abscess. Post-mortem specimen showing the autolytic appearance usually seen in this material. The section shows numerous amoebae, each surrounded by a clear halo indicating viability. The author is deeply indebted to Professor MSR Hutt who kindly provided the slides from which Figure 5.9 was prepared.

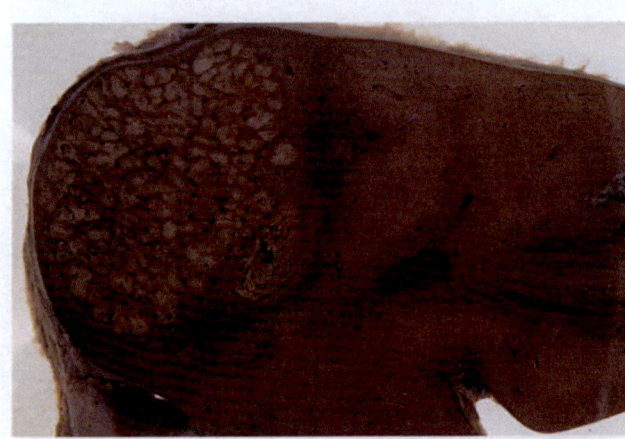

Figure 5.10 Actinomycosis of the liver. Multiloculate abscess found at post-mortem.

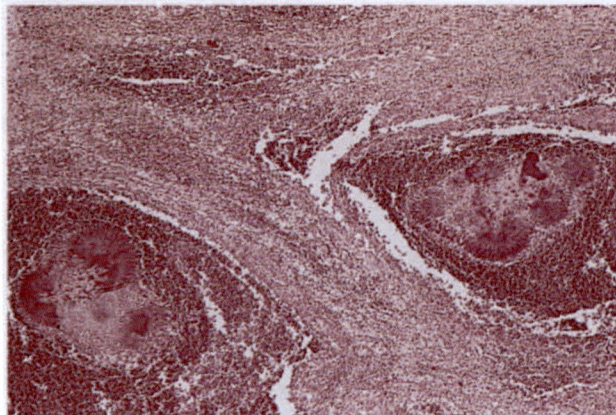

Figure 5.11 Actinomycosis of the liver. Same case as Figure 5.10, each locule contains colonies of organisms embedded in pus.

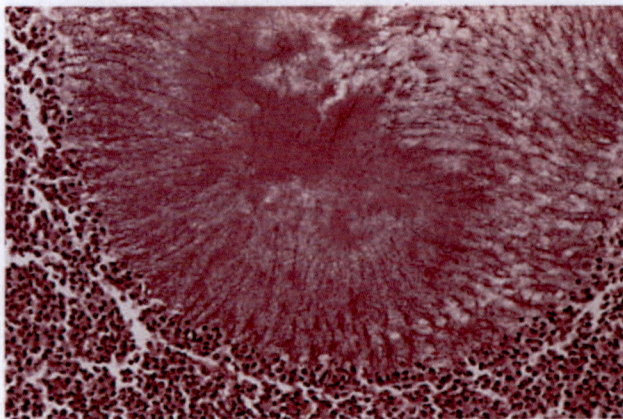

Figure 5.12 Actinomycosis. Same case as Figures 5.10 and 5.11, showing the organism in greater detail. A central core of eosinophilic material is surrounded by a fringe of basophilic fragments. Terminal clubs are not seen in this example.

almost any part of the body may be involved[10]. Although usually affected as part of systemic disease, the liver may he primarily involved[11]. Typically the abscess is composed of multiple small locules giving a honeycomb-like cut-surface, each containing soft granules embedded in thick pus (Figure 5.10).

Microscopically the hallmark of actinomyces infection is the organism, which is a distinctive filamentous bacterium with a tendency to aggregate into clumps of basophilic material surrounded by a fringe of eosinophilic clubs, each colony being some 300 μm in diameter (Figures 5.11 and 5.12). These are embedded in pus and surrounded by a wall of granulation tissue containing foam cells and occasional giant cells.

Nocardia asteroides, N. brasiliensis, and *N. caviae* are aerobic actinomycetes which also may rarely cause liver disease[12].

BOTRYOMYCOSIS

This is a suppurative condition cause by a variety of pyogenic bacteria, especially the pyogenic cocci and various enterobacteria, which is also known as bacterial 'pseudomycosis'. The abscess cavities contain structures resembling actinomycotic granules, which represent colonial aggregates of the causative organism[13].

TUBERCULOSIS

The liver is commonly found to be involved in serious and fatal tuberculosis. Miliary tuberculosis is the most common form of liver involvement and tuberculosis must always be seriously considered in any form of granulomatous liver disease, especially in a sick or pyrexial patient (Chapter 19). In the immunocompromised patient, especially those with AIDS, atypical mycobacteria should be considered in all liver biopsies, especially since the morphological changes may not be distinctive (Chapters 3 and 19).

Much less commonly, tuberculosis of the liver may take the form of a localized abscess or tuberculoma[14,15]. This is nevertheless important to recognize as it may be confused with a pyogenic abscess or a neoplasm. It is seen most often in children and in the black population, and more recently in patients with AIDS[16], and usually presents with fever and hepatic enlargement. There is nearly always active tuberculosis elsewhere in the body.

Macroscopically tuberculomas measure up to several centimetres in diameter and have an opaque white central core of caseous necrosis. Microscopically they show typical caseous tuberculosis with epithelioid and giant cells surrounding structureless eosinophilic caseation. Organisms are usually quite easily found with Ziehl-Nielsen stains.

REFERENCES

1. Donovan, A. J., Yellin, A. E. and Ralls, P. W. (1991). Hepatic abscess. World J. Surg., 15, 162–169
2. Silver, S., Weinstein, R. and Cooperman, A. (1979). Changes in the pathogenesis and detection of intrahepatic abscess. Am. J. Surg., 137, 608–610
3. Branum, G. D., Tyson, G. S., Branum, M. A. and Meyers, W. C. (1990). Hepatic abscess: changes in aetiology diagnosis and management. Ann. Surg., 212, 655–662
4. Foster, C. S. (1993). Infections and infestations of the liver. In Wight, D. G. D. (eds). Liver, Biliary Tract and Exocrine Pancreas. 11 pp. Edinburgh: Churchill Livingstone
5. Moore Gillon, J. C., Eykyn, S. J. and Phillips, I. (1981). Microbiology of pyogenic liver abscess. Br. Med. J., 283, 819–821
6. Perera, M. M., Kirk, A. and Noone, P. (1980). Presentation, diagnosis and management of liver abscess. Lancet, 2, 629–632
7. Lesesne, H. R., Holt, W. and Orringer, E. (1976). Is hepatic abscess a contraindication to percutaneous liver biopsy? Gastroenterology, 70, 297–298
8. Chaves, F. J. Z. C., Cruz, I., Gomes, C., Domingues, W., Marques de Silva, E. and Veloso, F. T. (1977). Hepatic amebiasis: analysis of 56 cases. 1 Clinical findings. Am. J. Gastroenterol., 68, 134–140
9. Maltz, G. and Knauer, C. M. (1991). Amebic liver abscess: a 15 year experience. Am. J. Gastroenterol., 86, 704–710
10. Brown, J. R. (1973). Human actinomycosis a study of 181 subjects. Hum. Pathol., 4, 319–330
11. Mongiardo, N., de Rienzo, B., Zonchetta, G., Lami, G. and Pellegrino, F. (1986). Primary hepatic actinomycosis. J. Infect., 8, 65–69
12. Palmer, D. L., Harvey, R. L. and Wheeler, R. L. (1974). Diagnostic and therapeutic considerations in Nocardia asteroides infection. Medicine, 53, 391–401
13. Greenblatt, M., Heredia, R., Rubenstein, L. and Alpert, S. (1964). Bacterial pseudomycosis ("botyromycosis") Am. J. Clin. Pathol., 41, 188–193
14. Leader, S. R. (1952). Tuberculosis of liver and gall bladder with abscess formation. A review and case report. Ann. Intern. Med., 37, 594–606
15. Zipser, R. D., Ran, J. E., Ricketts, R. R. and Bevans, L. C. (1976). Tuberculous pseudotumours of the liver. Am. J. Med., 61, 946–951
16. Moreno, S., Pacho, E., López-Herce, J. A., Rodríguez-Créixems, M., Martin-Scapa, C. and Bouza, E. (1988). Mycobacterium tuberculosis visceral abscesses in the acquired immunodeficiency syndrome (AIDS). [letter]. Ann. Intern. Med., 109, 437

Parasitic Infestations

6

PROTOZOA

Malaria

Malaria is a protozoan disease transmitted by Anopheline mosquitoes. It is extremely widespread in tropical climates and is still thought to account for over a million deaths per year in children under the age of four in Africa alone. More than any other disease, it is liable to be seen in non-endemic areas as a result of air travel. In hyperendemic areas, *Plasmodium falciparum* repeatedly reinfects virtually all children. As they become older resistance gradually increases, until by adolescence they may have no detectable parasites in the blood. The changes in the liver are identical in all forms of malaria, although they tend to be more severe in *P. falciparum* infection.

Although immediately after infection, during the pre-erythrocytic phase, multiplication of the parasite takes place exclusively in hepatocytes, this has no clinical effect and thus goes undetected. Transient jaundice, not due to haemolysis, and hepatomegaly, may be seen in up to half of all patients with primary malaria[1]. Biopsy in the early symptomatic phase reveals mainly sinusoidal changes, with striking hyperaemia and Kupffer cell hyperplasia; numerous parasitized red cells are seen both free in sinusoids and within sinusoidal lining cells[2], combined with fine pigment. Later in the disease, a picture rather similar to that seen in typhoid fever (Chapter 4) may develop. The malarial nodules resemble typhoid nodules and are composed of granulomatous collections of histiocytes and lymphocytes associated with hepatocyte necrosis. They are randomly distributed and found in about half of all cases.

The most common finding in the liver, however, is the presence of malarial pigment (Figure 6.1). This pigment, or haemozoin, is an acid haematin derived from the haem portion of haemoglobin as a result of action of the parasite. When red cells rupture, it is liberated into the bloodstream and then taken up by the phagocytes of the reticuloendothelial system in the spleen and bone marrow as well as in the liver. The pigment is brownish-black and distinctive in that it is birefringent (Figure 6.2), but negative with Perl's and PAS stains. Caution should be exercised with formalin fixation, since malarial pigment is virtually identical with formalin pigment even to the extent that it, too, is removed by alcoholic picric acid. The pigment is present in Kupffer cells which may be prominent. Although maximal in the acute phase the pigment does persist for some time after recovery. In recurrent infection there will also be pigment in portal tracts, the residue of previous attacks. The presence of lymphocytes in sinusoids may be an indication of an immunological response.

Tropical splenomegaly syndrome (TSS)

When sinusoidal lymphocytes are numerous, the spleen is usually enlarged and parasitaemia is absent. This syndrome has come to be termed *tropical splenomegaly syndrome* or *hyper-reactive malarial splenomegaly*. Affected individuals are usually children with splenomegaly, anaemia and occasionally other symptoms of hypersplenism, but no overt signs of malaria. There is sometimes a blood lymphocytosis. Liver biopsy shows a rather characteristic prominence of Kupffer cells with numerous lymphocytes in rows and small groups within sinusoids (Figure 6.3)[3]. The cells are predominantly T-lymphocytes[4]. Very occasionally the cells may include macrophages, eosinophils and even immature white cells. Similar cells may sometimes be present in portal tracts. There is no malarial pigment. The condition is thought to be an unusual immunological response to the malarial parasite, since it usually regresses with anti-malarial treatment.

The main differential diagnosis is from leukaemias. In TSS there is little correlation between the degree of sinusoidal infiltration and the number of lymphocytes in the blood, but morphologically the two conditions may be very similar. Distinction should be obvious when blood and bone marrow findings are taken into account.

Leishmaniasis

Visceral leishmaniasis or *kala-azar* is much less common than the other conditions discussed in this section and is much less likely to be encountered in developed countries. The parasite, *Leishmania donovani*, is transmitted by the sandfly and causes disease mainly as a result of proliferation within the cells of the reticuloendothelial system in spleen, liver and bone marrow. The proliferation may be massive, causing death, or may be chronic. In either case, the parasite, as so-called Leishman-Donovan bodies, is readily seen in hypertrophied Kupffer cells in the liver (Figure 6.4) and best confirmed with a Giemsa stain[5,6]. This appearance may be closely mimicked by disseminated histoplasmosis (Chapter 4). Here, too, Kupffer cells are hypertrophied and contain many organisms, of a size comparable to Leishmania, but they can be clearly distinguished with a PAS stain since histoplasmas will be strongly positive[7]. The latter is also more likely to be accompanied by hepatic necrosis. Diagnosis, when the condition is suspected clinically, is normally made by splenic aspiration or by serology[8].

Cryptosporidiosis

Cryptosporidia are increasing being encountered in the biliary tree during AIDS and other immunodeficiency syndromes[9,10]. The organisms are seen lining the epithelium of larger bile ducts (Figure 6.5), and may be part of a sclerosing cholangitis-like syndrome (Chapter 20).

Toxoplasmosis

Toxoplasma gondii is a protozoan parasite which was found originally in the liver of a North African rodent (the gondi). It is widely distributed through warm-blooded animals, and infection is acquired by eating raw infected meat or by ingestion of oocysts excreted, most commonly, by the domestic cat (sexual reproduction is confined to the cat family). Most infection is entirely asymptomatic in patients with normal immunity and hepatitis is extremely rare[11], but may be granulomatous[12,13]. Disseminated infection, including hepatic involvement (Figure 6.6), may occur in immunosuppressed patients[14]; both transplant patients (where the source of infection may be the donor organ)[15] and those with AIDS are occasionally affected[16].

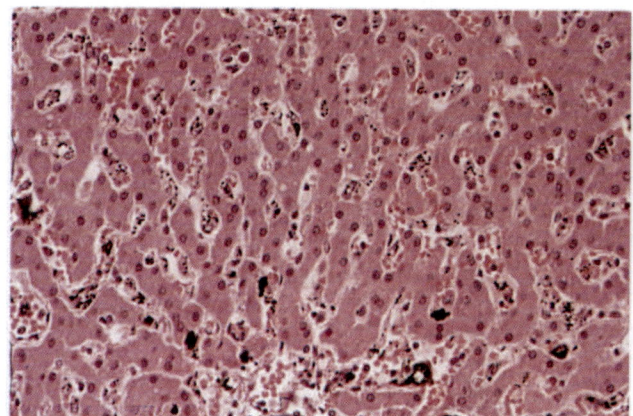

Figure 6.1 Malaria. Heavy brownish-black pigmentation of Kupffer cells, maximal in periportal regions.

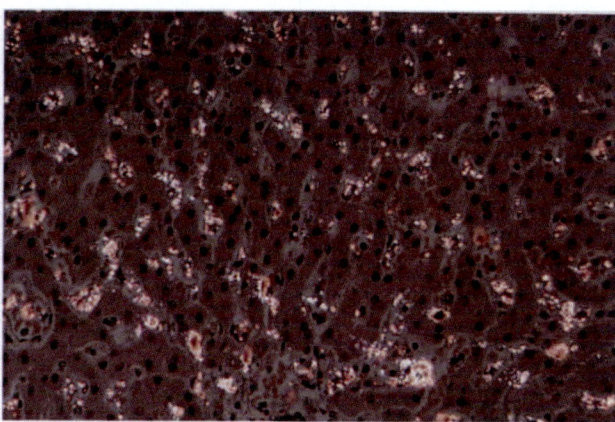

Figure 6.2 Malaria. Same section as Figure 6.1, viewed in polarized light showing that the pigment is birefringent.

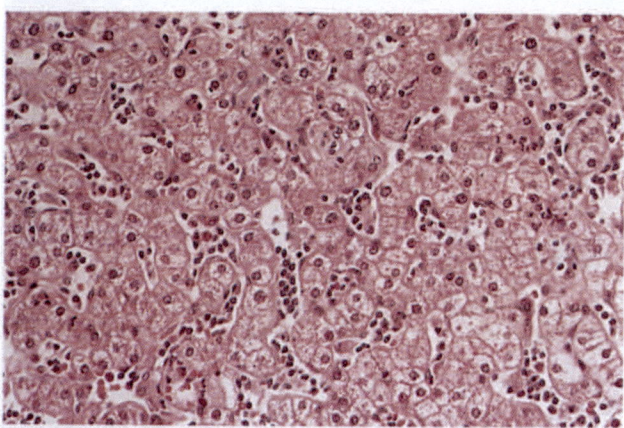

Figure 6.3 Tropical splenomegaly syndrome. Numerous lymphocytes are present in sinusoids and Kupffer cells are prominent, but there is no pigmentation.

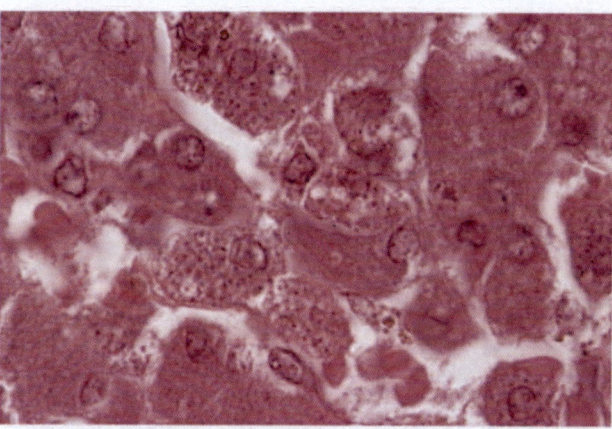

Figure 6.4 Kala-azar, Kupffer cells are enlarged and contain numerous granular basophilic Leishman-Donovan bodies as well as some golden-brown pigment.
The author is deeply indebted to Professor MSR Hutt who kindly provided the slides from which Figures 6.1-6.4 were prepared.

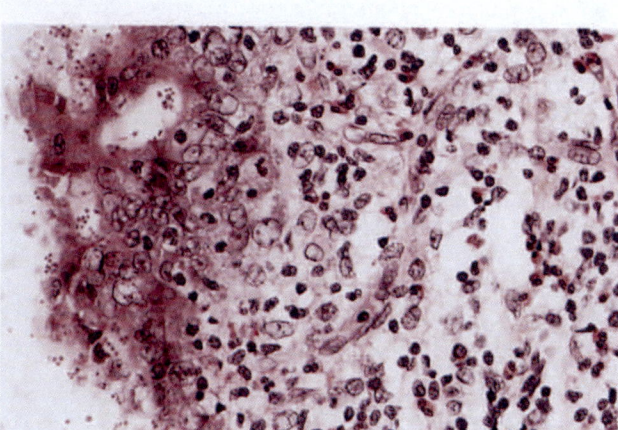

Figure 6.5 Cryptosporidiosis. Note the organisms adherent to the epithelial lining of a large bile duct. The epithelium is hyperplastic and there is some underlying chronic inflammation.

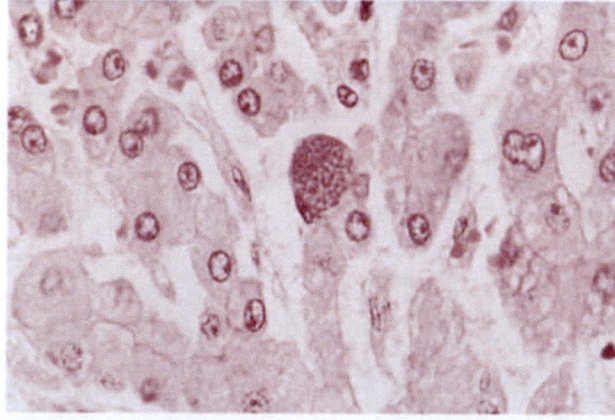

Figure 6.6 Toxoplasmosis. Disseminated infection following transplantation of a liver from an antibody-positive donor into an antibody-negative recipient. Numerous merozoites can be seen within and distending a Kupffer cell (a pseudocyst). Note the complete absence of inflammation or necrosis, the usual pattern in immunocompromised patients.

METAZOA

Schistosomiasis

There are three species of schistosome (blood flukes), all trematode flatworms, and together they are thought to infect over 200 million people in the world today. There is no direct spread from man to man, various species of freshwater snail act as the intermediate host, and thus, although travellers may bring the infection from endemic areas, there is no risk of transmission. The adult worms (about 1–2 cm in length) live in pairs, the female clasped by the male, in the vessels of the vesical or haemorrhoidal plexus. *Schistosoma haematobium* lays eggs predominantly in the bladder and they can be recognized by their terminal spines (Figure 6.7). However, rectal involvement is not rare and this may account for the access to the portal venous system and the occasional, but rarely severe, liver involvement. *Schistosoma mansoni* (ova with a subterminal spine, Figure 6.8) and *S. japonicum* (ova with a knob, which in contrast to the other two has a rather localized distribution in the Far East), are regularly found in the large bowel, and the liver is invariably affected to some degree. Embryonated ova, in the three weeks or so that they remain viable[17], excite an eosinophil response often with a few epithelioid cells, followed by a granulomatous response and vigorous scarring (Figure 6.9). The latter is often strikingly concentric and is thought to be the basic process in the so called pipe stem fibrosis described by Symmers in 1903[18] (Figure 6.10). Fibrosis of this degree is regarded as merely a function of numbers of ova and is found most often following *S. japonicum* infection, since this worm lays most eggs.

Macroscopically the major portal tracts radiate from the hilum of the liver as thick white fibrous scars resembling clay pipe stems (Figure 6.10). Microscopically, in addition to coarse fibrosis, there may be prominent nerves and bile duct proliferation. Inflammatory foci may be seen in the walls of portal veins and there is often an increased number of vessels, both arterioles and venules, the so-called 'angiomatoids' which are also seen in the lung. They are thought to represent arteriovenous communications. Pigment, morphologically very similar to malarial pigment, and thus also resembling formalin pigment, may be abundant in relationship to the portal tract ova, but may also be plentiful in Kupffer cells in the otherwise unaffected parenchyma. The pigment is birefringent and probably a complex porphyrin[19]. It has some distinctive ultrastructural features. Although the portal tract fibrosis is the most striking abnormality, there may also be thickening of the reticulin framework in the liver parenchyma due to capillarization of the sinusoids[20]. The cause of this is not known but it may be due to substances liberated by schistosomes or to an immunological response to them.

The advanced liver disease causes severe portal hypertension, but probably no more than some nodularity of the liver parenchyma. The accompanying true cirrhosis seen in up to 10% of cases is not thought to be directly related[21] but merely coincidental. Hepatitis B, for example, is a common cause of cirrhosis in schistosomal areas.

Liver flukes

Clonorchis sinensis and *Opisthorchis spp.* are common parasites in certain parts of the Far East–the post-mortem incidence reaching 80% in certain locations. The parasites have a complex life cycle, but infection is usually acquired by eating raw or under-cooked fish[17]. The metacercariae which hatch from the ingested cysts find their way to the biliary tree where they develop into adult worms which measure up to 2.5 cm in length. Here they live in the major bile ducts where they cause desquamation and

proliferation of the biliary epithelium which is eventually followed by the appearance of adenomatous hyperplasia. This is then thought to progress to typical cholangiocarcinoma (Chapter 24), often multifocal, in a significant proportion of cases[22]. Animal models have confirmed the hyperplastic changes, although not yet the progression to neoplasia, which has not been universally accepted. *Fasciola hepatica* is another fluke which infests man[23], but this is not thought to be followed by the development of tumours.

All the flukes may be associated with secondary infection and cholangitis or abscess formation. Biliary mud containing dead worms and ova as well as inflammatory debris is commonly found. The walls of the affected bile ducts may contain variable numbers of eosinophils. Diagnosis is best made by parasitological methods, in particular multiple examinations of stools for ova[24].

Liver flukes may be one cause of primary recurrent pyogenic cholangitis ('oriental cholangitis') which is seen so commonly in the Far East[25]. Opium addiction, through its effect on the sphincter of Oddi, may be an additional contributory factor.

Hydatid cyst

The dog tapeworm, *Echinococcus granulosus*, which measures only 2–3 cm in length, infects the upper small intestine. Eggs are shed into the faeces and consumed by cattle, sheep and other mammals. Man acts as an occasional intermediate host in a similar manner. The ingested ova hatch in the upper intestine and pass into the liver via the portal vein where most become arrested, whilst a few pass through and may settle in any organ. Here they gradually develop into classic hydatid cysts.

Over a period of many years they gradually enlarge until they may reach 25 cm or more. They have a thick white anucleate outer layer made up of numerous laminations. Internal to this is the germinal layer which gives rise to brood capsules, each of which contains many scolices or heads of the future tapeworms. With time, daughter cysts sprout as invaginations of the germinal layer and these too may give rise to more scolices and to grand–daughter cysts (Figure 6.11). Outside the cyst, the liver is compressed and may show a variable amount of inflammation and fibrosis.

Most patients with hepatic hydatid cysts have little in the way of symptoms[26]. Hepatomegaly may or may not be present and up to half show a blood eosinophilia. Diagnosis is best confirmed by ultrasound, which can show an absolutely pathognomonic picture. Suspicion of hydatid disease is an absolute contraindication to liver biopsy, since leakage of fluid (which can also occur spontaneously) may give rise to a fatal anaphylactic reaction. There are no characteristic changes in the adjacent liver. Loss of viability of the cyst is often followed by calcification.

Alveolar cyst is caused by *E. multilocularis*, the fox tapeworm, which has no outer cyst wall, and thus tiny daughter cysts spread progressively through the liver in a manner very comparable to the spread of a malignant neoplasm (Figure 6.12)[27]. Similarly, surgical resection of involved liver is the only means of treatment.

Other worms

Other worms, such as *Ascaris lumbricoides* and *Toxocara canis* may also affect the liver in endemic areas[28].

REFERENCES

1. Ramchandran, S. and Perera, M. V. F. (1976). Jaundice and hepatomegaly in primary malaria. J. Trop. Med. Hyg., 79, 207–210

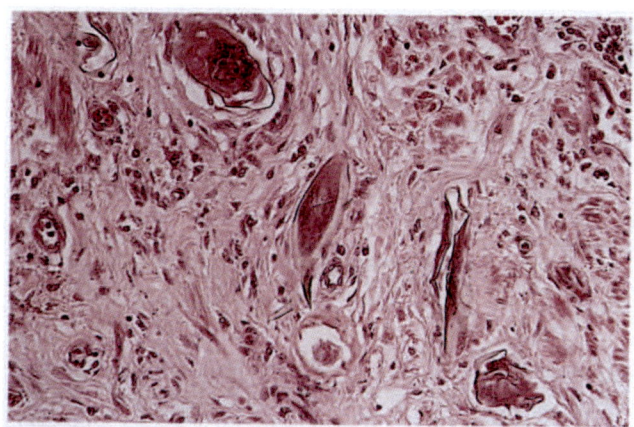

Figure 6.7 Schistosomiasis. Viable ova of *Schistosoma haematobium* (terminal spine) can be seen embedded in dense fibrous tissue within a portal tract. They are not exciting a granulomatous or foreign body reaction.

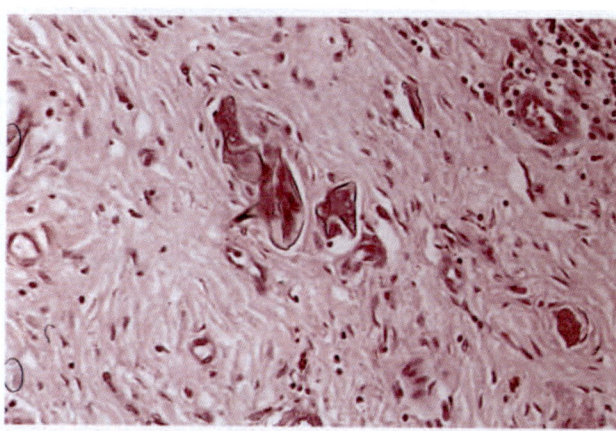

Figure 6.8 Schistosomiasis. Viable ova of *S. mansoni* (subterminal spine) embedded, as in Figure 6.5, in portal tract fibrous tissue and without a significant host cellular response.

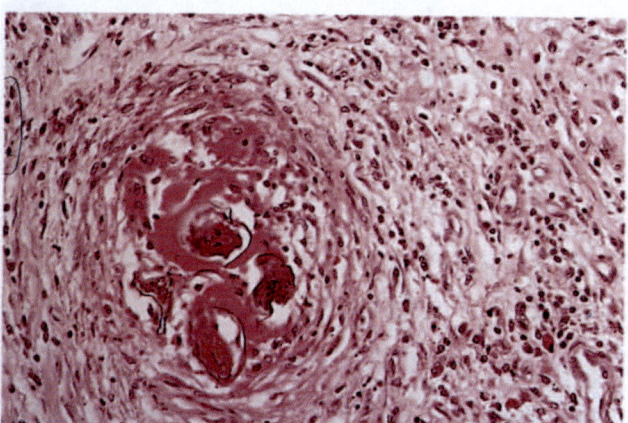

Figure 6.9 Schistosomiasis. Ova beginning to excite a granulomatous response, and surrounded by characteristic concentric fibrosis. Inflammatory cells are mainly lymphocytes and plasma cells. In other cases, the response may be much more sarcoid-like.

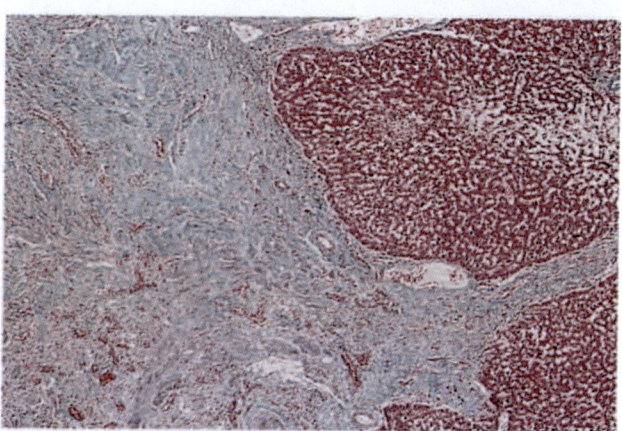

Figure 6.10 Schistosomiasis, pipe-stem fibrosis. Broad bands of relatively acellular fibrosis, based upon portal tracts, radiated from the hilum of the liver. The section shows the edge of one of these. In this case there is very little inflammation and no bile-duct proliferation. The hepatic architecture is otherwise normal. Masson trichrome.
The author is deeply indebted to Professor MSR Hutt who kindly provided the slides from which Figures 6.7–6.10 were prepared.

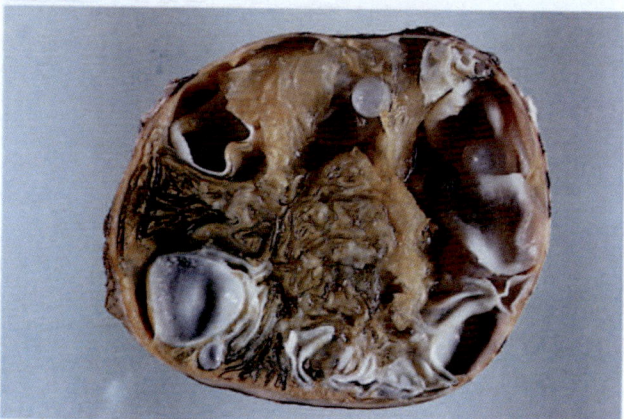

Figure 6.11 Hydatid cyst (*Echinococcus granulosus*). A bisected cyst 15 cm in diameter excised intact from the right lobe of the liver of a Cypriot patient who presented with hepatic enlargement. Daughter and grand-daughter cysts can be seen sprouting from the inner germinal layer.

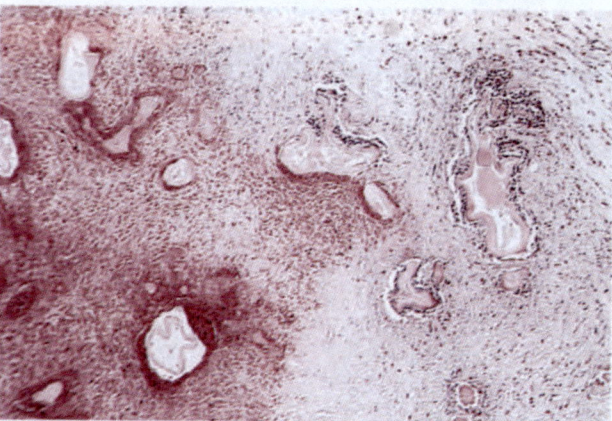

Figure 6.12 Alveolar cyst (*E. multilocularis*). In contrast to the hydatid cyst, there is no enveloping cyst wall. Multiple minute cysts spread through the liver, separated from one another and surrounded by fibrous tissue containing moderate numbers of eosinophils. Several of the cysts (left) are no longer viable and are exciting a foreign body reaction.

2. Warrell, D. A. and Francis, N. (1991). Malaria. In McIntyre, N., Benhamou, J.-P., Bircher, J., Rizetto, M. and Rodes, J. (eds). Oxford Textbook of Clinical Hepatology. pp. 701–706. Oxford: Oxford University Press

3. Hutt, M. S. R. (1985). Idiopathic tropical splenomegaly in Uganda (big spleen disease). In Sommers, S. C. (eds). Haematologic and Lymphoid Pathology Decennial, l966-1975,. pp. 31–44. NewYork: Appleton-Century-Crofts

4. Marsh, K. and Greenwood, B. M. (1986). The immunopathology of malaria. In Stricland, G. T. (eds). Clinics in Tropical Medicine and Communicable Disease. pp. 91–125. London: W B Saunders

5. Daneshbod, K. (1976). Visceral leishmaniasis (kala-azar) in Iran: a pathologic and electron microscopic study. Am. J. Clin. Pathol., 57, 156–166

6. Duarte, M. I. S. and Corbet, C. E. P. (1987). Histopathological patterns of the liver involvement in visceral leishmaniasis. Rev. Inst. Med. Trop. S. Paolo., 29, 131–136

7. Ridley, D. S. (1974). The laboratory diagnosis of tropical diseases with special reference to Britain: a review. J. Clin. Pathol., 27, 435–444

8. Bryceson, A. D. M. (1991). Visceral leishmaniasis. In McIntyre, N., Benhamou, J.-P., Bircher, J., Rizetto, M. and Rodes, J. (eds). Oxford Textbook of Clinical Hepatology. pp. 707–711. Oxford: Oxford University Press

9. Hasan, F. A., Jeffers, L. J., Dickinson, G., Otraki, C. L., Greer, P. J., Reddy, C. R. and Schiff, E. R. (1991). Hepatobiliary cryptosporidiosis and cytomegalovirus infection mimicking metastatic cancer to the liver. Gastroenterology, 100, 1743–1748

10. Cappell, M. S. (1991). Hepatobiliary manifestations of the acquired immune deficiency syndrome. Am. J. Gastroenterol., 86, 1–15

11. Frankel, J. K. and Remington, J. S. (1980). Hepatitis in toxoplasmosis [letter]. N. Engl. J. Med., 302, 178

12. Weitberg, A. B., Alper, J. C., Diamond, I. and Fligiel, Z. (1979). Acute granulomatous hepatitis due to acquired toxoplasmosis. N. Engl. J. Med., 300, 1093–1096

13. Marazuela, M., Moreno, A., Yebra, M., Cerezo, E., Gomez, G. C. and Vargas, J. A. (1991). Hepatic fibrin-ring granulomas: a clinicopathologic study of 23 patients. Hum. Pathol., 22, 607–13

14. Oksenhendler, E., Cadranel, J., Sarfati, C., Katlama, C., Datry, A., Marche, C., Wolf, M., Roux, P., Derouin, F. and Clauvel, J. P. (1990). Toxoplasma gondii pneumonia in patients with the acquired immunodeficiency syndrome. Am. J. Med., 88, 18–21

15. Wreghitt, T. G., Hughes, M. and Calne, R. Y. (1987). A retrospective study of viral and Toxoplasma gondii infection in 54 liver transplant recipients received in Cambridge. Serodiag. Immun., 1, 219–229

16. Holliman, R. E. (1988). Toxoplasmosis in the acquired immunodeficiency syndrome. J. Infect., 16, 121–128

17. Warren, K. S. (1991). Blood flukes (schistosomes) and liver flukes. In McIntyre, N., Benhamou, J.-P., Bircher, J., Rizetto, M. and Rodes, J. (eds). Oxford Textbook of Clinical Hepatology. pp. 714–721. Oxford: Oxford University Press

18. Symmers, W. S. C. (1903). Note on a new form of liver cirrhosis due to the presence of the ova of Bilharzia haematobia. J. Pathol. Bacteriol., 9, 237–239

19. Moore, G., Homewood, C. R. and Gilles, H. M. (1975). A comparison of pigment from S. mansoni and Plasmodium berghei. Ann. Trop. Med. Parasitol., 69, 373–374

20. Grimaud, J. A. and Borojevic, R. (1977). Chronic human schistosomiasis mansoni. Pathology of Disse's space. Lab. Invest., 36, 268–273

21. Kamel, I. R., Elwi, A. M., Cheever, A. W., Mosimann, J. E. and Danner, R. (1978). Schistosoma mansoni and haematobium infections in Egypt. IV Hepatic lesions. Am. J. Trop. Med. Hyg., 27, 931–938

22. Hou, P. C. (1956). The relationship between primary carcinoma of the liver and infestation with Clonorchis sinensis. J. Pathol. Bacteriol., 72, 239–246

23. Acosta-Ferreira, W., Vercelli-Retta, J. and Falconi, L. M. (1979). Fasciola hepatica human infection. Histopathological study of 16 cases. Virchows Arch. [A]., 383, 319–328

24. Hou, P. C. and Pang, L. S. C. (1964). Clonorchis sinensis infestation in man in Hong Kong. J. Pathol. Bacteriol., 87, 245–250

25. King, M. S. (1971). Biliary tract disease in Malaya. Br. J. Surg., 58, 829–832

26. Joske, R. A. (1974). The changing pattern of hydatid disease, with special reference to hydatid of the liver. Med. J. Austr., 1, 129–132

27. Miguet, J. P. and Bresson-Hadni, S. (1989). Alveolar echinococcosis of the liver. J. Hepatol., 8, 373–379

28. Ong, G. B. (1992). Helminthic diseases of the liver and biliary tract. In Millward-Sadler, G. H., Wright, R. and Arthur, M. J. P. (eds). Wright's Liver and Biliary Disease. pp. 1540–1574. London: W B Saunders

'There can be few subjects that have received more attention in the last few years yet remain among "the most confused and confusing areas in medicine"[1]'–thus began the chapter on chronic hepatitis in the first edition of this book. Some at least of the confusion has been cleared following the characterization of the main causes of acute viral hepatitis. It is clear that hepatitis A and hepatitis E (epidemic NANB hepatitis)', whatever the morphological features seen in biopsies, progress to chronic hepatitis only extremely rarely[2] (Chapter 3), whilst infections with hepatitis B sometimes, and those with hepatitis D or hepatitis C frequently progress. These developments have greatly improved the position with regard to diagnosis and management of chronic hepatitis.

DEFINITION OF CHRONIC HEPATITIS

It is now widely accepted that a minimum period of 6 months of continuous or remittent disease is necessary for the diagnosis of chronic hepatitis[3]. It may follow overt or subclinical viral hepatitis, especially hepatitis D, B and C, exposure to certain drugs, or have no known cause. The main outstanding problem with the diagnosis is that the time of onset of the condition is not always known, and thus if it is insidious the disease process may have been present for longer than clinically apparent. The diagnosis of chronic hepatitis is normally taken to imply infection with one of the hepatitis viruses, or autoimmune or drug-related hepatitis. By convention, other diseases which may closely simulate chronic hepatitis both clinically and morphologically, such as primary biliary cirrhosis, Wilson's disease, alcoholic liver disease and α_1-anti-trypsin deficiency, are normally excluded from the definition. They will, however, have to be considered in the differential diagnosis of chronic hepatitis. There is also often some difficulty in deciding whether or not cirrhosis has supervened. When cirrhosis is present it may be inactive, with little or no continuing necrosis and inflammation, or active, which implies superimposed chronic hepatitis.

Biopsy is essential for the diagnosis of chronic hepatitis. It cannot be accurately assessed on the basis of clinical and biochemical features alone. Conversely, it may be impossible to distinguish chronic from acute hepatitis on purely morphological grounds without a knowledge of the clinical features, particularly the duration of the illness.

CLASSIFICATION

The current standard classification of chronic hepatitis is shown in Table 7.1. The terms chronic persistent and chronic aggressive hepatitis were first proposed by De Groote et al.[4] and became widely adopted. These authors felt that a distinction should be made between a morphological diagnosis of chronic aggressive hepatitis and a clinical diagnosis of chronic active hepatitis, particularly since they felt that the two conditions do not always completely correspond. However, since the diagnosis of any form of chronic hepatitis requires biopsy this difference is more apparent than real, and so chronic active hepatitis (CAH) tends now to be used in either context. Further support for this practice was given by the international group[3].

Table 7.1 Classification of chronic hepatitis

Chronic persistent hepatitis	(portal hepatitis)
Chronic active hepatitis	
without BHN	(periportal CAH)
with BHN	(subacute hepatic necrosis)
Chronic lobular hepatitis	(unresolved viral hepatitis)

A third term–chronic lobular hepatitis (CLH)–was added by Popper and Schaffner in 1971[5]. The international group preferred 'unresolved' or 'protracted' hepatitis because of the generally much better prognosis of these cases as compared to CAH with lobular involvement. A fourth type–chronic septal hepatitis[6]–has not gained wide acceptance because it probably is no more than a result of necrosis and inflammation in any kind of hepatitis[7].

Because all these morphological forms of chronic hepatitis can be found at the same time in an individual patient, it seems likely that this classification may well gradually become overtaken by events, particularly since it is now so much easier to identify the precise cause of the hepatitis[8].

CLINICAL AND MORPHOLOGICAL FEATURES

The major difference between chronic persistent hepatitis (CPH) and chronic active hepatitis (CAH) is the location of the inflammatory infiltrate. In CPH it is confined to the portal tracts whilst in CAH it extends into the periportal parenchyma or beyond.

CHRONIC PERSISTENT HEPATITIS

This condition may be clinically silent or associated with easy fatiguability or other rather vague symptoms. The liver may be enlarged. Biochemical abnormalities are usually restricted to elevated or fluctuating levels of transaminases. Gamma globulins and alkaline phosphatase are normal. Without a preceding attack of hepatitis the diagnosis is much more difficult in view of the other conditions which may simulate CPH (see below). The condition may resolve or remain static for many years but the ultimate prognosis is regarded as good. However, a few patients may progress to CAH even in the presence of normal biochemistry[9]. Biopsy is thus necessary to monitor progress.

CPH is predominantly a portal lesion (Figure 7.1). The overall liver architecture is preserved, although there may be occasional thin, short, straight fibrous septa radiating from portal tracts (Figure 7.2). The cellular infiltrate is composed mainly of lymphocytes (Figure 7.3) with a few plasma cells and macrophages and even occasional eosinophils and neutrophils, often in the form of compact aggregates. There may be associated irregularities of bile duct epithelium. The limiting plate is generally well preserved; an important point in the distinction from CAH. Occasionally the distinction may be blurred by spillover of inflammatory cells from portal tracts into the parenchyma, also seen in acute hepatitis, particularly amongst drug-users, and can usually be distinguished from piecemeal

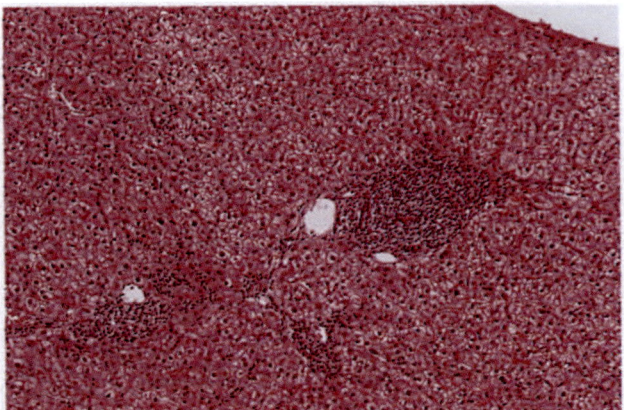

Figure 7.1 Chronic persistent hepatitis. This male drug addict had persistent minor abnormalities of liver function tests one year after acute hepatitis B. Liver biopsy shows fairly intense chronic inflammatory cell infiltration of all portal tracts, but no extension of the process into the parenchyma.

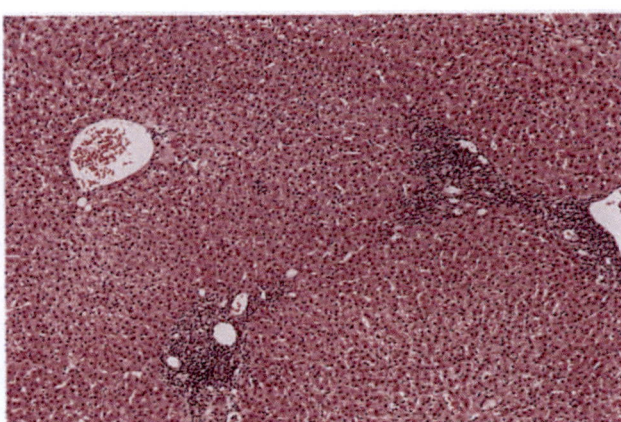

Figure 7.2 Chronic persistent hepatitis (known chronic hepatitis C). Note the lymphoid aggregates confined to portal tracts which are linked to one another by thin fibrous septa.

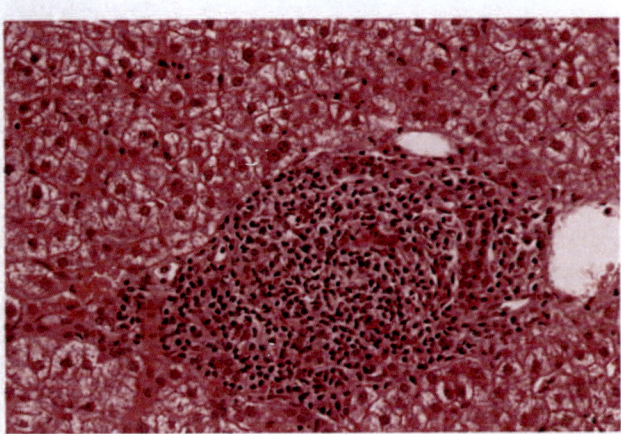

Figure 7.3 Chronic persistent hepatitis. Same biopsy as Figure 7.1. Higher magnification shows that the cells are almost exclusively lymphocytes, and confirms that the limiting plates are intact.

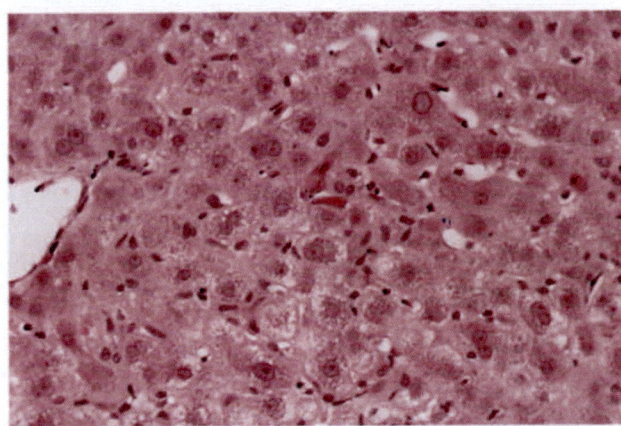

Figure 7.4 Chronic lobular hepatitis (known chronic hepatitis C). Note the low-grade hepatitis with an occasional acidophil body and a few sinusoidal lymphocytes.

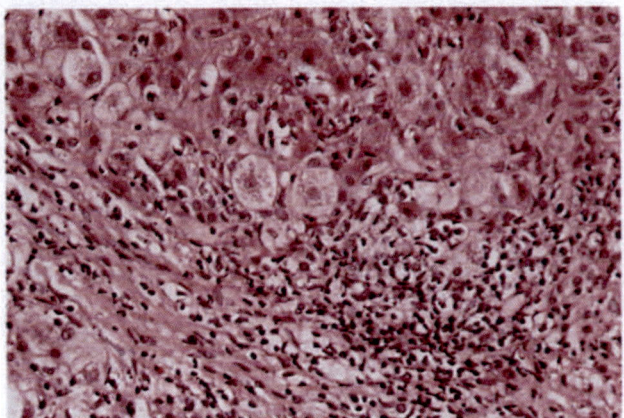

Figure 7.5 Chronic active hepatitis, piecemeal necrosis. This biopsy, from a patient with HBsAg-negative CAH, shows chronic inflammatory cells, mainly lymphocytes and plasma cells, aggressively destroying the limiting plate (which runs horizontally across the field) and apparently attacking periportal hepatocytes which show ballooning degeneration.

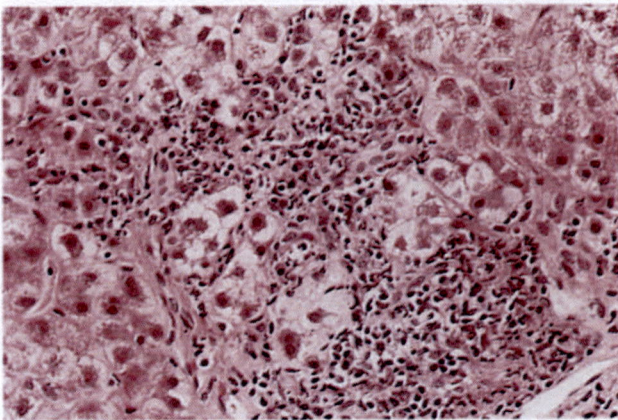

Figure 7.6 Chronic active hepatitis, piecemeal necrosis. Another example of autoimmune CAH in which the changes are even more severe. The liver cells at the centre of this field are showing advanced degenerative changes and are surrounded by inflammatory granulation tissue.

necrosis by the absence of liver cell necrosis. Not all parts of the liver are equally affected by the inflammation, but in general the smaller the portal tract the more conspicuous the inflammation. Indeed, if most small portal tracts are not inflamed the diagnosis is probably not CPH[10]. Larger tracts may show merely peripheral inflammation or inflammation localized to only one part. Bile duct proliferation is usually trivial or non-existent. There is often some parenchymal inflammation, including occasional focal necrosis, acidophil bodies and Kupffer cell proliferation, amounting to a low-grade lobular hepatitis (Figure 7.4)—most such cases will probably prove to be due to chronic hepatitis C[11–13]. In carriers of hepatitis B ground glass cells containing HBsAg may be plentiful but their distribution is haphazard.

Differential diagnosis of CPH

In practice, there may be some difficulty in differentiating CPH from residual acute hepatitis on the one hand and from mild CAH on the other. There is no clear morphological distinction between CPH and resolving acute hepatitis. All cases of AVH probably pass through a similar morphological phase and thus a knowledge of the time scale is essential. If there was no recognized acute attack, diagnosis may be more problematical and the other causes of portal hepatitis listed below should be considered. However, it should be re-emphasized that many such cases can now be easily resolved by serum virus markers.

Other causes of portal hepatitis

Chronic active hepatitis

There may be some problems at the interface between very mild chronic active hepatitis (CAH) (defined as showing piecemeal necrosis of limiting plates) and CPH, but in these circumstances the CAH is mild and therefore the distinction is probably of little significance[7]. Treated autoimmune CAH may be indistinguishable from CPH (see below).

Non-specific reactive hepatitis

This is seen in association with a variety of non-hepatic diseases or in relationship to space occupying lesions within the liver (Chapter 21). Portal tract inflammation may be quite similar to that in CPH but is usually less uniform with uninvolved portal tracts present in the same microscopic field. There is usually no architectural disturbance and lobular inflammation takes the form of focal necroses, occasionally with granuloma-like collections of mononuclear cells. NSRH is extremely common in post–mortem material.

Primary biliary cirrhosis

In its early stages PBC may be very similar to CPH, in the absence of bile duct lesions or granulomas (Chapter 17). Stains for copper are unlikely to be helpful at this early stage and thus the distinction is probably best made by the almost invariable presence of antimitochondrial antibody in the serum in PBC.

Lymphoreticular disorders

Chronic lymphatic leukaemia and other lymphoreticular disorders may be associated with portal infiltration, but the cellular infiltrates are usually denser, more compact and less pleomorphic than in CPH.

CHRONIC LOBULAR HEPATITIS

As originally defined, chronic lobular hepatitis has no or only a minimal portal inflammatory component[14,15]. There is focal parenchymal necrosis, acidophil body formation with or without confluent necrosis, and therefore may be confused with acute hepatitis. It is vital therefore always to be in full possession of all the clinical data. It is probably most often associated with chronic hepatitis B, when it should be possible to detect HBsAg containing hepatocytes, or with chronic hepatitis C (Figure 7.4).

CHRONIC ACTIVE HEPATITIS (CHRONIC AGGRESSIVE HEPATITIS)

Chronic active hepatitis (CAH) is defined as an inflammatory condition in which there is piecemeal necrosis of the hepatocytes of the limiting plates which form the boundary between portal tract and hepatic parenchyma[16]. Similar changes may affect peripheries of nodules in established cirrhosis. The limiting plates often have a moth-eaten appearance due to the fact that some liver cells have disappeared, others are swollen and hydropic, often with granular PAS positive material in their cytoplasm. Single cells, or often small groups of cells, some swollen, others shrunken, may be apparently trapped within portal tracts (Figures 7.5 and 7.6). The groups often take the form of rosettes or acini of cells with a central bile canaliculus (Figure 7.7). They can be distinguished from rather similar acini seen in cholestasis by the presence of a peripheral collagenous basement membrane around the former (Figure 7.8)[17]. These are the appearances of classic or lymphocytic piecemeal necrosis, which must be distinguished from biliary and other types of piecemeal necrosis seen in chronic cholestatic conditions (Chapter 16). Periportal liver cell loss cannot always be readily distinguished from portal tract expansion in routine sections. Connective tissue stains, such as elastic van Gieson (EVG) or orcein[18], are often very helpful in that they clearly delineate the hard collagen and the elastic of the original portal tract (Figure 7.9). The inflammatory cells are mainly lymphocytes and macrophages, but plasma cells may be quite numerous[10]. There is bile duct proliferation and here, too, as in other situations, this may be associated with infiltration by a few neutrophil or eosinophil polymorphs. The inflammatory changes tend to be more severe in the smaller portal tracts.

CAH with bridging hepatic necrosis

The original definition of CAH[4], recognized that CAH might have differing degrees of severity. CAH can be subdivided into two groups (Table 7.1). In some cases, the inflammation is confined to the portal tract and periportal parenchyma (Figure 7.10), whilst in others it is more extensive and is accompanied by bridging hepatic necrosis (BHN) (Figures 7.11 and 7.12)[19,20] (see Chapter 2). The key to the significance of BHN seems to be whether or not piecemeal necrosis spreads from the portal tract to the surviving cells lining the portal to central bridge[10]. When it does so, the inflammatory infiltrate migrates into the liver parenchyma, replacing some liver cells and surrounding others. The reticulin framework collapses, the sinusoids in the bridge acquire basement membranes and become capillaries, so called 'passive' septa. The consequence has been extension of the piecemeal necrosis from the periportal region to involve the whole lobule with the development of portal systemic shunts. Thus the combination of BHN with piecemeal necrosis has extremely damaging consequences. One without the other may be much less harmful. For example, this degree of necrosis in otherwise uncomplicated viral

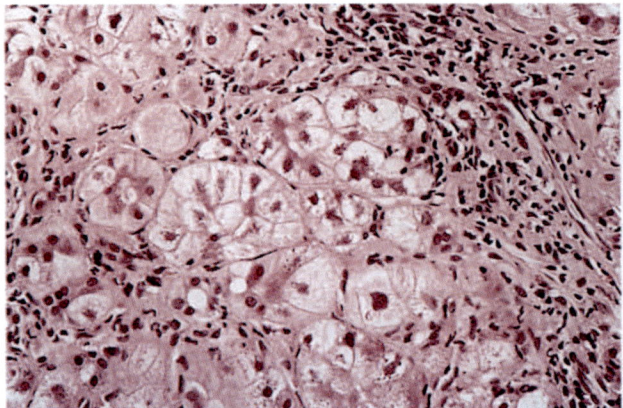

Figure 7.7 Chronic active hepatitis, rosette formation. Autoimmune CAH showing periportal piecemeal necrosis with rosette formation.

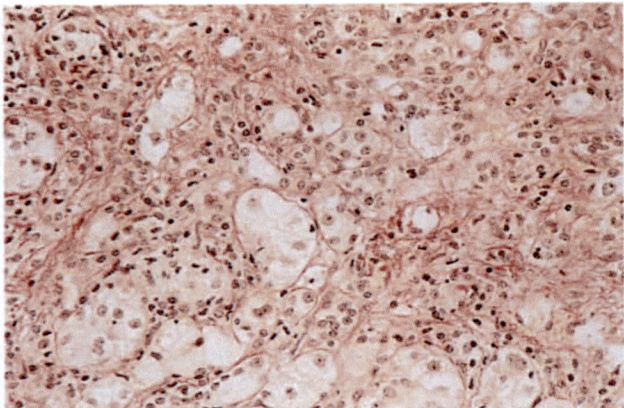

Figure 7.8 Chronic active hepatitis, rosette formation. Another case showing that each is surrounded by a collagenous basement membrane. Elastic van Gieson.

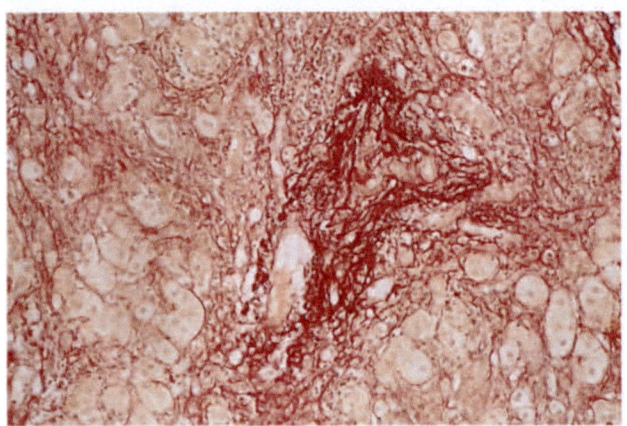

Figure 7.9 Chronic active hepatitis. Another case of HBsAg-negative CAH showing periportal liver cell loss. The pre-existing portal tract can be seen at the centre of the field, stained a deep red colour. Surrounding this is a network of much finer collagen, formed following periportal hepatocellular necrosis. Elastic van Gieson.

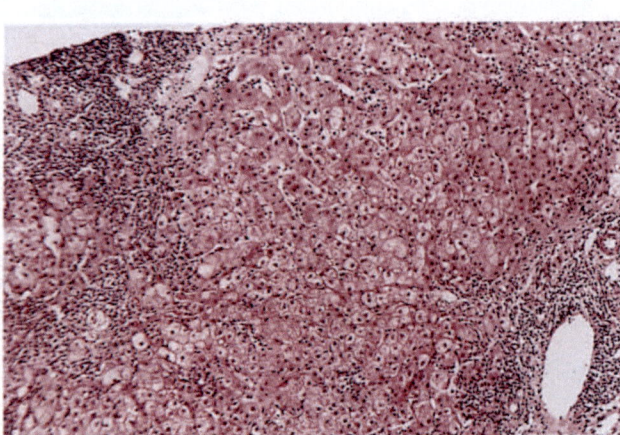

Figure 7.10 Periportal chronic active hepatitis. Autoimmune CAH showing intense portal tract chronic inflammation with piecemeal necrosis and extension of inflammation into the periportal parenchyma. The remainder of the lobule is normal and there is no bridging hepatic necrosis.

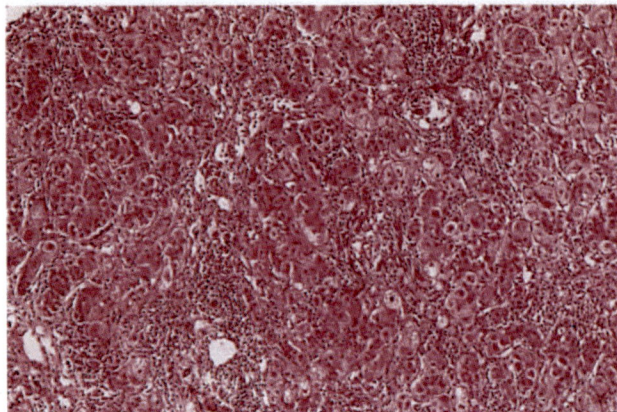

Figure 7.11 Chronic active hepatitis with bridging hepatic necrosis. Autoimmune CAH showing complete disruption of the normal architecture due to BHN. The surviving liver cells are subjected to piecemeal necrosis so that the liver is reduced to single cells and groups of cells separated and surrounded by inflammatory fibrous tissue.

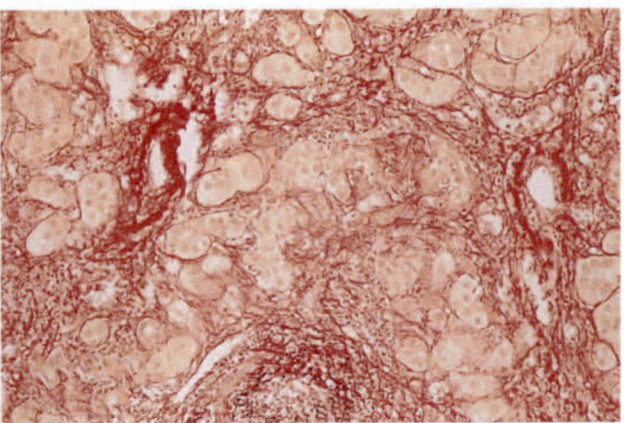

Figure 7.12 Chronic active hepatitis with bridging hepatic necrosis. Same case as 7.11. This connective tissue stain demonstrates the architectural disruption. There is a central vein to left and right and a portal tract centre bottom. Bridging necrosis links the two central veins (convex upwards) through the nodal point of Mall, and the central veins with the portal tract. Elastic van Gieson.

hepatitis may be followed by complete recovery[21]. Similarly, CAH without BHN has a much more favourable prognosis (see below). More extensive necrosis than so far described, extending into zone II and even zone I of the acinus, will have the same sort of significance. That is to say, if the persisting liver cells are subject to piecemeal necrosis there is likely to be progression to cirrhosis. If there is no piecemeal necrosis, as will always be the case if all the cells in a lobule are destroyed (called multilobular necrosis by some authors), then that part of the liver may be reduced to an insignificant scar. Widespread multilobular necrosis often causes dramatic shrinkage of the left lobe (Figures 11.11 and 11.12).

Microscopically in CAH with BHN the changes of piecemeal necrosis and chronic inflammation are no longer confined to the portal regions (Figures 7.11 and 7.12). Broad septa dissect the lobules, corresponding to the portal to central bridges described above. Narrower septa radiate from these into the adjacent liver parenchyma where they separate and surround small groups of liver cells. Acinus formation, hydropic swelling, new basement membranes and collagen are all found as in periportal piecemeal necrosis, but now throughout the lobule causing complete disruption of the hepatic architecture. In cases following hepatitis B, ground glass cells may be seen (Figure 7.13). Their absence in a biopsy does not rule out hepatitis B since their distribution is very irregular (Figure 7.13).

Cholestasis is an occasional complication of CAH[22] possibly due to mechanical interference with bile flow at the damaged limiting plate. When it occurs it may be accompanied by the usual secondary phenomena such as feathery degeneration and multinucleation (Figure 7.14) (Chapter 16). Clinically it may be associated with pruritis.

Small interlobular bile ducts, especially those in the central part of portal tracts, may show epithelial abnormalities in CAH (Figure 7.15)[23]. Characteristically there is multilayering of the epithelium which typically only affects part of the circumference of the duct. This change can usually be distinguished from that in PBC where multilayering is unusual but duct rupture and granuloma formation are common[24]. There may be an increased tendency to the development of cirrhosis[25] in its presence, almost certainly because most of these cases would have been examples of hepatitis C which has a high risk of chronicity (see below, although the case shown in Figure 7.15 was due to autoimmune CAH and responded fully to steroids, the patient being disease-free 30 years later).

Differential diagnosis of CAH

There is probably a continuous histological spectrum from CPH through CAH and CAH with BHN to cirrhosis. Although this will usually be mirrored to some extent by clinical and biochemical parameters this is not always the case. Thus histological changes may be either more or less marked than expected clinically, which may partly be due to sampling error (Figure 7.16)[26]. It may be difficult to define the exact moment of onset of cirrhosis, particularly in severe CAH with BHN. Laparoscopic evidence of the presence or absence of nodules may be very helpful in this context. Once cirrhotic nodules have appeared they may continue to be attacked by piecemeal necrosis around their periphery, so called activity, or the process may become quiescent with subsidence of the inflammation. As already stated, it is often difficult to assess the significance of lobular and periportal changes after acute viral hepatitis (q.v.). It may be necessary to wait several months and repeat the biopsy.

SPECIFIC FEATURES OF CHRONIC HEPATITIS
Viral causes

As already stated, the main viruses responsible for chronic hepatitis are hepatitis B, with or without co- or superinfection with hepatitis D, and hepatitis C. The appearances of chronic hepatitis B are well described, but those of chronic hepatitis C are only now being fully documented.

Chronic hepatitis B
Persistence of hepatitis B
There are wide fluctuations in the geographic incidence of hepatitis B. It appears to be common in Mediterranean countries, Africa and the Middle and Far East, but much less prevalent in Britain and North America. Population screens similarly reveal a wide variation in the incidence of asymptomatic carriers, ranging from 20% amongst the Casinawah Indians of Peru to 0.1% in the US and UK. Some estimates have put the total number of carriers in the world as high as 200×10^6. Many of these surveys have been done upon blood donors and can thus be considered to have excluded patients with a history of jaundice; however, this is not invariably the case.

Persistence of HBV after acute infection may occur in from 5 to 95% of individuals. Persistence is unusual after overt clinical hepatitis, suggesting that clearance of the virus requires an active hepatitic illness. Conversely, persistence is more likely to follow asymptomatic or subclinical infection, especially if the virus is acquired perinatally.

The failure to eradicate HBV reflects an inadequate response to virus, but the precise mechanism has not been fully defined. There are probably at least several possibilities[27]. In the neonatal period, when the risk of persistence is highest, it may be due to specific immunological tolerance to HB antigens and/or a modulating effect of maternal antibody to HBcAg. In older patients, other possible defects include: a failure of anti–HBsAg, possibly due to high levels of HBsAg inducing tolerance; enhancement caused by anti–HBcAg masking the target antigen on hepatocytes; and a failure of interferon production and thus of upregulation of class I HLA molecules on the hepatocyte surface.

In chronic hepatitis, the mechanism of hepatocyte damage is thought to be the same as in acute hepatitis (Chapter 3), namely a T-lymphocyte mediated attack upon HBcAg in the cell membrane, and the outcome in an individual patient depends upon the fate of the virus. If virus replication continues for long periods, then there will be progressive liver cell damage with scarring and ultimately cirrhosis. If, on the other hand, the virus can be eliminated or, alternatively, partially contained, then there will be less chronic liver damage. One way in which viral replication can become contained is for virus to become fully integrated into the genome. When this happens, HBsAg continues to be transcribed but HBcAg and HBeAg do not because the process of integration destroys the HB core gene[28]. If integration occurs speedily, there may not yet be significant liver damage–the so-called 'healthy' carrier. If, secondly, integration becomes complete after the development of cirrhosis, the disease process may then become inactive. Finally, viral replication may continue unabated and thus the cirrhosis continues to show active hepatitis.

Histological features of chronic hepatitis B
Ground glass cells and hepatitis B surface antigen Cells with a uniform finely granular eosinophilic cytoplasm, often with a peripheral clear space and a displaced nucleus, were first described in the German literature and

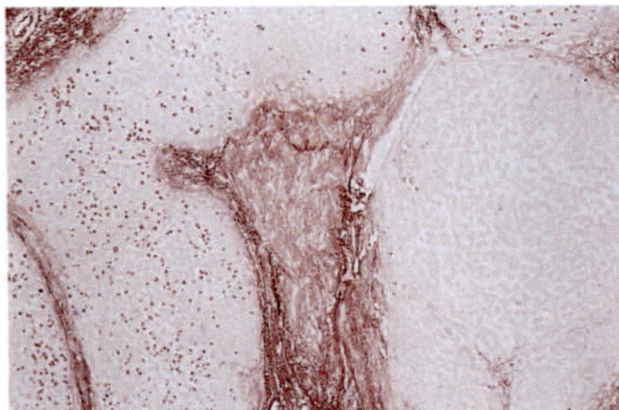

Figure 7.13 Chronic active hepatitis, cirrhosis. HBsAg-positive CAH showing the irregular distribution of orcein-positive hepatocytes. The nodule to the left contains numerous positive cells, that on the right, none. Orcein.

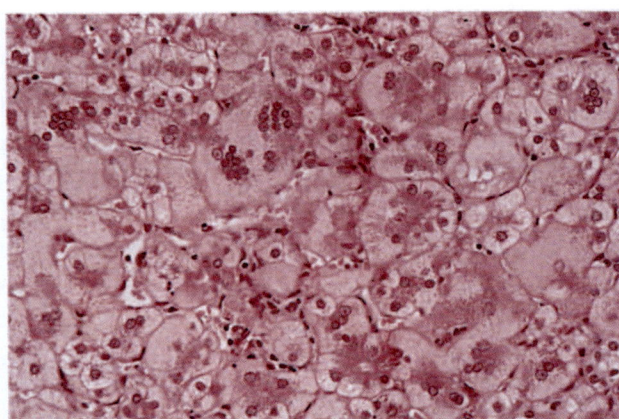

Figure 7.14 Chronic active hepatitis with cholestasis. Autoimmune CAH with striking biochemical cholestasis in a young adult female patient. Note the presence of a number of multinucleate hepatocytes as well as the other features of CAH. This is probably attributable to the cholestasis, although bile retention is not visible in this field.

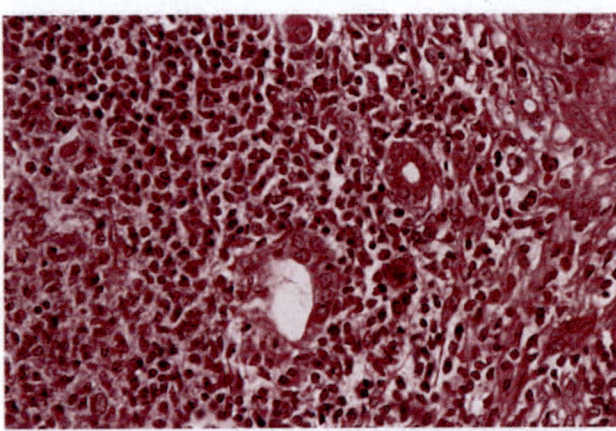

Figure 7.15 Chronic active hepatitis with atypical bile duct epithelium. Same biopsy as Figures 7.11 and 7.12. This portal tract contains a dense infiltrate of chronic inflammatory cells, mostly lymphocytes and plasma cells. the bile duct below centre shows epithelial abnormalities in the form of multilayering (upper right) and partial disruption. The latter is more characteristic of primary biliary cirrhosis that CAH.

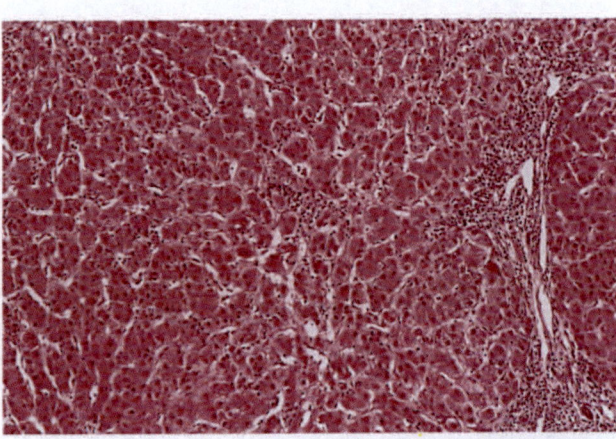

Figure 7.16 Chronic active hepatitis. This shows another part of the same generous surgical wedge biopsy as Figure 7.11, 7.12 and 7.15, illustrating how variable the disease may be from one place to another. Here the chronic inflammation is more or less confined to portal tracts and thus resembles CPH. The only change visible in the parenchyma is regenerative activity in the form of twinning of liver cell plates.

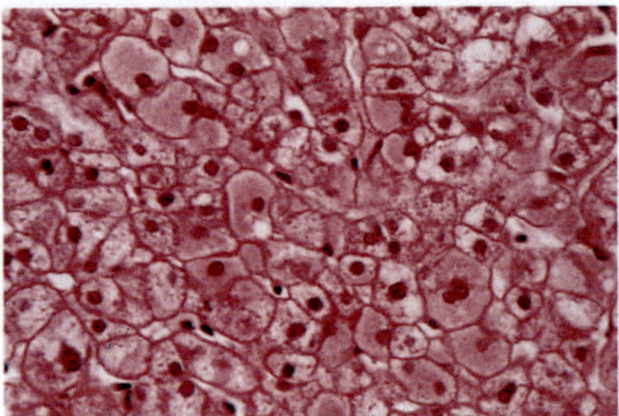

Figure 7.17 Ground glass cells. HBsAg carrier. Note the cells with a very uniform homogeneous eosinophilic cytoplasm. Some also have a characteristic clear space around the cytoplasmic membrane.

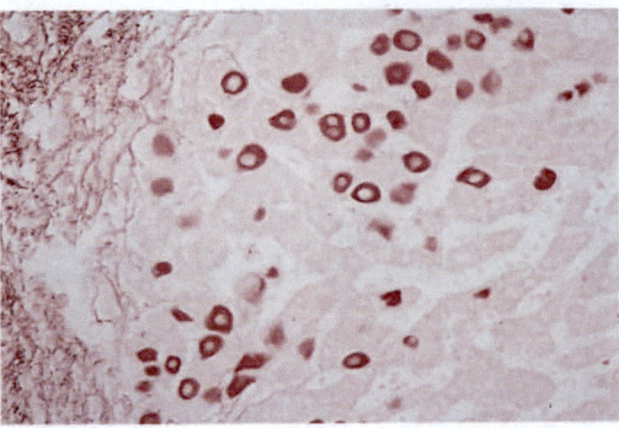

Figure 7.18 HBsAg carrier, orcein-positive cells are stained brown. Orcein.

related to induction of smooth endoplasmic reticulum (SER) by drugs such as chlorpromazine and rifampicin (Figure 10.1)[29,30]. Similar 'induced' ground glass cells are also quite frequently seen in cholestasis and alcoholic injury[31]. Subsequently, similar cells in the livers of carriers of hepatitis B (Figure 7.17) were shown, by immuno-fluorescence techniques, to contain cytoplasmic HBsAg[32]. Shikata noticed that both orcein (Figure 7.18) and alde-hyde fuchsin stained these HBsAg containing cells (but not those due to other causes) and that the stains could easily be applied both prospectively and retrospectively to ordinary paraffin embedded material[33]. Similar results are obtained with trichrome[34] and Victoria blue[35] stains. This is thus a useful method for the demonstration of HBsAg in sections, and it is relatively specific although not as sensitive as the immunological techniques[36].

Viral antigens are not detected in the acute phase of viral hepatitis, because virus-containing cells are elimin-ated, and thus orcein positive cells are also absent. Orcein cannot therefore help to distinguish hepatitis B from other types of hepatitis in the acute phase. In the carrier state, however, orcein positive ground glass cells are common. In general, there tends to be an inverse relationship between their number and the presence of inflammation (see below). Their distribution tends to be very irregular and thus there is a considerable sampling error in needle biopsies (Figure 7.13)[37]. Whenever possible at least five blocks should be examined before a case is labelled HBsAg negative[38].

The aldehyde fuchsin method can also be successfully applied to epoxy sections[39]. Immunoperoxidase methods, using specific antibody, are also technically straightfor-ward at least on paraffin sections, although horseradish peroxidase does appear to bind non-immunologically, rather like orcein itself, to HBsAg containing liver cells[40]. This is thus a potential source of error when applying this method to other antigens in liver tissue.

Histologically, a great range of appearances may be found in chronic HB, ranging from the presence of ground-glass HBsAg containing cells in an otherwise normal liver, through CPH, CLH to mild or severe CAH with or without cirrhosis. Since the mechanism of liver cell damage is the same as that in the acute hepatitis, cytotoxic T-lymphocytes continue to play a central role and are seen in close contact with hepatocytes in areas of liver cell damage[7,41]. A variety of other cells may also be found in portal tracts, including dendritic cells, T-helper cells and plasma cells[42]. The diagnosis is very much dependent upon finding HB markers in serum and/or tissues.

Clinico-pathological correlations

Carriers of HBV, whose disease is usually asymptomatic for long periods, fall into two main groups, those with continuing viral replication and therefore HBV-DNA in the serum and those without – both groups have persist-ence of serum HBsAg.

Continuing virus replication. This is a heterogeneous group which contains a high proportion of young males, drug addicts and clients of venereal disease clinics. Estimates of the proportion of those who will develop chronic hepatitis and cirrhosis vary widely, but, as already stated, this is thought to be more likely to follow a mild or inapparent acute infection. Two recent studies have put the risk at about 10%[43], although, especially in patients who acquire the infection very early in life, it may be as high as 50%[44]. Biochemically the only abnormality is often a slight elevation of serum transaminases, yet the biopsy may reveal much more severe liver damage than expected[45]. These patients generally have expression of

both HBcAg and HBsAg in roughly equal amounts. As well as HBsAg and HBV-DNA, most patients also have HBeAg, whose presence always means active viral repli-cation, in the blood. Conversely, the absence of HBeAg generally means that there is no active replication. The only exception to this rule is a small group (about 5% overall) who are infected by a virus with a mutation in the precore region of the genome[44].

A distinct group is formed by the immunosuppressive carriers. These patients may be receiving formal thera-peutic immunosuppression for transplantation or inflam-matory disease or may be spontaneously immunosup-pressed as a result of lymphoreticular or other disease. They often show little evidence of morphological abnor-mality in their livers, however some will show CPH or CAH. Immunological studies reveal generalized expression of HBcAg in a great proportion of liver cell nuclei as well as some cytoplasmic expression (Figure 7.19)[29]. In addition a few cells show cytoplasmic HBsAg and there is often a honeycomb-like pattern of HBsAg in liver cell membranes[46]. Orcein positive ground glass cells are present but rather scarce; occasionally orcein, too, produces predominantly membranous staining. Dane par-ticles are present in the serum and these patients have a high infectivity as attested by the numerous serious outbreaks of hepatitis, often with high mortality, amongst the staff in dialysis units before regular antigen screen-ing[47]. A unique pattern of expression has been described in liver transplant patients and termed *fibrosing cholestatic hepatitis*[48]. This is associated with rapidly progressive disease and characterized by slender bands of fibrous tissue radiating into the parenchyma, and mixed with proliferating ductules (Figure 7.20). There is also usually strong diffuse expression of HBsAg (cytoplasmic and membranous) and HBcAg and HBeAg (mainly nuclear).

No continuing viral replication–healthy carriers: These patients are usually discovered following blood donor surveys. On liver biopsy, they show a very low percentage of changes regarded as significant[49]. Most cases show only ground glass cells, minor inflammatory changes, fatty change or no abnormality at all (Figure 7.17). Only 7% show CPH and one patient out of 167 (0.6%) actually was cirrhotic. Family studies have shown a high incidence of more than one case, with the highest prevalence amongst siblings and parents and the lowest between spouses. These findings suggest a significant genetic component or a very early age of first infection. Immuno-logical studies on these livers demonstrate an excess of cells containing HBsAg corresponding to the ground glass cells seen on haematoxylin and eosin staining; orcein gives similar results. These are sometimes very numerous, but because of the great variability from one part of the liver to another may not always be conspicuous in a biopsy. In contrast, there is virtually no expression of HBcAg[29]. The infectivity of these patients is generally considered to be low since HBV-DNA is not usually found in the blood, probably, as explained above, because the virus is now fully integrated. The incidence of signifi-cant liver disease is so low that biopsy is probably not justified[50,51]

Chronic hepatitis C

It is clear (Chapter 2) that a significant proportion of patients infected by HCV progress to chronic disease. Furthermore, it may be difficult on morphological grounds to distinguish acute from chronic hepatitis[11]. Many cases of HCV infection resemble the classic descriptions of CPH[8], and may indeed account for most such cases. The features noted in Chapter 2, acidophilic degeneration, acidophil body formation, microvesicular fat and lobular

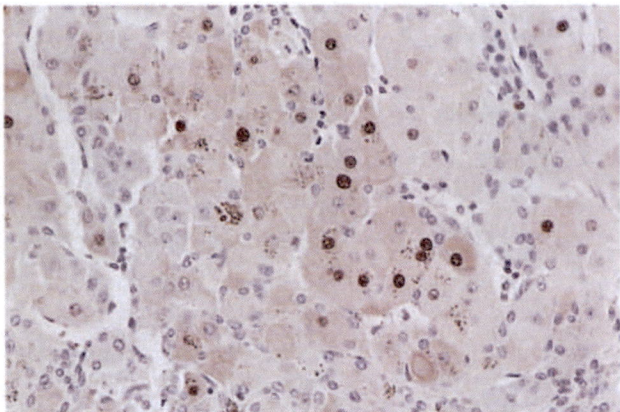

Figure 7.19 Chronic hepatitis B, immunosuppressive type. Note the extensive positive staining for HBcAg, which is mainly but not exclusively nuclear. There was little associated inflammation. Immunoperoxidase.

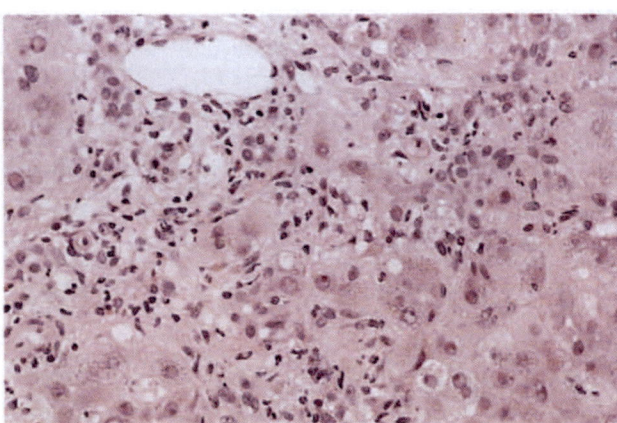

Figure 7.20 Fibrosing cholestatic hepatitis–due to recurrent hepatitis B after liver transplantation. This patient had received a graft for end-stage chronic hepatitis B about three months before this biopsy. Note the mixture of inflammatory cells and bile ductules invading the parenchyma at the limiting plate. There was very widespread expression of both HBsAg and of HBcAg.

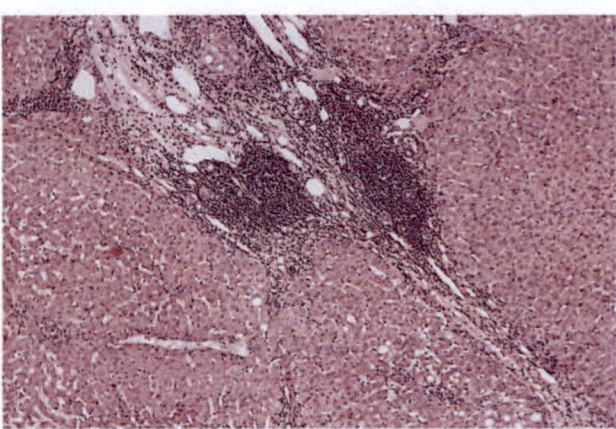

Figure 7.21 Chronic hepatitis C. This liver was removed at transplantation for end-stage disease. Note the compact aggregates of lymphocytes within the fibrous septa of this cirrhotic liver.

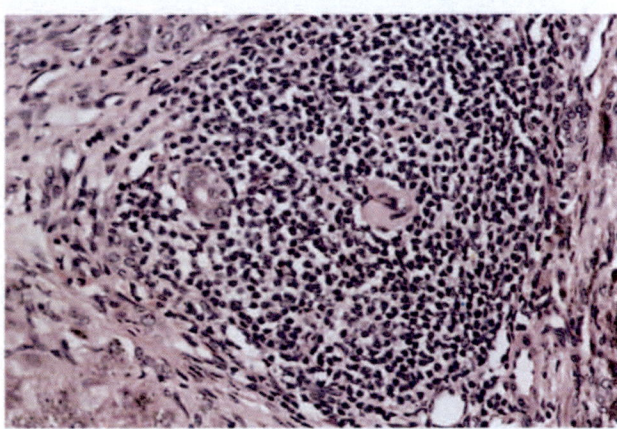

Figure 7.22 Chronic hepatitis C. Another case, similar to that shown in Figure 7.21, also treated by liver transplantation. Note that this dense lymphoid aggregate contains a small bile duct (to left of centre) which shows some nuclear irregularities.

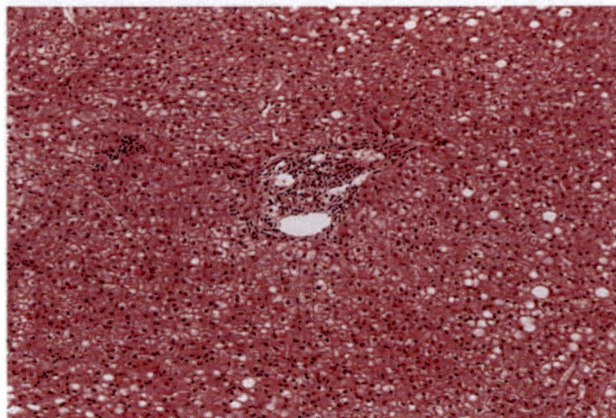

Figure 7.23 Autoimmune chronic active hepatitis in remission. This patient had been under treatment with steroids for 5 years. The section shows changes indistinguishable from those of CPH, plus a few parenchymal foci of fat, but no active inflammatory destruction of hepatocytes or fibrosis.

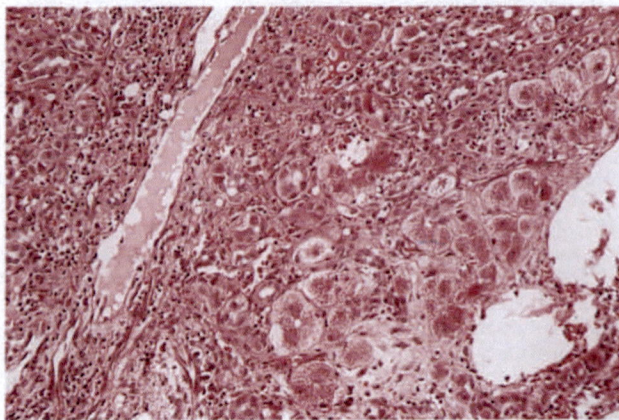

Figure 7.24 Wilson's disease. This 12-year-old girl presented with a typical syndrome of 'lupoid hepatitis', but copper studies showed conclusively that she had Wilson's disease. The section shows that Wilson's disease can be morphologically indistinguishable from CAH.

inflammation may all be seen in the chronic phase. However, the most distinctive feature, present in about 60% of cases, is the presence of portal lymphoid aggregates, often surrounding or at the side of damaged bile ducts (Figures 7.21 and 7.22)[8]. The changes may affect only part of the circumference and consist of vacuolation and lymphocytic infiltration of the epithelium. Despite the histologically rather mild changes, there is no doubt that there is a high risk of the development of cirrhosis, but probably only after many years[7]. The pathogenesis of the chronic liver disease remains unknown.

Autoimmune chronic active hepatitis (AICAH)

There is a group of patients in whom the chronic hepatitis is thought to be autoimmune[52]. Originally described as particularly affecting young women who also often had a positive LE cell test, it was termed 'lupoid hepatitis'. It also affects other age-groups and commonly presents with hepatosplenomegaly. Patients often have other auto-immune disorders, and they often have other autoantibodies, especially anti-actin smooth muscle antibodies. These patients regularly have IgG antibodies in high titre to a variety of common viral antigens and a high frequency of HLA antigens A1, B8, DR3 and DRW3. There is usually also an increase in the peripheral CD4 to CD8 ratio and a suppressor T-cell defect reversible by prednisolone *in vitro*. Viral markers are consistently negative. One probable target antigen on the hepatocyte is the asialoglycoprotein receptor protein[53], although other subgroups may have different mechanisms.

In general, the histological features of AICAH are similar to those produced by the viruses, although lacking viral markers, and have a tendency to be severe, i.e. usually CAH (Figures 7.11 and 7.12). Liver-cell rosettes are often prominent (Figure 7.7). Treatment with corticosteroids may result in complete remission of disease or be indistinguishable from CPH (Figure 7.23)[54], and there are no histological features by which one can predict continuing remission or subsequent relapse. Regular biopsy would therefore seem to be essential in these cases.

Wilson's disease (Chapter 15)

This should always be considered in the presence of CAH (Figure 7.24). Although this is an unusual presentation of a rare disease, the therapeutic implications are so great that it must not be missed. The patients are usually under 30 years and the presence of nuclear glycogen vacuoles, focal fatty change, peripheral hyaline and cytoplasmic copper may all be helpful features, but ultimately chemical measurement of the total hepatic copper will be necessary in cases of doubt.

Primary biliary cirrhosis (PBC)

This may have a periportal component in addition to the typical portal tract changes (Chapter 17) but rarely extends to involve the whole lobule. Apart from the bile duct lesions mentioned above and discussed in detail in Chapter 17, lymphoid aggregates, sparse bile ducts, ductular proliferation, abundant orcein positive copper protein all favour PBC.

Malignant lymphomas

These may occasionally cause problems in diagnosis but are not usually associated with significant piecemeal necrosis.

Drugs

Enquiry should be made in every case for a history of drugs, particularly those known to cause CAH, such as methyldopa (Chapter 10). Evidence of drug abuse should also be sought. There is some evidence that drug abusers have more advanced disease, yet a better prognosis than non-addicts. Clues to drug abuse may be given by the occasional presence of starch grains in portal tracts where they may even excite a granulomatous response[55].

Alcoholic liver disease

This disease can usually be recognized by the presence of typical lobular changes (Chapter 13). However there seems no doubt that alcoholism may be associated with CAH indistinguishable from that described above and completely lacking the more usual features of alcohol related disease[56]. This may well be more common than previously appreciated.

α_1-Anti-trypsin deficiency

This condition can be excluded by the absence of the typical PAS-positive inclusions in periportal liver cells (Figure 8.24).

TREATMENT AND PROGNOSIS OF CHRONIC HEPATITIS

The prognosis of chronic hepatitis is largely determined by its cause. Corticosteroids are effective in the treatment of AICAH, but not following hepatitis B[57]. Whilst there has been much interest in the use of interferon-α as a means of clearing virus, in all cases there appears to be a high rate of relapse on discontinuation of therapy[44].

REFERENCES

1. Conn, H. O. (1976). Chronic hepatitis, reducing an iatrogenic enigma to a workable puzzle. Gastroenterology, 70, 1182–1184
2. McDonald, G. S. A., Courtney, M. G., Shattock, A. G. and Weir, D. G. (1989). Prolonged IgM antibodies and histopathological evidence of chronicity in hepatitis A. Liver, 9, 223–228
3. Leevy, C. M., Popper, H. and Sherlock, S. (1976). Diseases of the liver and biliary tract, Standardization of nomenclature, diagnostic criteria, diagnostic methodology. Washington: U S Government Printing Office (1976). (Fogarty International Center Proceedings No. 22), DHEW publication No. (NIH) 76–725,
4. De Groote, J., Desmet, V. J., Gedigk, P., Korb, G., Popper, H., Poulsen, H., Scheuer, P. J., Schmid, M., Thaler, H., Uehlinger, E. and Wepler, W. (1968). A classification of chronic hepatitis. Lancet, 2, 626–628
5. Popper, H. and Schaffner, F. (1971). The vocabulary of chronic hepatitis. N. Engl. J. Med., 280, 1154–1156
6. Gerber, M. A. and Vernace, S. (1974). Chronic septal hepatitis. Virchows Arch. [A], 363, 303–309
7. Scheuer, P. J. (1993). Chronic hepatitis. In Wight, D. G. D. (ed). Liver, Biliary Tract and Exocrine Pancreas. Vol. 11. Systemic Pathology. Symmers, W. S. C. Series ed. 3rd edn. Edinburgh: Churchill Livingstone
8. Gerber, M. A. (1992). Chronic hepatitis C: the beginning of the end of a time-honored nomenclature. Hepatology, 15, 733–734
9. Chadwick, R. G., Galizzi, J., Heathcote, J., Lyssiotis, T., Cohen, B. J., Scheuer, P. J. and Sherlock, S. (1979). Chronic persistent hepatitis; hepatitis B virus markers and histological follow up. Gut, 20, 372–377
10. Popper, H. and Schaffner, F. (1976). Chronic hepatitis taxonomic, etiologic and therapeutic problems. In Popper, H. and Schaffner, F. (eds). Progr. Liver Dis. V. pp. 531–557. Baltimore: Grune and Stratton
11. Scheuer, P. J., Ashrafzadeh, P., Sherlock, S., Brown, D. and Dusheiko, G. (1992). The pathology of hepatitis C. Hepatology, 15, 567–571
12. Bach, N., Thung, S. N. and Schaffner, F. (1992). The histological features of chronic hepatitis C and autoimmune chronic hepatitis: a comparative analysis. Hepatology, 15, 572–577

13. Gerber, M. A., Krawczynski, K., Alter, H. J., Sampliner, R. E., Margolis, H. S. and Sentinel counties chronic non-A non-B hepatitis study team. (1992). Histopathology of community acquired chronic hepatitis C. Mod. Pathol., in press,

14. Wilkinson, S. P., Portmann, B., Cochrane, A. M. G., Tee, D. E. H. and Williams, R. (1978). Clinical course of chronic lobular hepatitis. Quart. J. Med., 47, 421–429

15. Liaw, Y.-F., Chu, C.-M., Chen, T.-J., Lin, D.-Y., Chang-Chien, C.-S. and Wu, C.-S. (1982). Chronic lobular hepatitis: a clinico-pathological and prognostic study. Hepatology, 2, 258–262

16. Popper, H., Paronetto, F. and Schaffner, F. (1965). Immune processes in the pathogenesis of liver disease. Ann. N. Y. Acad. Sci., 120, 781–799

17. Nagore, N., Howe, S., Boxer, L. and Scheuer, P. J. (1989). Liver cell rosettes: structural differences in cholestasis and hepatitis. Liver, 9, 43–51

18. Scheuer, P., J and Maggi, G. (1980). Hepatic fibrosis and collapse: histological distinction by orcein staining. Histopathology, 4, 487–490

19. Boyer, J. L. and Klatskin, G. (1970). Pattern of necrosis in acute viral hepatitis. Prognostic value of bridging (subacute hepatic necrosis). N. Engl. J. Med., 283, 1063–1071

20. Bianchi, L., De Groote, J., Desmet, V. J., Gedigk, P., Korb, G., Popper, H., Poulsen, H., Scheuer, P. J., Schmid, M., Thaler, H. and Wepler, W. (1977). Acute and chronic hepatitis revisited. Lancet, 2, 914–919

21. Summerskill, W. H. J. (1974). Chronic active liver disease re examined: prognosis hopeful. Gastroenterology, 66, 450–464

22. Shouval, D. (1970). Chronic active hepatitis with cholestatic features. II. A histopathological study. Am. J. Gastroenterol., 72, 551–555

23. Christoffersen, P., Dietrichson, O., Faber, V. and Poulsen, H. (1972). The occurrence and significance of abnormal bile duct epithelium in chronic aggressive hepatitis. Acta Pathol. Microbiol. Scand. [A], 80, 294–302

24. Christoffersen, P., Poulsen, H. and Scheuer, P., J. (1972). Abnormal bile duct epithelium in chronic aggressive hepatitis and primary biliary cirrhosis. Hum. Pathol., 3, 227–235

25. Poulsen, H. and Christoffersen, P. (1972). Abnormal bile duct epithelium in chronic aggressive hepatitis and cirrhosis. A review of morphology and clinical, biochemical and immunologic features. Hum. Pathol., 3, 217–225

26. Soloway, R. D., Baggenstoss, A. H., Schoenfield, L. J. and Summerskill, W. H. J. (1971). Observer error and sampling variability tested in evaluation of hepatitis and cirrhosis by liver biopsy. Am. J. Dig. Dis., 16, 1082–1086

27. Sylvan, S. P. E. (1991). Cellular immune response to hepatitis B virus antigens in man. Liver, 11, 1–23

28. Dejean, A. (1985). Specific hepatitis B virus integration in hepatocellular carcinoma DNA through a viral 11-base-pair direct repeat. Proc. Natl. Acad. Sci. USA, 81, 5350–5358

29. Gudat, F., Bianchi, L., Sonnabend, W., Thiel, G., Aenishaenslin, W. and Staider, G. A. (1975). Pattern of core and surface expression in liver tissue reflects state of specific immune response in hepatitis B. Lab. Invest., 32, 1–9.

30. Popper, H. (1975). The ground glass hepatocyte as a diagnostic hint. Hum. Pathol., 6, 517–520.

31. Thomsen, P., Poulsen, H. and Petersen, P. (1976). Different types of ground glass hepatocytes in human liver biopsies: morphology, occurrence and diagnostic significance. Scand. J. Gastroenterol., 11, 113–119

32. Hadziyannis, S., Gerber, M. R., Vissoulis, C. and Popper, H. (1973). Cytoplasmic hepatitis B antigen in 'ground–glass' hepatocytes of carriers. Arch. Pathol., 96, 327–330

33. Shikata, T., Uzawa, T., Yoshiwara, N., Akatsuka, T. and Yamazaki, S. (1974). Staining methods of Australia antigen in paraffin sections. Detection of cytoplasmic inclusion bodies. Jpn. J. Exp. Med., 44, 25–36

34. Gubetta, L., Rizzetto, M., Crivelli, O., Verme, G. and Arico, S. (1977). Trichrome stains for intrahepatic localization of hepatitis B surface antigen (HBsAg). Histopathology, 1, 277–288

35. Tanaka, K., Mori, W. and Suwa, K. (1981). Victoria blue nuclear fast red stain for HBs antigen detection in paraffin sections. Acta Pathol. Jpn., 31, 93–98

36. Clausen, P. P. and Thomsen, P. (1978). Demonstration of hepatitis B surface antigen in liver biopsies. Acta Pathol. Microbiol. Scand. A, 86, 383–388

37. Deodhar, K. P., Tapp, E. and Scheuer, P. J. (1975). Orcein staining of hepatitis B antigen in paraffin sections of liver biopsies. J. Clin. Pathol., 28, 66–70

38. Sumithran, E. (1977). Methods for the detection of HBsAg in paraffin sections of liver; a guideline for their use. J. Clin. Pathol., 30, 460–463

39. Shamoto, M., Nishio, H., Katoh, Y., Senba, H. and Ito, M. (1977). Selective staining of HBsAg in thick epoxy sections of liver. Stain Technol., 52, 285–289

40. Omata, M., Liew, G. T., Ashcavai, M. and Peters, R. L. (1980). Non immunologic binding of horseradish peroxidase to HBsAg. A possible source of error in immunohistochemistry. Am. J. Clin. Pathol., 73, 626–632

41. Dienes, H. P. (1989). Morphologic and pathogenetic aspects of cell damage in hepatitis with potential chronicity. Stuttgart: Gustav Fischer Verlag

42. van den Ord, J. J., de Vos, R., Facchetti, F., de Wolf-Peeters, C. and Desmet, V. J. (1990). Distribution of non-lymphoid, inflammatory cells in chronic HBV infection. J. Pathol., 160, 223–230

43. Nielsen, J. O., Dietrichson, O., Elling, P. and Christoffersen, P. (1971). Incidence and meaning of persistence of Australia antigen in patients with acute viral hepatitis development of chronic hepatitis. N. Engl. J. Med., 285, 1157–1160

44. Jacyna, M. R., Millward-Sadler, G. H. and Thomas, H. C. (1992). Chronic hepatitis. In Millward-Sadler, G. H., Wright, R. and Arthur, M. J. P. (eds). Wright's Liver and Biliary Disease. 3rd edn. pp. 787–820. London: W B Saunders

45. Sampliner, R. E. (1979). The liver histology and frequency of clearance of HBsAg in chronic carriers. Am. J. Med. Sci., 277, 17–22

46. Ray, M. B., Desmet, V. J., Fevery, J., De Groote, J., Bradburne, A. F. and Desmyter, J. (1976). Distribution patterns of HBsAg in the liver of hepatitis patients. J. Clin. Pathol., 29, 94–100

47. Leading article. (1972). Hepatitis hazard in regular haemodialysis. Br. Med. J., 4, 501

48. Davies, S. E., Portmann, B. C., O'Grady, J. G., Aldis, P. M., Chaggar, K., Alexander, G. J. and Williams, R. (1991). Hepatic histological findings after transplantation for chronic hepatitis B virus infection, including a unique pattern of fibrosing cholestatic hepatitis. Hepatology, 13, 150–7

49. Schrago, S. S., Auslander, M. O. and Gitnick, G. L. (1977). Hepatic pathologic condition in asymptomatic Australia antigen carriers. A light microscopical study of 26 cases and review of the literature. Arch. Pathol. Lab. Med., 101, 648–651

50. Koretz, R. L., Lewin, K. J., Rebhun, D. J. and Gitnick, G. L. (1978). HBsAg carriers to biopsy or not to biopsy. Gastroenterology, 75, 860–863

51. Piccinino, F., Sagnelli, E., Manzillo, G. and Pasquale, G. (1977). Liver histology in 34 HBsAg long term healthy carriers. Acta Hepato-Gastroenterol., 23, 148–154

52. Meyer zum Büschenfelde, K.-H. (1992). Autoimmune Hepatitis. Semin. Liver Dis., 11, No 3 (whole issue)

53. Poralla, T., Treichel, U., Löhr, H. and Fleischer, B. (1992). The asialoglycoprotein receptor as target structure in autoimmune liver diseases. Semin. Liver Dis., 11, 215–222

54. Czaja, A. J., Ludwig, J., Baggenstoss, A. H. and Wolf, A. (1981). Corticosteroid treated CAH in remission. Uncertain prognosis of CPH. N. Engl. J. Med., 304, 5–9

55. Molos, M. A., Litton, N. and Schubert, T. T. (1987). Talc liver. J. Clin. Gastroenterol., 9, 198–203

56. Goldberg, S. J., Mendenhall, C. L., Connell, A., M. and Chedid, A. (1977). 'Non-alcoholic' chronic hepatitis in the alcoholic. Gastroenterology, 72, 598–604

57. Wright, E. C., Seeff, L. B., Berk, P. D., Jones, A. and Plotz, P. H. (1977). Treatment of chronic active hepatitis. Analysis of three controlled trials. Gastroenterology, 73, 1422–1430

Neonatal and Structural Disease

Unconjugated bilirubinaemia is extremely common in the neonatal period and is usually physiological. However, unconjugated bilirubinaemia of any degree occurring in the first 24 hours of life is pathological. Haemolysis is probably the most common cause, and the others too are mostly non-hepatological, including conditions such as infection, hypoxia and hypoglycaemia. Galactosaemia and fructosaemia (Chapter 9) are rare treatable conditions which should always be sought (by the detection, initially, of non-glucose reducing substances in the urine).

Conjugated hyperbilirubinaemia, in contrast, is always pathological and can be broadly classified into those conditions having structural defects of the biliary tree (extrahepatic causes) and those showing hepatocellular damage (intrahepatic)[1]. Clinical and morphological evidence of cholestasis is found whatever the basic cause. It should be borne in mind, however, that bile plugs may be found in the liver of any sick baby in the first months of life. In addition to the changes of cholestasis and all the secondary phenomena described in Chapter 16, giant cell transformation of hepatocytes is a common finding.

GIANT CELL TRANSFORMATION

A variable number of liver cells are enlarged and contain anything from four or five up to 40 or more nuclei, often clustered together in one part of the cell (Figure 8.1). The cell cytoplasm is frequently abundant and often rarefied with granules of bilirubin and/or iron pigment. The cell borders are indistinct and the cell may become detached from its neighbours. Glycogen and cytoplasmic enzymes may be increased. These cells are found in any part of the acinus but are most often seen in the perivenular zone 3.

This change seems to be a response primarily of the neonatal liver and is thus rare after the age of 1 year. It may occur to some extent in any of the cholestatic syndromes and so of itself is of little diagnostic value. In particular the presence of giant cells does not distinguish between biliary atresia on the one hand and neonatal hepatitis on the other. 'Small giant' cells are sometimes found in older children and adults[2], usually in association with cholestasis but also a variety of other conditions (Figure 8.2). The pathogenesis is unclear although it has been claimed that some at least may be a manifestation of paramyxovirus infection[3].

EXTRAHEPATIC AND STRUCTURAL DISEASE
Biliary Atresia

Biliary atresia is the most common of the extrahepatic malformations and is present in about 50% of infants with prolonged cholestasis, accounting in all for some 1:8000 live births. The condition is defined as complete obstruction of bile flow due to obliteration of part or all of the extrahepatic biliary tree. The whole extrahepatic biliary tree may be abnormal or there may merely be segmental involvement, which is maximal at the junction of the cystic and hepatic ducts[2]. The gallbladder may be normal or small or absent.

Serial sections of the biliary remnants reveal three basic patterns[4-6], consisting of: (a) a cord of concentrically arranged connective tissue with no epithelial components (Type 1); (b) connective tissue with glands only (Type 2); or (c) connective tissue with a central duct and peripheral gland remnants (Type 3). There are two basic corrective operations. If there is a residual bile duct at the porta hepatis (and bile is visible in its lumen)[7] the duct can be anastomosed to a Roux loop of jejunum. If there is no extrahepatic bile duct (often called 'uncorrectable' atresia, which encompasses about 80–95% of all cases[8]) hepato–portoenterostomy or Kasai's operation is employed. Here the biliary tree remnant is excised intact and a Roux loop of jejunum is brought up to the porta hepatis. Provided the operation is performed within 60 days of birth, bile drainage can be established in up to 90% with a 5-year survival of 40% many of whom are alive and well[9] at up to 24 years. Bouts of ascending cholangitis and portal hypertension are the main complications in survivors. Without operation, the development of biliary cirrhosis is inevitable and usually appears within 1–6 months; most patients dying by the age of 3 years (Figure 8.6), or becoming candidates for liver transplantation[10]. It should be stressed that the single most important determinant for successful outcome after Kasai's procedure is the time at which the operation is performed[11] – 86% of infants treated before eight weeks became jaundice-free, whilst only 41% of those operated on between eight and twelve weeks did so. Accurate early diagnosis is thus vital.

Clearly it is vital to distinguish between biliary atresia and the various forms of hepatocellular damage (see below) which may be accompanied by reduced bile secretion and often a narrowed but still patent biliary tree (perhaps due to a process of 'disuse atrophy')[12].

The main diagnostic tools are biopsy[13], radioisotope scan using a ^{99m}Tc tagged derivative of iminodiacetic acid to test for bile duct patency, cholangiography and ultrasound, perhaps combined with laparoscopy[14]. Each of these investigations on its own may be misleading but taken together the error rate is very low[12]. Some authors feel that surgical exploration and open biopsy are always indicated[15], whilst others are equally convinced that unnecessary surgery should always be avoided where possible[13] and indeed, can be misleading in as many as 20% of cases[12]. Thus each case should probably be managed on its own merits.

Histological findings

The histological changes are profoundly influenced by the age of the patient. The *earliest stage*, from about one to four weeks, is characterized by non-specific features of canalicular cholestasis with occasional degenerate hepatocytes. Giant cell transformation is often present but not marked at this stage, and the changes overall are not diagnostic. In the *second stage*, from about four to seven weeks, the portal tract changes come to acquire the typical characteristics of large bile duct obstruction (Chapter 16). Typically, there is rounding and oedema of the portal tract with marginal ductular proliferation (Figure 8.3). Special stains, such as trichrome, may demonstrate bile duct proliferation beautifully, but the extent can easily be exaggerated and thus over emphasized[13]. Equally important from a diagnostic point of view are degenerative changes in portal bile ducts[16]. These show inflammation and degenerative changes comparable to those seen in the extra-hepatic duct remnants, and thus indicate a similar process in the intrahepatic ducts. Alagille[15] performed a discriminant analysis of 21 clinical, biochemical and histological features, and whilst confirming the importance of bile duct proliferation found that various clinical features, such as stool colour and birth-weight ranked next in importance. Babies with large duct obstruction are more likely to have completely acholuric stools at an earlier age but are less likely to have a low birth weight than babies with hepatocellular disease. Portal fibrosis and bile thrombi within portal tract ductules were also more common in atresia. With these combined features he claimed an accuracy of diagnosis of 85%.

Bile thrombi are at first centrilobular but eventually become periportal (Figure 8.4) and, by about 3 months, more chronic features such as bile lakes may be seen. With the passage of time, portal tracts expand and show progressive fibrosis and loss of bile ducts, leading to the inevitable development of a large green, ultimately nodular, liver (Figures 8.5 and 8.6)[17]. By this stage the inflammatory infiltration tends to recede, as the number of interlobular bile ducts also declines in most but not all cases. Surviving ducts may show periductal fibrosis, irregular narrowing of the lumen and atrophy of the lining epithelium.

In about 20% of cases, there is some overlap of appearances with congenital hepatic fibrosis[18] (see below). This was well-described by Brough & Bernstein, although not recognized as such[13]. They found elongated and tortuous proliferating interlobular ducts which appeared to have many interconnections in the plane of section (Figure 8.7), apparently representing flattened cisterns. It is clear that the authors were describing what is now considered to be a ductal plate malformation. It has been postulated that these changes represent a dysplasia or developmental abnormality of the portal tracts in response to early severe extra-hepatic obstruction which began in utero[16]. The long-term fate of this subgroup is very similar to that of the majority of cases.

Pathogenesis of atresia

Tthe distinction between extrahepatic biliary atresia and intrahepatic disorders (see below) is not always clearcut and this has led a number of authors to postulate a common aetiology under the generic term 'infantile obstructive cholangiopathy'[19].

Apart from the giant cell transformation, which is most unusual in cholestasis from other causes[20], the other changes already described, namely abnormalities of the bile duct epithelium (both degenerative and proliferative) and inflammatory changes, are seen not only in portal tracts but also in the extrahepatic bile duct remnants[21].

These suggest a continuing process which persists even after surgical correction[22] and, together with the irregular distribution of bile duct remnants, argue in favour of an obliterative inflammation rather than a true atresia. This, too, would be in accord with the observation that most infants with atresia are born with bile-stained meconium.

The underlying cause of the inflammatory process remains unknown, but the possibilities include infection, ischaemia or toxic injury. Organisms under suspicion include hepatitis B and non-A, non-B, cytomegalovirus, rubella and reoviruses, but none is yet proved to have a role[23]. The evidence in favour of toxic injury is no better[16]. Vascular insufficiency during development of the biliary tree is the most popular current explanation and this also has a certain amount of experimental support[21]. Genetic defects, such as trisomy 18 and α_1 antitrypsin deficiency

(see below) may also cause a similar picture. The majority of cases, however, have no known predisposing cause.

Non-parasitic hepatic cysts

Various classifications have been used, but the most logical is that shown in Table 8.1[24].

Table 8.1 Classification of non-parasitic hepatic cysts†

Solitary

Polycystic

Non-communicating

   Adult polycystic disease

Communicating with ductal plate malformation (DPM)

   Congenital hepatic fibrosis
   Infantile polycystic disease
   Malformation syndromes
   Congenital hepatic fibrosis–nephronophthisis

Communicating without DPM

   Caroli's disease

Systemic biliary dilatation

   With/without choledochal cyst

Others

† After Witzelben, C. L. (1990). Cystic disease of the liver. In Zakim, D. and Boyer, T. D. (eds). *Hepatology. A Textbook of Liver Disease*. 3rd edition. pp. 1395–1411. Philadelphia: W B Saunders

Solitary cyst

Solitary cysts of the liver are an incidental finding at post-mortem in less than 1% of autopsies[25], although they are now recognized more frequently in life with the widespread use of ultrasound[24]. 'Solitary' cysts may sometimes be multiple, in which case it is necessary to look for evidence of cysts in other organs, to exclude the possibility that the patient belongs to one of the genetic groups. They usually cause no symptoms and have no significance. Occasionally a large cyst may give rise to pressure problems or it may perforate or bleed.

Polycystic disease

Only the polycystic diseases are heritable, multiple and have manifestations in other organs often including the kidney. There are three principal subgroups (Table 8.1) – non-communicating cysts, of which adult polycystic disease is the main example; communicating cysts with various malformations of the ductal plate; and Caroli's syndrome.

Adult polycystic disease

This syndrome is inherited as an autosomal dominant. About one-third of patients with adult polycystic renal disease also have one or more cysts of the liver[26], whereas about half of all patients with polycystic disease of the liver also have polycystic disease of the kidneys. The liver condition usually causes no significant liver dysfunction and, as in infantile polycystic disease, the ultimate course is determined largely by the renal lesion when present. About 5% of patients have cysts in other organs such as pancreas, spleen and the internal genitalia. There is also an increased prevalence of berry aneurysms in the subarachnoid arteries[24]. Although this group of patients is usually distinct from the next, occasionally there is evidence of ductal plate malformation coexisting with the typical non-communicating cysts[27].

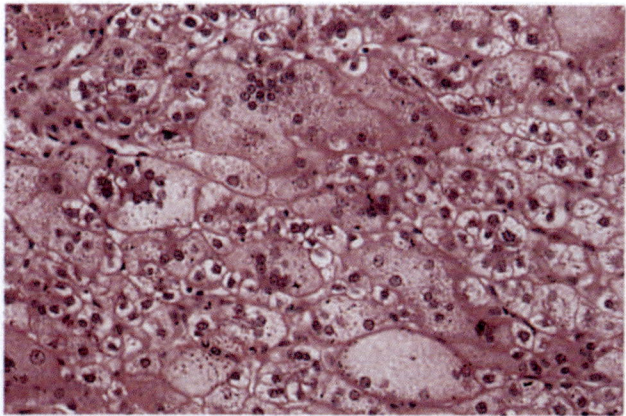

Figure 8.1 Giant cell hepatitis, which was found for the first time at autopsy on a 1-day-old full-term infant who was not jaundiced. The biliary tree was patent and no cause could be found. Note the great variation in liver cell size with some forming large syncytia with multiple nuclei. No cholestasis is visible in this instance.

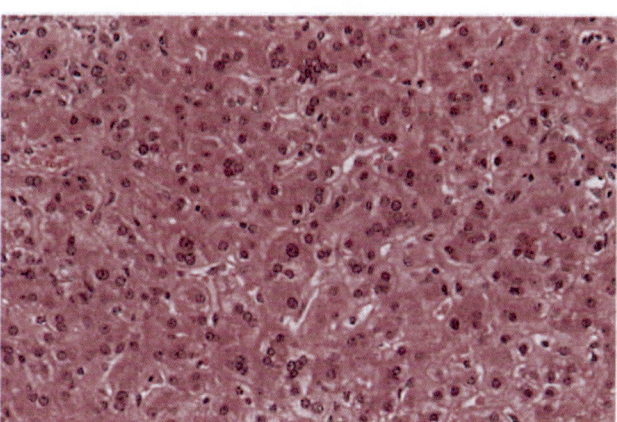

Figure 8.2 Giant cell transformation attributed to erythromycin estolate. A 54-year old female patient developed cholestatic jaundice which was related to treatment with this drug and rapidly cleared on its withdrawal. Biopsy shows cholestasis and numerous hepatocytes containing up to ten nuclei.

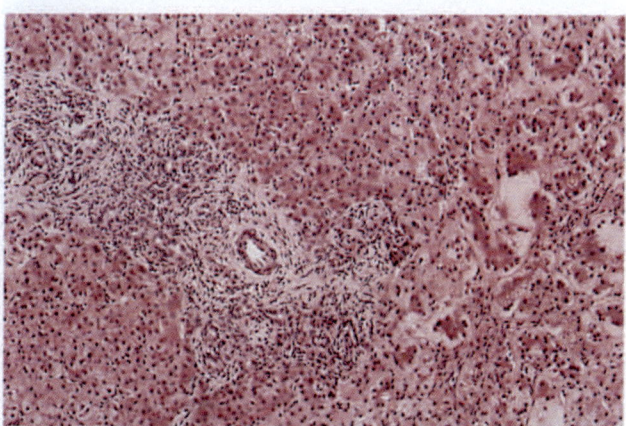

Figure 8.3 Biliary atresia. An 11-week-old infant with progressive obstructive jaundice. Biopsy shows expansion of portal tracts with some marginal bile duct proliferation, and patchy giant cell transformation.

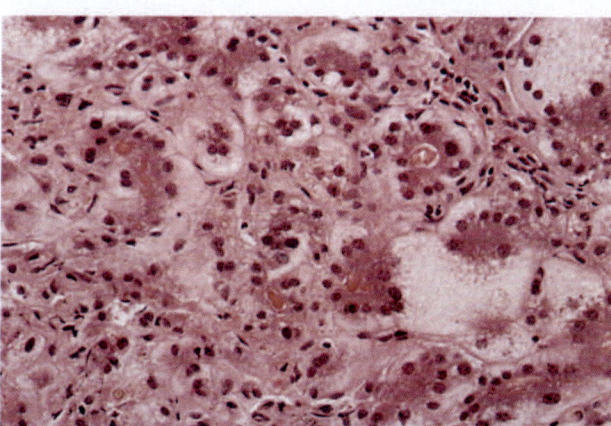

Figure 8.4 Biliary atresia. Same case as Figure 8.3. Striking giant cell transformation which is also associated with prominent cholestasis. Note that several of the distended bile canaliculi appear to be in the centre of giant cells.

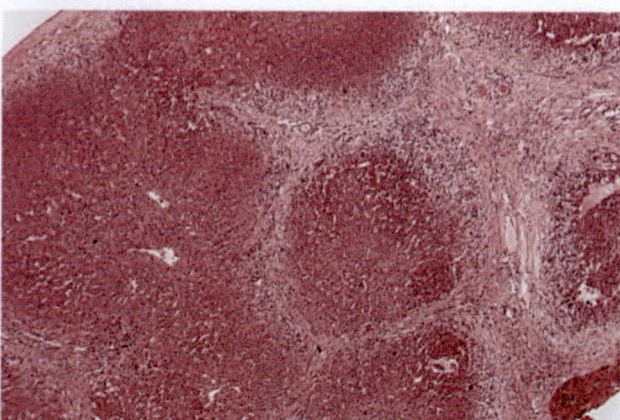

Figure 8.5 Biliary atresia. A 6-month-old infant with progressive jaundice. Biopsy shows developing biliary cirrhosis with linkage of expanded portal tracts, but, as yet, preservation of architecture within the parenchyma.

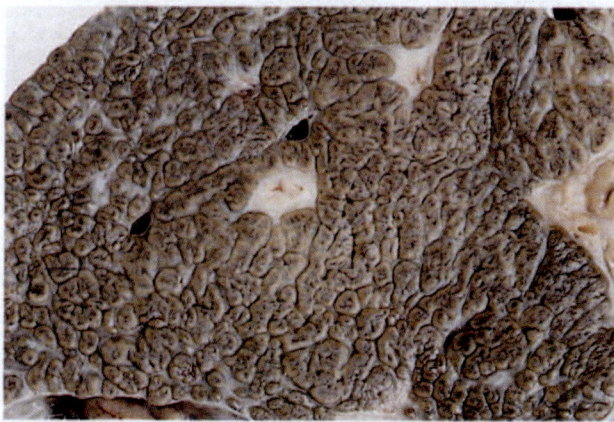

Figure 8.6 Biliary atresia. Macroscopic view of established biliary cirrhosis in which the nodules are outlined by a pale rim, which corresponds to the zone of oedematous connective tissue seen microscopically in all advanced biliary cirrhosis (see Chapter 16).

Patients with clinical liver involvement most often present in the fifth or sixth decade with hepatic enlargement. The cysts may be very numerous, ranging in size from the barely visible to 10 or more centimetres in diameter (Figure 8.8). Occasionally the liver may reach weights as great as 15 kilograms, necessitating treatment by liver transplantation[10]. Microscopically the cysts have a flattened epithelial lining and there is little supporting connective tissue. Some portal areas may contain typical bile duct hamartomas or von Meyenburg complexes[27] (Chapter 22), considered to be the precursor lesion in adult polycystic disease; others are entirely normal (Figure 8.9).

Ductal plate development

During early development the intrahepatic bile ducts arise by a process of transformation of liver cell plates[28]. In embryos of 20–30 mm size, the hepatocytes adjacent to the mesenchyme surrounding the branches of the portal vein take on the cytokeratin profile of biliary epithelium[29]. A second layer is then formed followed by a lumen, so that the portal tract connective tissue becomes encased by a tubular structure, the ductal plate. Subsequently the plate is invaded by connective tissue and as a result of progressive remodelling an anastomosing system of bile ducts links parenchymal canaliculi with the extrahepatic bile ducts.

Communicating polycystic disease with ductal plate malformation

In this group of conditions, which are inherited as autosomal recessive conditions, the development of the ductal plate becomes arrested. As well as being related, the conditions show some clinical and pathological overlap with one another[29]. The overlap between some case of extrahepatic biliary atresia and congenital hepatic fibrosis has already been mentioned.

Infantile polycystic disease

Although this has been subdivided into a number of different categories, all are regularly associated with liver abnormalities, and there is good morphometric evidence[30] that the perinatal, neonatal and infantile types are all one disease. The liver may be normal macroscopically or slightly enlarged, but all the portal tracts are always abnormal microscopically (Figure 8.10). The biliary channels are more or less dilated, and are increased in number, often in the form of a more or less confluent channel around the periphery of the portal tract–persistence of the ductal plate. (Figure 8.11) They show extensive branching and anastomosis, often with papillary projections into the lumen[31]. These are lined by columnar or cuboidal epithelium and often extend into the parenchyma where the bile duct epithelium may lie in direct contact with liver cell plates (Figure 8.12). The amount of connective tissue accompanying these biliary cisterns is very variable. When abundant, the appearances merge with those of congenital hepatic fibrosis (q.v.). The prognosis in childhood polycystic disease is uniformly poor and determined entirely by the renal changes (dilatation of collecting tubules).

Liver cysts may also be encountered in a number of other quite well-defined clinical syndromes, such as Meckel-Gruber syndrome[31], Jeune's syndrome and tuberose sclerosis[30], although in the liver the appearances are not diagnostic.

Congenital hepatic fibrosis

This syndrome is sporadic or inherited as an autosomal recessive characteristic[32] and as stated above it tends to merge and overlap with infantile polycystic disease and with Caroli's disease[33]. Different members of a single family may even show different degrees of involvement of the liver and kidney. In its pure form it tends to present in childhood as an enlarged liver or in adolescence or adult life with established portal hypertension. The liver is enlarged and firm, and on section the portal tracts stand out as anastomosing fibrous bands of variable thickness. Microscopically numerous irregular small bile ducts are scattered evenly through the fibrous septa (Figure 8.13), but careful search often reveals typical ductal plate malformations[34]. The lumina often contain concretions of bile, and microcysts are quite common (Figure 8.14). The presence of larger cysts, especially if accompanied by significant inflammation attributable to cholangitis, should prompt a search for one of the varieties of Caroli's syndrome. The fibrous bands may surround one or more islands of liver parenchyma which for a long time preserve their normal architecture with normal efferent veins (Figure 8.13). Eventually, portal hypertension is inevitable, possibly because of compression of intrahepatic branches of the portal vein[35] Even when advanced, the changes remain characteristic; in no other condition is there such a regular arrangement of bile ducts with a significant lumen in fibrous tissue septa. Treatment by porto-caval anastomosis may produce significant benefit[32]. Cystic disease of the kidney is found in about half of all patients, but is much more common in familial than sporadic cases. Both cystic disease and congenital hepatic fibrosis have a small increased risk of bile duct carcinoma (Chapter 24).

Caroli's syndrome[36]

The malformation, which is four times as common in females, may affect any part of the intra- or extra-hepatic biliary tree. In contrast to biliary atresia and choledochal cyst, it does not usually draw attention to itself until adult life, when cholangitis (Fig 8.15) is the most common presenting symptom. Younger patients are more likely to present with pain, jaundice and hepatic enlargement in any combination.

The cysts range up to 5 cm in diameter and can be separated by completely normal intervening duct. They often contain soft bilirubin calculi[37]. Caroli describes two types, both of which may be seen in the same family[38]. The first and rarer type consists solely of dilatations of the biliary tree with no accompanying sclerosis (Figure 8.16). This has a relatively favourable prognosis with stasis and infection being the main complications. The second type shows marked portal fibrosis imparting a cirrhotic texture to the liver and is associated with the development of portal hypertension (Figure 8.17). It is this second category which may show some overlap with congenital hepatic fibrosis.

Biopsy in Caroli's syndrome may merely show secondary changes, particularly those of biliary obstruction with the diagnosis being made by other means, such as cholangiography, isotope or CT scan. Because of the frequent occurrence of ascending infection, inflammatory changes within portal tracts are also common (Figure 8.15). The cysts are lined by columnar or cuboidal epithelium which is often ulcerated. In type two, as well as abundant portal fibrosis, there are often collections of numerous dilated bile ductules giving almost an angiomatous appearance.

Apart from infection, other complications include stone formation, perforations, pancreatitis and secondary biliary cirrhosis. There also appears to be a small risk of bile duct carcinoma (Figure 8.18). Surgical treatment can greatly

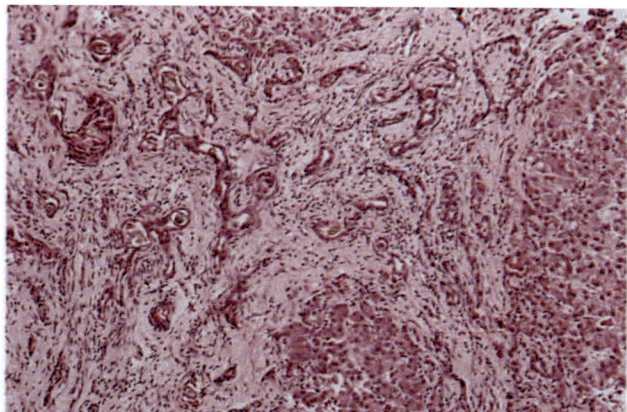

Figure 8.7 Biliary atresia. A 3-month-old infant with progressive jaundice. Biopsy shows expanded portal tracts with striking bile duct proliferation. Note that many of the ducts are cut longitudinally and many contain concretions of bile within their lumina.

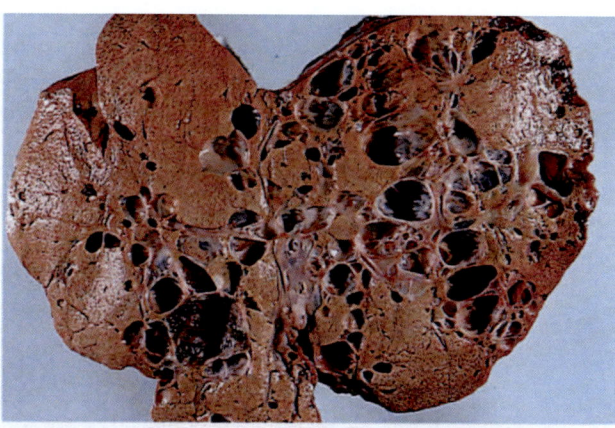

Figure 8.8 Adult polycystic renal disease. This patient presented in her fifth decade with massive hepatomegaly followed by chronic renal failure of which she died aged 49. At autopsy, the liver was massively enlarged (weight 6500 g) with many cysts measuring up to 10 cm in diameter.

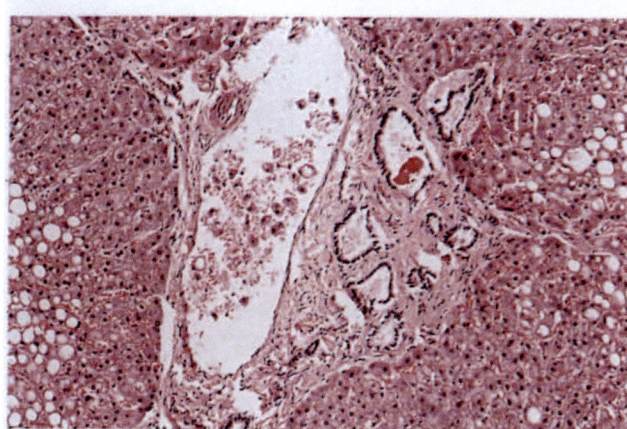

Figure 8.9 Adult polycystic renal disease. Post-mortem section of the more usual liver lesion associated with this condition. Many portal tracts were normal, others contained a group of dilated bile ducts each lined by a single layer of cuboidal epithelium and often containing biliary casts. Note the close resemblance to a von Meyenburg complex.

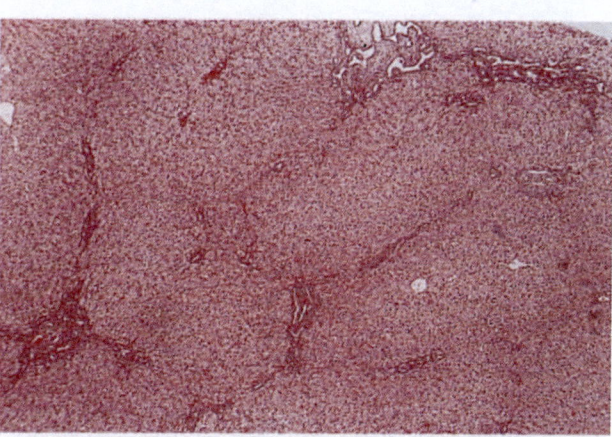

Figure 8.10 Infantile polycystic renal disease. A 3-month-old child with bilateral cystic kidneys. Liver biopsy shows that every portal tract is abnormal and they are tending to link up with one another. Note the general similarity with congenital hepatic fibrosis (Figure 8.13) and Caroli's syndrome (Figure 8.17).

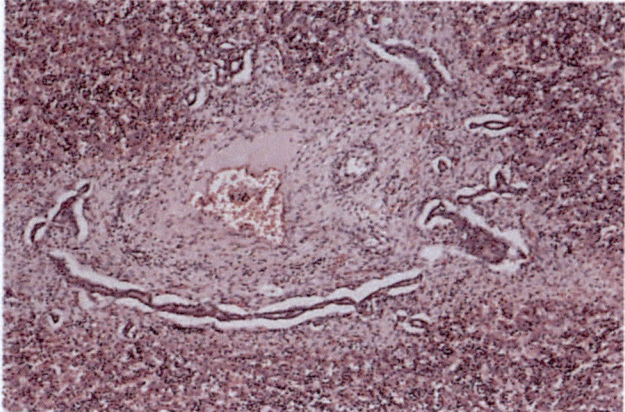

Figure 8.11 Ductal plate malformation in an eighteen–week fetus with infantile polycystic renal disease. Note the circular profile of the bile duct which surrounds the portal tract.

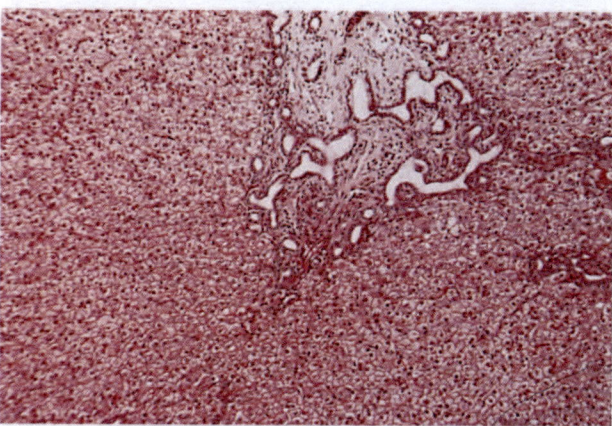

Figure 8.12 Infantile polycystic renal disease. Same case as Figure 8.10. Portal tract showing the typical intercommunicating bile ducts. Note that there is little increase in connective tissue in this case. One or two bile ducts completely devoid of connective tissue can be seen embedded in the parenchyma below the portal tract.

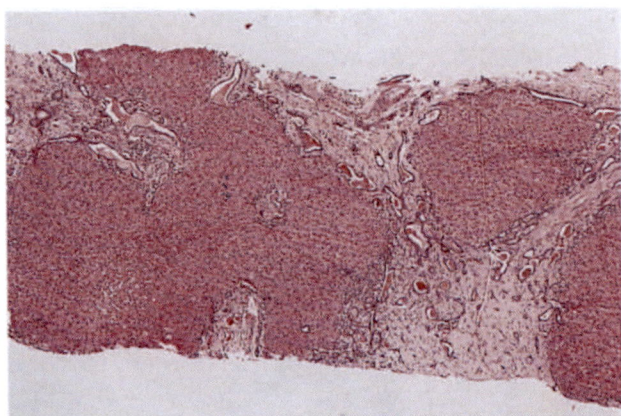

Figure 8.13 Congenital hepatic fibrosis. This 10-year-old child presented with hepatosplenomegaly. Investigations revealed portal hypertension with oesophageal varices. Liver biopsy shows the very characteristic picture of broad bands of fibrous tissue intercommunicating with one another, but surrounding liver parenchyma which has retained its normal architecture.

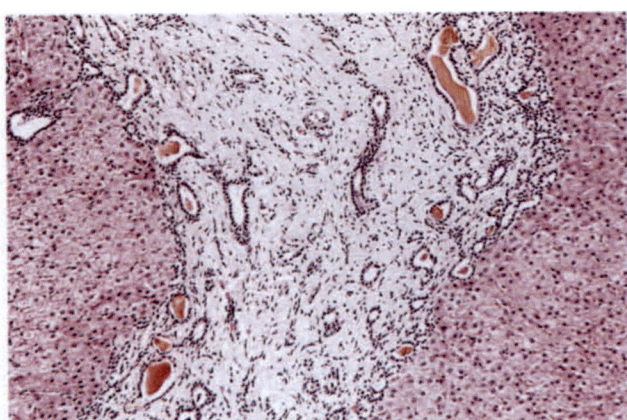

Figure 8.14 Congenital hepatic fibrosis. Same case as Figure 8.13. Higher magnification shows the proliferating bile ductules within the portal connective tissue. Many contain concretions of yellow bile pigment.

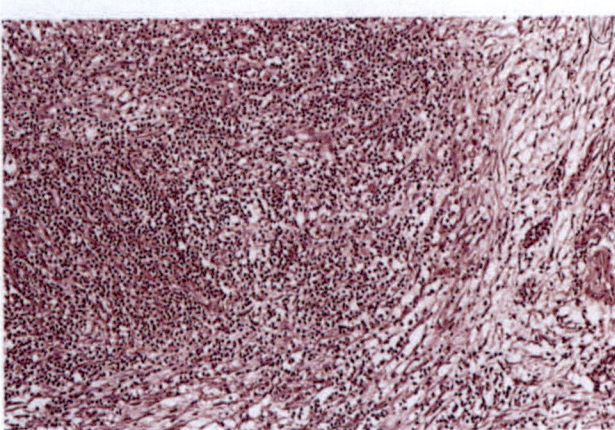

Figure 8.15 Caroli's syndrome, with cholangitis showing an abscess centred upon a portal tract. Coliform organisms were cultured from the blood at the time of the biopsy.

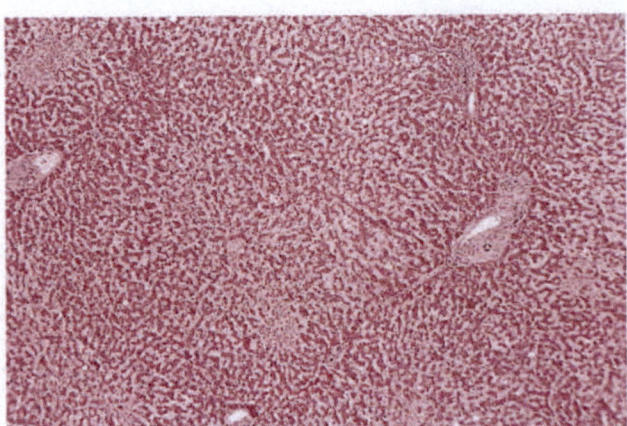

Figure 8.16 Caroli's syndrome (type 1). This section shows an entirely normal liver, with unremarkable portal tracts, thus random biopsy cannot be relied upon to detect this condition.

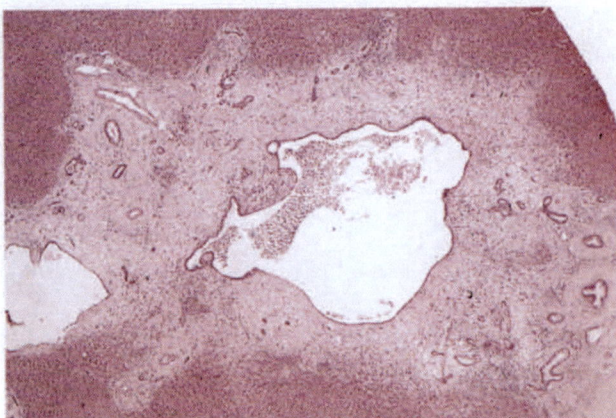

Figure 8.17 Caroli's syndrome (type 2). A 57-year-old male presented with pyrexia. Investigations revealed classic cystic dilatation of the biliary tree. Biopsy showed that most portal tracts contained abnormal bile ducts. Note the central dilated bile duct surrounded by oedematous connective tissue containing ductules.

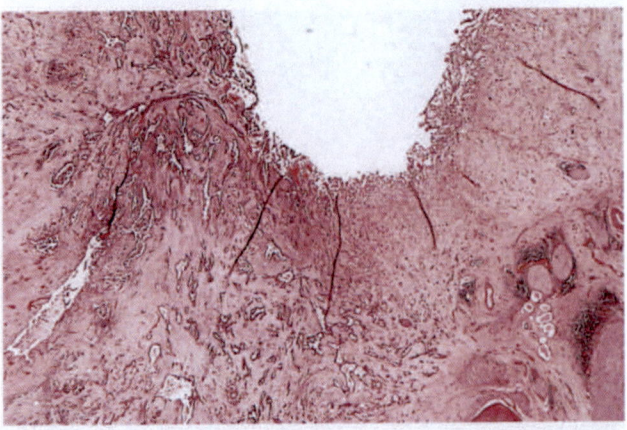

Figure 8.18 Caroli's syndrome (type 1) with cholangiocarcinoma. A 57-year-old female who died of pulmonary embolism. Multiple dilatations of the biliary tree discovered for the first time at autopsy. One of these was the seat of a cholangiocarcinoma. The dilated duct has lost its epithelial lining and well differentiated tubular adenocarcinoma can be seen infiltrating its wall.

reduce the mortality and morbidity. Both types of Caroli's syndrome are probably inherited as autosomal recessive conditions and are frequently associated with infantile medullary sponge kidney.

Choledochal cyst

Choledochal cyst, where the common bile duct is replaced by an often very large cystic space devoid of epithelial lining, may present with the same clinical and biopsy findings as atresia[39], although they can present at any age. When the cyst is large, however, it is readily palpable at the lower edge of the liver. This is not a heritable condition, although it may be associated with dilatations of the intrahepatic biliary tree[40]. The pathogenesis is not known[24], but it may have an obstructive basis.

INTRAHEPATIC AND HEPATITIC DISEASE
Paucity of intrahepatic bile ducts

There is considerable debate as to whether this is a homogeneous group and whether it is a developmental or acquired condition[41]. Alagille[15] found evidence of two distinct subgroups. One was familial, probably autosomal dominant with incomplete penetrance, and associated with other developmental anomalies, such as a characteristic facies, vertebral arch defects and cardiac murmurs (often now termed *Alagille's syndrome*, or less commonly syndromatic hepatic ductular hypoplasia or arteriohepatic dysplasia)[42]. The other was sporadic, occurring in infants of low birth weight and associated with α_1-anti-trypsin deficiency or viral infection in a proportion of cases.

Instead of the normal ratio of approximately one bile duct to one portal tract (range 0.9–1.8), this is reduced to 0–0.4 (Figure 8.19). The portal tracts themselves may be reduced in number[43] but otherwise they show little abnormality. In particular, fibrosis is not significant and even when present tends not to progress. There may or may not be parenchymal evidence of hepatitis with giant cells or of cholestasis and secondary changes. The latter may be more prominent in the first year of life.

Both groups are associated with severe pruritis which is relieved by cholestyramine. The ultimate prognosis of the liver disease is in general quite favourable with complete resolution in a proportion of cases[44].

Without loss of intrahepatic ducts
Inspissated bile syndrome

This is a cholestatic syndrome which typically presents with prolonged jaundice in the neonatal period[45]. It is particularly associated with haemolytic syndromes, for example in rhesus incompatibility (Figure 8.20). Histologically there is centrilobular cholestasis, often with no other changes. A similar picture may be seen following total parenteral nutrition[46].

Neonatal hepatitis (giant cell hepatitis)

Neonatal hepatitis forms a heterogeneous group which includes a number of metabolic disorders, including α_1-antitrypsin deficiency (see below), galactosaemia and cystic fibrosis; a range of viral infections, including hepatitis B rubella, cytomegalovirus, herpes simplex, varicella, coxsackie and echo viruses; and a substantial group where no cause is found[18]. Whatever the cause, the picture appears to be essentially one of cholestasis with hepatitis. Giant cell transformation is usual and may be marked (Figure 8.21). There may also be ballooning degeneration, acidophil bodies, persistent extramedullary haemopoiesis and portal inflammation and fibrosis. In the majority of cases, no firm viral aetiology is obtained and the condition must simply be labelled giant cell hepatitis

by default. It is obviously important to differentiate neonatal hepatitis from biliary atresia, where early surgery may be indicated. The prognosis seems to be variable. Where no underlying cause is established, as many as 60% of children may recover[47], although the outlook is much worse if the condition is familial[14].

Inborn errors of metabolism
α_1-Anti-trypsin deficiency

This is the commonest of the metabolic disorders of the liver and has an approximate incidence of 1:1500 live births[48]. α_1-Anti-trypsin (α_1AT) is the major protease inhibitor in normal serum and there are a number of different phenotypes. That associated with liver disease has been called PiZZ, in which the serum levels are only about 15% of normal.

The possession of this phenotype alone does not appear to determine the outcome in an individual patient. Some patients present in the neonatal period with cholestatic liver disease, others in late childhood or adolescence with established cirrhosis, whilst others seek medical attention in young adult life with premature and severe chronic bronchitis or emphysema. This last group, too, may or may not have cirrhosis of the liver.

The livers of all these patients show characteristic changes. Variable numbers of liver cells contain inclusion bodies which stain a vivid magenta colour with PAS after diastase digestion (Figure 8.22). The inclusions are globular and range in size from 1 to 40 μm. Individual cells may contain variable numbers (in the range 1–20) and they are found most often in periportal hepatocytes or at the periphery of nodules in established cirrhosis. Some authors[49] have had difficulty in detecting inclusions before 3 months of age, whilst others have found them to be present as early as 1 month. Numerous studies have shown that they are antigenically identical with α_1AT (Figure 8.23)[50]. Ultrastructurally the material accumulates in distended endoplasmic reticulum, maximally adjacent to the Golgi apparatus.

Neonatal jaundice occurs in about 10% of patients with the PiZZ phenotype[48] and, according to one retrospective survey of the literature[51], accounts for up to 40% of all cases of neonatal hepatitis. It is cholestatic in type and usually appears within a few weeks of birth. It may persist for many weeks but usually clears spontaneously by about 8 months. There is often an accompanying elevation of serum enzymes. Histologically there is cholestasis with a variable degree of giant cell hepatitis and other secondary changes, such as ballooning degeneration and acidophil bodies[49,52]. The characteristic inclusions are difficult to see in routine H&E preparations but should always be readily visible with the PAS stain. A proportion of these children will show paucity of intrahepatic bile ducts (see above), others bile duct proliferation[53]. A chronic active hepatitis-like histological picture is also sometimes seen[54] (Chapter 7).

After an asymptomatic interval there may be a recurrence of liver disease in late childhood due to the development of cirrhosis, which ultimately proves fatal[55]. About 10% of homozygotes may present for the first time as adults with fully developed cirrhosis (Figure 8.24)[56]. The cirrhosis may be macro- or micronodular and microscopically contains the characteristic inclusion bodies. Occasionally periportal cells contain Mallory's hyalin and orcein stains for copper protein are often positive (Chapter 15). There also appears in this group to be an increased risk of primary hepatic carcinoma[56]. The same PAS-positive inclusions are found in the tumour cells of between 10 and 50% of all cases of hepatocellular carcinoma[57], and rather less often in the non-tumorous liver[58].

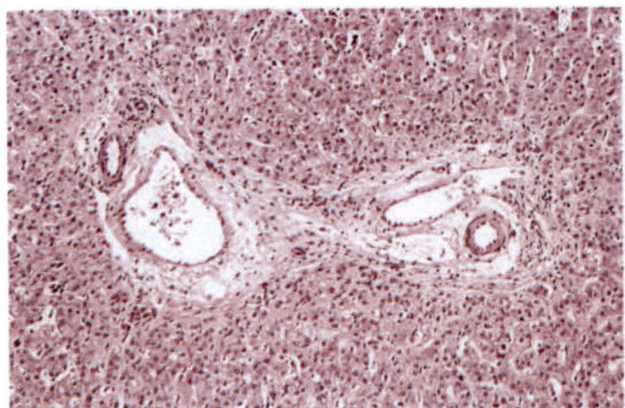

Figure 8.19 Alagille's syndrome (syndromatic paucity of intrahepatic bile ducts). The biopsy from a four-year-old child who also had congenital heart disease shows a complete absence of bile ducts.

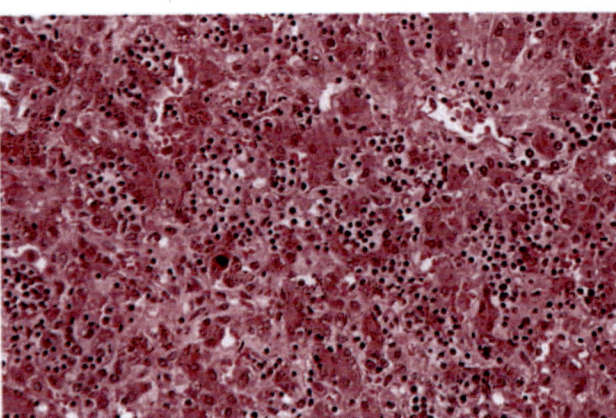

Figure 8.20 Inspissated bile syndrome, haemolytic disease of the new-born. An infant with rhesus incompatibility born at 34 weeks of gestation remained jaundiced despite several exchange transfusions. Died of respiratory disease. Post-mortem liver shows prominent extra-medullary haemopoiesis and a number of large bile plugs.

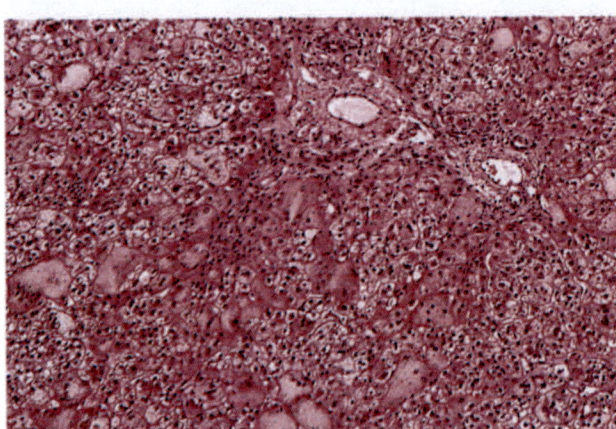

Figure 8.21 Giant cell hepatitis. A 6-week-old infant with a hepatic syndrome and normal biliary tree. No virus was isolated. Biopsy shows striking giant cell transformation of the parenchyma with occasional foci of extramedullary haemopoiesis (top right). No cholestasis. Portal tracts are normal with normal numbers of bile ducts.

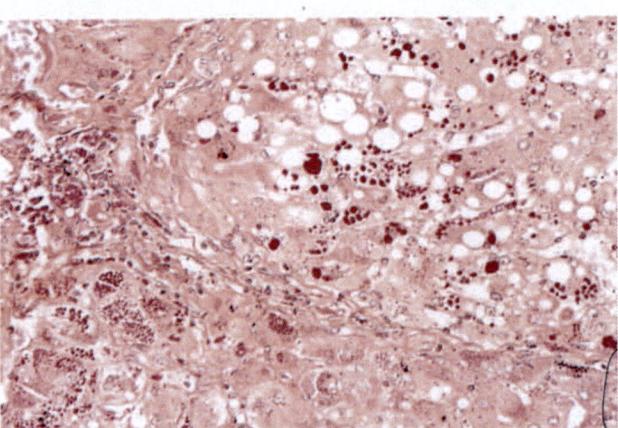

Figure 8.22 α_1-Anti-trypsin deficiency. An advanced case at post-mortem showing the magenta-coloured globules of α_1-anti-trypsin of varying size and most numerous in the periportal liver cells. PAS diastase.

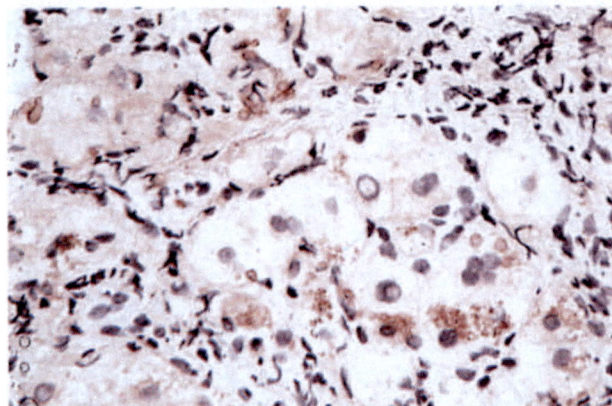

Figure 8.23 α_1-Anti-trypsin deficiency. Another advanced case (male of 15 years with established cirrhosis) showing that the globules are indeed composed of α_1-anti-trypsin. Note that in the larger globules the brown staining is denser around the periphery. Specific immuno-peroxidasemethod.

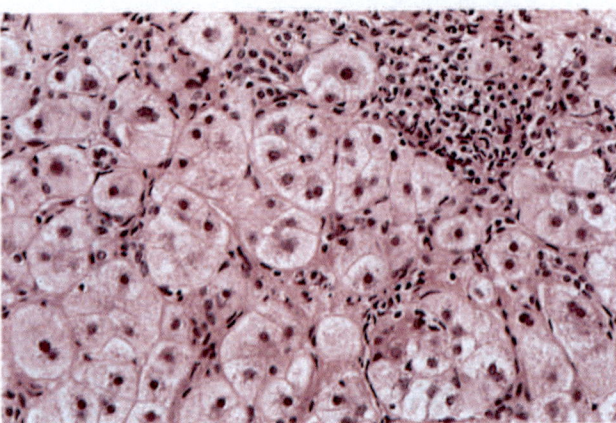

Figure 8.24 α_1-Anti-trypsin deficiency, chronic active hepatitis. A 40-year-old female who presented with hepatosplenomegaly. Liver biopsy shows an aggressive hepatitis with piecemeal necrosis, indistinguishable in this section from idiopathic CAH. However, PAS staining revealed numerous PAS-positive globules and she was subsequently shown to be a homozygote.

The prognosis of neonatal cholestasis due to α_1AT deficiency is not as grave as was once suspected[59]. In particular, the patients with hepatocellular damage may have a relatively better outcome[53] as compared with those in whom portal fibrosis and bile duct proliferation are marked. It is, however, difficult or impossible to predict future progress in any individual patient.

PAS-positive inclusions have been found in cirrhotic livers of patients who are heterozygotes (PiMZ), an association regarded as fortuitous by some[60] but significant by others[61], since in a large series of consecutive biopsies there was a close link between α_1AT globules and fibrosis and micronodular cirrhosis. More puzzling is their occasional presence in livers of normal people (PiMM)[62] and in alcoholic cirrhosis[63], and thus, although their presence is usually an indication of the PiZZ phenotype, this is not invariably the case. Similarly, not all PAS-positive globules are composed of α_1AT[64]. Immunoglobulin G, for example, may have a superficially similar appearance and thus, where appropriate, a specific technique should be used to confirm α_1AT. α_1AT globules are frequently accompanied by orcein positive granules, particularly when there is also cirrhosis[65], and, indeed, the latter may even be themselves faintly positive.

Pathogenesis of α_1AT deficiency Whilst the pathogenesis of emphysema is easily explicable on the basis of diminished availability of antiproteases in the lung to combat proteases liberated by neutrophils[66], the explanations for the development of liver disease and its very varied manifestations have been far from satisfactory. However, as a first step, the mechanism of accumulation of α_1AT within the endoplasmic reticulum is now clearer[67]. The abnormal PiZ protein has an amino acid substitution at position 342, which is important in the normal PiM protein as a hinge region. The mutation results in polymerization of molecules to form long chains which cannot be exported from the cell. Since this is an equilibrium process, some 15% remains monomeric and can be exported normally. Polymerization is temperature dependent, occurring at a greater rate at 41°C than at 37°C. Furthermore, since α_1AT is an acute phase reactant, synthesis is greatly increased at times of stress, and thus the variability of clinical expression might be a function of the number of episodes of intercurrent infection, and thus fevers, sustained by the individual patient. The mechanism whereby the accumulated protein damages the liver is much less clear[55], although it seems likely that it is due to the accumulated protein rather than the lack of antiprotease activity in the serum[68].

Other inborn errors of metabolism

Other inborn errors which might present in the neonatal period or be associated with cholestasis are much less common[69]. Byler's disease is a rare familial recessive condition, sometimes called 'malignant', characterized by the early onset of a progressive cholestasis[15]. Fibrosis occurs early and death from cirrhosis usually occurs in early childhood. Galactosaemia and hereditary fructose intolerance (Chapter 9) may also present as a cholestatic syndrome. Both must be recognized because of their relatively favourable prognosis with correct dietary restriction. Finally, other disorders, such as cystic fibrosis and Niemann Pick disease, may present with a cholestatic syndrome (Chapter 9).

Differential diagnosis of neonatal cholestasis

It would be foolish to place too much reliance on a single investigation such as liver biopsy in such a difficult diagnostic area. Thus interpretation of the biopsy must be made in the full light of the clinical history, ultrasound and radiological findings. The aim is to distinguish those conditions potentially amenable to surgical treatment, such as biliary atresia and choledochal cyst, and where possible to avoid surgery in the remainder. The characteristic bile duct proliferation, when present in every portal tract in the biopsy, is the single, most important indicator of large duct obstruction. Giant cells alone have no significance, since they may be seen in any condition. The presence of fat, however, is unusual and a reliable pointer to metabolic disorders such as galactosaemia and fructose intolerance (Chapter 9). α_1AT globules should be present in all cases of α_1AT deficiency.

REFERENCES

1. Ishak, K. G. and Sharp, H. L. (1987). Developmental abnormalities and liver disease in childhood. In MacSween, R. N. M., Anthony, P. P. and Scheuer, P. J. (eds). Pathology of the Liver. 3rd edn. pp. 66–98. Edinburgh: Churchill Livingstone
2. Lau, J. Y. N., Koukoulis, G., Mieli-Vergani, G., Portmann, B. C. and Williams, R. (1992). Syncytial giant-cell hepatitis–a specific disease entity? J. Hepatol., 15, 216–219
3. Phillips, M. J., Blendis, L. M., Poucell, S., Patterson, J., Petric, M., Roberts, E., Levy, G. A., Superina, R. A., Greig, P. D., Cameron, R., Langer, B. and Purcell, R. H. (1991). Syncytial giant-cell hepatitis. Sporadic hepatitis with distinctive pathological features, a severe clinical course, and paramyxoviral features. N. Engl. J. Med., 324, 455–460
4. Gautier, M., Jehan, P. and Odievre, M. (1976). Forty eight cases of extrahepatic biliary atresia. Correlation with postoperative bile flow restoration. J. Pediatr., 89, 704–709
5. Chandra, R. S. and Altman, R. P. (1978). Ductal remnants in extrahepatic biliary atresia. A histopathological study with clinical correlation. J. Pediatr., 93, 196–200
6. Mujano, T., Suruga, A., Tsuchiya, A. and Suda, K. (1977). A histopathological study of the remnants of extrahepatic bile duct in so-called 'non-correctable' biliary atresia. J Pediatr. Surg., 12, 19–25
7. Psacharopoulos, H. T., Howard, E. R., Portmann, B. and Mowat, A. P. (1980). Extrahepatic biliary atresia; pre operative assessment and surgical results in 47 consecutive cases. Arch. Dis. Child, 55, 851–856
8. Howard, E. R. and Davenport, M. (1992). Paediatric liver disease: surgical aspects. In Millward-Sadler, G. H., Wright, R. and Arthur, M. J. P. (eds). Wright's Liver and Biliary Disease. 3rd edn. pp. 1208–1232. London: W B Saunders
9. Howard, E. R., Driver, M., McClement, J. and Mowat, A. P. (1982). Results of surgery in 88 consecutive cases of extrahepatic biliary atresia. J. R. Soc. Med., 75, 408–413
10. Wight, D. G. D. (1993). The pathology of liver transplantation. In Wight, D. G. D. (ed.). Liver, Biliary Tract and Exocrine Pancreas. Vol. 11. Systemic Pathology. Symmers, W. S. C. (series ed.) Vol 11. Edinburgh: Churchill Livingstone
11. Mieli-Vergani, G., Howard, E. R., Portmann, B. and Mowat, A. P. (1989). Later referral for biliary atresia–missed opportunities for effective surgery. Lancet, 1, 421–423
12. Hays, D. M., Woolley, M. M., Snyder, W. H., Reed, G. B., Gwinn, J. L. and Landing, B. H. (1967). Diagnosis of biliary atresia, Relative accuracy of percutaneous liver biopsy, open biopsy and operative cholangiography. J. Pediatr., 71, 598–607
13. Brough, A. J. and Bernstein, J. (1974). Conjugated hyper bilirubinaemia in early infancy. A reassessment of liver biopsy. Hum. Pathol., 5, 507–516
14. Mieli-Vergani, G. and Mowat, A. P. (1992). Paediatric liver disease: medical aspects. In Millward-Sadler, G. H., Wright, R. and Arthur, M. J. P. (eds). Wright's Liver and Biliary Disease. 3rd Edn., pp. 1138–1154. London: W. B. Saunders
15. Alagille, D. (1979). Cholestasis in the first 3 months of life. In Popper, H. and Schaffner, F. (eds). Progress in Liver Disease VI. pp. 471–485. New York: Grune and Stratton
16. Desmet, V. J. (1991). Embryology of the liver and intrahepatic biliary tract, and an overview of malformations of the bile duct. In McIntyre, N., Benhamou, J.-P., Bircher, J., Rizetto, M. and Rodes, J. (eds). Oxford Textbook of Clinical Hepatology, pp. 497–519. Oxford: Oxford University Press
17. Desmet, V. J. (1987). Cirrhosis: aetiology and pathogenesis: chol-

estasis. In Boyer, J. L. and Bianchi, L. (eds). Liver Cirrhosis, pp. 101–118. Lancaster: MTP Press

18. Desmet, V. J. (1990). Cholestatic syndromes of infancy and childhood. In Zakim, D. and Boyer, T. D. (eds). Hepatology. A Textbook of Liver Disease, pp. 1355–1395. Philadelphia: W B Saunders

19. Landing, B. H. (1974). Consideration of the pathogenesis of neonatal hepatitis, biliary atresia and choledochal cyst. The concept of infantile obstructive cholangiopathy. Prog. Pediatr. Surg., 6, 113–119

20. Landing, B. H., Mahnovski, V. and Dahms, B. (1979). Considerations of certain aspects of the pathogenesis of neonatal hepatitis and biliary atresia. In Javitt, N. B. (eds). Neonatal Hepatitis and Biliary Atresia. pp.79–1296. 315–321 US Dept Health Education Welfare, NIH

21. Witzleben, C. L., Buck, B. E., Schnanfer, L. and Brzosko, W. J. (1978). Studies in the pathogenesis of biliary atresia. Lab. Invest., 38, 525–532

22. Haas, J. E. (1978). Bile duct and liver pathology in biliary atresia. World J. Surg., 2, 561–569

23. Witzleben, C. L. (1976). Etiologies of infantile obstructive cholangiopathy. J. Pediatr., 88, 909–910

24. Witzleben, C. L. (1990). Cystic diseases of the liver. In Zakim, D. and Boyer, T. D. (eds). Hepatology. A Textbook of Liver Disease. 3rd edn. pp. 1395–1411. Philadelphia: W B Saunders

25. Henson, S. W., Gray, H. K. and Dockerty, M. B. (1956). Benign tumours of the liver. III. Solitary cysts. Surg. Gynecol. Obstet., 103, 607–612

26. Milutinovic, J., Fialkow, P. J., Rudd, T. G., Agoda, L. Y., Phillips, L. A. and Bryant, J. I. (1980). Liver cysts in patients with autosomal dominant polycystic kidney disease. Am. J. Med., 68, 741–744

27. Grunefeld, J.-P., Albouze, G., Junger, P., Landais, P., Dana, A., Droz, D., Moynot, A., Lafforgue, B., Boursztyn, E. and Franco, D. (1985). Liver changes and complications in adult polycystic renal disease. Adv. Nephrol., 14, 1–20

28. Desmet, V. J. (1992). Congenital diseases of intrahepatic bile ducts: variations on the theme 'ductal plate malformation'. Hepatology, 16, 1069–1083

29. MacSween, R. N. M. and Burt, A. D. (1989). Pathology of the intrahepatic bile ducts. In Anthony, P. P. and MacSween, R. N. M. (eds). Recent Advances in Histopathology. 14. pp. 161–184. Edinburgh: Churchill Livingstone

30. Landing, B. H., Wells, T. R. and Claireaux, A. E. (1980). Morphometric analysis of liver lesions in cystic diseases of childhood. Hum. Pathol., 11, 549–560

31. Adams, C. M., Danks, D. M. and Campbell, P. E. (1974). Comments upon the classification of infantile polycystic diseases of the liver and kidney, based upon three dimensional reconstruction of the liver. J. Med. Genet., 11, 234–243

32. Summerschild, H. C., Langmark, F. and Maurseth, K. (1973). Congenital hepatic fibrosis; report of two new cases and review of the literature. Surgery, 73, 53–58

33. Desmet, V. J. (1992). What is congenital hepatic fibrosis? Histopathology, 20, 465–477

34. Desmet, V. J. (1985). Intrahepatic bile ducts under the lens. J. Hepatol., 1, 545–559

35. Nonomura, A., Ohta, G., Yoshida, K., Kurachi, M., Matsubara, F. and Takazakura, E. (1978). Congenital hepatic fibrosis. A case report with study of three-dimensional reconstruction of serial sections of the liver. Acta Pathol. Jpn., 28, 949–956

36. Caroli, J. (1973). Disease of the intrahepatic biliary tree. Clin. Gastroenterol., 2, 147–161

37. Mercadier, M., Chigot, J. P., Clot, J. P., Langlois, P. and Lansieux, P. (1984). Caroli's disease. World J. Surg., 8, 22–29

38. Hadad, A. R., Westbrook, K. C., Campbell, F. T. and Morris, W. D. (1976). Congenital dilatation of the bile ducts. Am. J. Surg., 132, 799–804

39. Khobayashi, A. and Ohbe, Y. (1977). Choledochal cyst in infancy and childhood: analysis of 16 cases. Arch. Dis. Child., 52, 121–128

40. Todani, T., Watanabe, Y., Narusue, M., Tabuchi, K. and Okajima, K. (1977). Congenital bile duct cysts. Classification, operative procedures, and review of thirty-seven cases including cancer arising from choledochal cyst. Am. J. Surg., 134, 263–269

41. Perrault, J. (1981). Paucity of interlobular bile ducts: Getting to know it better. Dig. Dis. Sci., 26, 481–484

42. Berman, M. D., Ishak, K. G., Schaefer, E. J., Barnes, S. and Jones, E. A. (1981). Syndromatic hepatic ductular hypoplasia (arteriohepatic dysplasia). A clinical and hepatic histologic study of three patients. Dig. Dis. Sci., 26, 485–497

43. Hadchouel, M., Hugon, R. N. and Gautier, M. (1978). Reduced ratio of portal tracts to paucity of intrahepatic bile ducts. Arch.

Pathol. Lab. Med., 102, 402

44. Alagille, D., Estrada, A., Hadchouel, M., Gautier, M., Odievre, M. and Dommergues, J. P. (1987). Syndromatic paucity of interlobular bile ducts (Alagille syndrome or arteriohepatic dysplasia). J. Pediatr., 110, 195–200

45. Emery, J. L. (1974). Pathology with reference to the bile retention syndrome. Postgrad. Med. J., 50, 344–347

46. Klein, S. and Nealon, W. H. (1988). Hepatobiliary abnormalities associated with total parenteral nutrition. Semin. Liver Dis., 8, 237–246

47. Chang, M. H., Hsu, H. C., Lee, C. Y. et al. (1987). Neonatal hepatitis: a follow-up study. J. Pediatr. Gastroenterol. Nutr., 6, 203–207

48. Sveger, T. (1976). Liver disease in α_1-antitrypsin deficiency detected by screening 200,000 infants. N. Engl. J. Med., 294, 1316–1321

49. Talbot, I. C. and Mowat, A. P. (1975). Liver disease in infancy: histological features and relationship to α_1-antitrypsin deficiency. J. Clin. Pathol., 28, 559–563

50. Callea, F., Brisigotti, M., Faa, G., Lucini, L. and Eriksson, S. (1991). Identification of PiZ gene products in liver tissue by a monoclonal antibody specific for the Z mutant of α_1-antitrypsin. J. Hepatol., 12, 372–376

51. Aägenaes, O., Henriksen, T. and Sorland, S. (1976). Hereditary neonatal cholestasis with vascular malformation. In Berenberg, S. R. (eds). Liver Diseases in Infancy and Childhood. pp. 198–206. Baltimore: Williams and Wilkins

52. Ghishan, F. K. and Greene, H. L. (1988). Liver disease in children with PiZZ alpha$_1$ antitrypsin deficency. Hepatology, 8, 307–310

53. Hadchouel, M. and Gautier, M. (1976). Histopathological study of the liver in the early cholestatic phase of α_1-antitrypsin deficiency. J. Pediatr., 89, 211–215

54. Scheuer, P. J. (1993). Chronic hepatitis. In Wight, D. G. D. (eds). Liver, Biliary Tract and Exocrine Pancreas. Vol. 11. Systemic Pathology. Symmers, W. S. C. Series ed. 3rd edn. Edinburgh: Churchill Livingstone

55. Perlmutter, D. H. (1991). The cellular basis for liver injury in α_1-antitrypsin deficency. Hepatology, 13, 172–185

56. Eriksson, S., Carlson, J. and Velez, R. (1986). Risk of cirrhosis and primary liver cancer in alpha$_1$-antitrypsin deficiency. N. Engl. J. Med., 314, 736–739

57. Thung, S. N., Gerber, M. A., Sarno, E. and Popper, H. (1979). Distribution of five antigens in hepatocellular carcinoma. Lab. Invest., 41, 101–105

58. Palmer, P. E. and Wolfe, H. J. (1976). α_1-Anti-trypsin deficiency in primary hepatic carcinomas. Arch. Pathol. Lab. Med., 100, 232–236.

59. Sveger, T. (1988). The natural history of liver disease in α_1-antitrypsin deficiency. Acta .Paediatr. Scand., 77, 847–851

60. Morin, T., Martin, J.-P., Geldmann, G. D., Benhamou, J.-P. and Ropartz, C. (1975). Heterozygous α_1 anti-trypsin deficiency and cirrhosis in adults, a fortuitous association. Lancet, 1, 250–251

61. Clausen, P. P. (1980). α_1Anti-trypsin globules in liver biopsies. Acta Pathol. Microbiol. Scand A, 88, 225–230

62. Bradfield, J. W. B. and Blenkinsopp, W. K. (1977). α_1-Anti-trypsin globules in the liver and Pi M phenotype. J. Clin. Pathol., 30, 464–466

63. Pariente, E.-A., Degott, C., Mastin, J., Feldmann, G., Potet, F. and Benhamou, J.-P. (1981). Hepatocytic PAS-positive diastase resistant inclusions in the absence of α_1-anti-trypsin deficiency high prevalence in alcoholic cirrhosis. Am. J. Clin. Pathol., 76, 299–302

64. Qizilbash, A. and Youn-Pong, O. (1983). Alpha$_1$-antitrypsin disease: differential diagnosis of PAS positive, diastase resistant globules in liver cells. Am. J. Clin. Path., 79, 697–702

65. Callea, F., Ray, M. B. and Desmet, V. J. (1981). α_1-Anti-trypsin and copper in the liver. Histopathology, 5, 415–424

66. Carrell, R. W. (1987). α_1-Antitrypsin deficiency. In Weatherall, D. J., Ledingham, J. G. G. and Warrell, D. A. (eds). Oxford Textbook of Medicine. 2nd edn. pp. 9.44–9.46. Oxford: Oxford University Press

67. Lomas, D. A., Evans, D. L., Finch, J. T. and Carrell, R. W. (1992). The mechanism of Z α_1-antitrypsin accumulation in the liver. Nature, 357, 605–607

68. Curiel, D. T., Holmes, M. D., Okayama, H., Brantly, M. L., Vogelmeier, C., Travis, W. D., Stier, L. E., Perks, W. H. and Crystal, R. G. (1989). Molecular basis of the liver and lung disease associated with the alpha$_1$-antitrypsin deficiency allele Mmalton. J. Biol. Chem., 264, 13938–13945

69. Portmann, B. C. (1993). Paediatric liver disease. In Wight, D. G. D. (ed). Liver, Biliary Tract and Exocrine Pancreas. Vol. 11. Systemic Pathology. Symmers, W. S. C., series ed. 3rd edn. Edinburgh: Churchill Livingstone

Many of the inherited metabolic disorders affect the liver. However, outside specialist centres, most pathologists will see only a handful of cases in a working lifetime and thus only the commonest and best defined morphologically will be discussed in any detail in this section. More detailed accounts of these and rarer disorders are available elsewhere[1-4].

In many of these conditions the ultimate diagnosis depends upon the demonstration of either the specific enzyme defect biochemically or characteristic ultrastructural features. Thus if any of these conditions is suspected prior to biopsy or at post-mortem, material should be preserved in the appropriate fixative for electron microscopy and another sample set aside at $-20°C$ or below for subsequent chemical assessment. Both these investigations may more appropriately be carried out in a specialist referral centre.

INBORN ERRORS OF LIPID METABOLISM
Gaucher's disease

Gaucher's disease is a lysosomal storage disease in which a deficiency of the enzyme glucosylceramide β-glycosidase leads to accumulation of glucosylceramide, a glucocerebroside, in the cells of the reticuloendothelial system. It is inherited as an autosomal recessive condition and is encountered most often in Ashkenazi Jews. It has been classified into three different types on the basis of the age of onset and other clinical features. The common type I affects adults who usually present with hepatosplenomegaly and minor abnormalities of liver function tests.

Histologically the hallmark of the disease is the Gaucher cell. This is of histiocytic origin and measures $70-100\ \mu m$ in diameter. It has one or more rather densely staining nuclei and a characteristic wrinkled or striated cytoplasm (Figure 9.1). The striations are best demonstrated with either PAS stain after diastase digestion or a trichrome stain. The cells are auto-fluorescent and often also contain a little stainable iron.

Typically the cells are found in the centrilobular regions, but random foci are also common (Figure 9.2). They tend to distend sinusoids and are regularly accompanied by degenerative changes in hepatocytes as well as perisinusoidal fibrosis[5]. Rarely Gaucher's disease is complicated by portal hypertension or cirrhosis.

Niemann–Pick disease

Niemann–Pick disease is associated with deficiency of the catabolic enzyme sphingomyelinase leading to accumulation of sphingomyelin in most tissues of the body[1]. Although five types have been recognized, most have an autosomal recessive inheritance and affect Jews most often. The commonest, type A, presents in infancy with hepatosplenomegaly and failure to thrive, and leads to death in $1-2$ years.

In the liver, sphingomyelin accumulates first in Kupffer cells and subsequently in liver cells. Affected cells measure $20-40\ \mu m$ in diameter and have a vacuolated cytoplasm (Figures 9.3 and 9.4). In frozen sections, they stain with Oil-red-O and Luxol fast blue and are birefringent under polarized light. In paraffin sections some are PAS-positive

due to a rather variable quantity of ceroid or lipofuscin. Sometimes the latter are stained a sea-blue colour with Giemsa, one variety of sea blue histiocytosis[6]. As sphingomyelin accumulates in liver cells they become progressively less eosinophilic and more vacuolated until they become indistinguishable from abnormal Kupffer cells.

Occasionally Niemann–Pick disease is associated with neonatal cholestasis and a type of giant cell hepatitis. The accumulating cells cause variable degrees of atrophy of liver cells and perisinusoidal fibrosis, but cirrhosis is rare.

Fabry's disease

This condition principally affects the kidneys and the cardiovascular system. There may be accumulation of strongly PAS-positive diastase-resistant ceramide trihexoside in Kupffer cells and portal macrophages[7]. Frozen sections reveal that the same cells contain cholesterol in addition. Liver cells are unaffected.

Cholesterol ester storage disease and Wolman's disease

Both conditions are due to deficiency of acid esterase and are associated with the accumulation of cholesterol and cholesterol esters in the liver, bone marrow, spleen, adrenals and intestines, which are often yellow–orange in colour[8]. In the liver, both Kupffer cells and hepatocytes are vacuolated, but only Kupffer cells and portal macrophages contain cholesterol, recognized by its characteristic birefringent crystals on frozen sections. Liver cells contain neutral lipid. There is variable pericellular fibrosis and bile duct proliferation, particularly in Wolman's disease which has a poor prognosis, with death in the first few months of life the rule.

Lipid-filled foam cells may also be encountered in the liver in a number of other conditions, such as familial high-density lipoprotein deficiency (Tangier disease)[9] and familial hyperlipoproteinaemias. Here the lipid accumulation is often more conspicuous in organs other than the liver and the diagnosis is rarely possible on the liver picture alone. The lipid accumulation is usually confined to macrophages which are PAS-negative and, on frozen sections, strongly sudanophilic.

MUCOPOLYSACCHARIDOSES

This is a group of seven disorders, closely related to one another but each with a genetically determined deficiency of specific lysosomal enzymes involved in the degradation of mucopolysaccharide (glycosaminoglycans)[10]. When there is a block in the removal of a terminal sugar, the remainder of the polysaccharide chain is not further degraded, resulting in its accumulation within lysosomes in various tissues and organs, often resulting in severe somatic and neurological disease. Each syndrome can be recognized by its clinical manifestations and by demonstration of the specific enzyme deficiency, but there is some inconsistency with regard to terminology. Only five of the seven disorders affect the liver and these include Hurler's syndrome, Hunter's syndrome (the only one which is sex-linked), Sanfillippo's disease and Morquio's syndrome.

The liver is enlarged, firm or hard and is pale in colour. Fibrosis may be extensive and cirrhosis is common. Mucopolysaccharide accumulates in both parenchymal cells and Kupffer cells, both of which are swollen with pale or vacuolated cytoplasm (Figure 9.5). Ideally, tissues should be fixed in dioxane picrate solution[1] since acid mucopolysaccharide is soluble in formalin. The latter is best demonstrated with colloidal iron and staining is removed by prior digestion with hyaluronidase. It is also weakly PAS positive and diastase-resistant.

Fucosidosis causes an essentially similar gross and microscopic picture[1].

MUCOLIPIDOSES

These are rare lysosomal storage diseases in which there are multiple defects of mucopolysaccharide lipid and glycoprotein metabolism, but the specific enzyme defects are, as yet, uncharacterized[11]. Histologically there is accumulation of mucopolysaccharide and lipid in both hepatocytes and Kupffer cells imparting a foamy or vacuolated and often empty appearance to the respective cells in sections.

INBORN ERRORS OF CARBOHYDRATE METABOLISM
Glycogen storage disease

All forms of glycogen storage disease other than types V and VII involve the liver where there is excessive or abnormal accumulation of glycogen. Skeletal and cardiac muscle are also involved in a number of these and the different forms can only be definitively characterized by enzyme analysis performed on the appropriate tissue. However, hepatic morphology, particularly when taken in context with clinical and biochemical findings, is often reasonably distinctive[12]. From the patient's point of view, the critical abnormality is usually an inability to release enough glucose from liver or muscle in response to need.

Soluble glycogen is present in the normal liver in abundance, thus the diagnosis of glycogen storage disease depends on factors other than the mere presence of glycogen.

Type I (von Gierke's disease-deficiency of glucose-6-phosphatase) and Type III (Cori's disease-debrancher enzyme, amylo-1,6 glucosidase deficiency) are similar to one another clinically. They may be associated with hypoglycaemia, metabolic acidosis and hepatomegaly (but, in contrast to the lipidoses, no splenomegaly). Both appear to improve with the passage of time, although Type I is often fatal in childhood.

Histologically they are rather similar and show a universal and uniform distension of liver cells with associated collapse of sinusoids leading to a mosaic pattern. Liver cells stain palely and have well-defined plasma membranes and central nuclei, giving a plant-like appearance (Figure 9.6). Glycogen vacuolation of liver cell nuclei is often very prominent, particularly in periportal regions (Figure 9.7). Lipid vacuoles are frequently seen in liver cells of Type I, but not Type III. Conversely, thin fibrous septa often radiate from portal tracts in Type III, but are not seen in Type I disease. Type I disease may rarely be complicated by the development of liver cell adenoma or even hepatocellular carcinoma[13].

Type II disease (Pompe's disease—acid maltase deficiency) occurs in a number of different forms which may become manifest in infancy, childhood or adult life. Although clinically muscle may be affected more than the liver, which is not usually very large, the liver changes are often characteristic. Liver cells are only mildly enlarged and sinusoids are not obliterated, but there is a uniform hazy microvacuolation due to lysosomal accumulation of glycogen. There are no vacuolated nuclei and there is no accumulation of lipid.

Type IV (amylopectinosis, brancher enzyme, amylo-1,4 1,6-transglucosidase deficiency) is very rare but histologically virtually pathognomonic. Periportal liver cells contain large pale inclusions of abnormal glycogen which displace the nucleus. These are intensely PAS-positive but only partly digested by diastase. This disease is associated with progressive fibrosis and ultimately cirrhosis. In the late stage the inclusions may not be easy to distinguish from those of α_1-antitrypsin deficiency.

The remaining types of glycogen storage disease that affect the liver (VI, VIII, IX and X) are all rather similar and characterized principally by unequal glycogen accumulation within the liver so that a mosaic is built up of cells of different sizes, especially in the periportal regions. There may also be slight fibrosis and fine droplets of fat.

Galactosaemia

This autosomal-recessive disease is due to a deficiency of the specific enzyme galactose-1-phosphate-uridyl transferase, whose absence results in the accumulation in tissues of toxic quantities of galactose-1-phosphate particularly in the liver, kidneys and lens of the eye[14]. The incidence varies from 1:12 000 to 1:187 000 live births.

The clinical symptoms are directly related to the ingestion of galactose and presentation usually occurs with jaundice, diarrhoea and failure to thrive in the first week of life. The first abnormality to appear in the liver is fatty change, which may be marked, followed by bile ductular proliferation and cholestasis. Later pseudoglandular transformation, siderosis and fibrosis supervene, all of which may be well established by 6 weeks (Figures 9.8 and 9.9).

It is important to make the diagnosis as early as possible, since further deterioration can be prevented by a galactose-free diet. Reducing substances are present in the urine, but definitive diagnosis requires demonstration of the specific enzyme defect in red cells[15].

Hereditary fructose intolerance

This condition is very comparable to galactosaemia, both in its manifestations and the implications for therapy. Here the enzyme defect is a deficiency of fructose-1-phosphate aldolase, and deterioration is arrested by the institution of a fructose free diet[16]. The morphological manifestations associated with chronic exposure are similar to those seen in galactosaemia, with cirrhosis being the end result. Acute exposure can, however, lead to acute hepatic necrosis and death from fulminant liver failure (Figure 9.10)[17]. Accumulation of fructose-1-phosphate apparently causes the major manifestations of the disease through the inhibition of other enzymic reactions[4]. Once affected children are old enough to choose, they usually develop a profound aversion to sweet foods, which may produce vomiting within hours, and may thus survive to lead a normal life.

Mannosidosis

This is another rare autosomal recessive disease characterized by the accumulation of mannose-rich oligosaccharides due to deficiency of acidic alpha mannosidase. In the liver, both hepatocytes and reticuloendothelial cells contain faintly PAS-positive vacuoles (Figure 9.11)[9].

INBORN ERRORS OF PROTEIN METABOLISM
Hereditary tyrosinaemia

Although there are several other disorders of amino acid metabolism, only this one (type 1 or hepatorenal type of

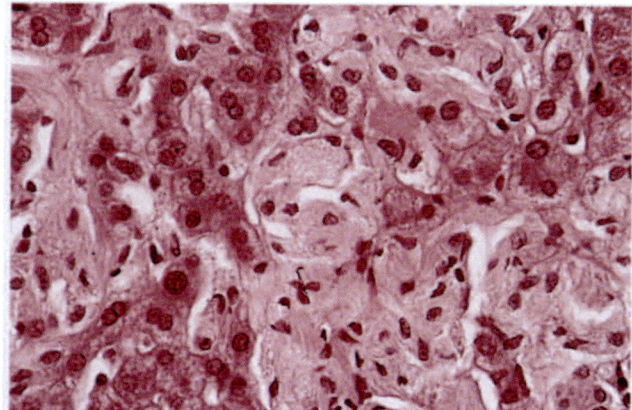

Figure 9.1 Gaucher's disease. A 17-year-old male presented with hepatomegaly. High magnification shows that the cells are quite distinct from liver cells and that they have small dense nuclei and characteristic striated cytoplasm which is even more apparent with PAS stain.

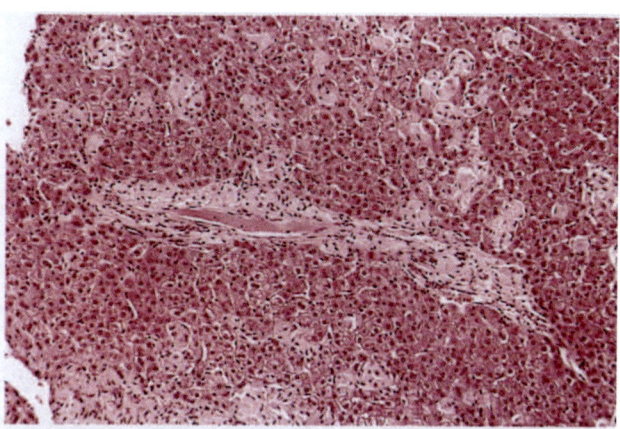

Figure 9.2 Gaucher's disease. Same case as Figure 9.1. Biopsy shows the classic appearances with large pale histiocytic cells grouped around the central venule and scattered in clusters throughout the remainder of the lobule.

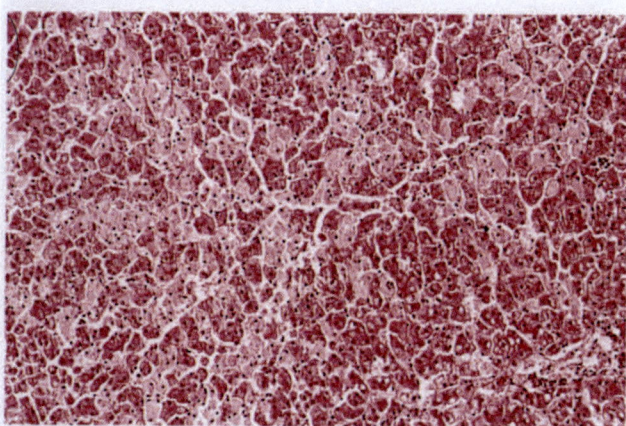

Figure 9.3 Niemann-Pick disease. Failure to thrive and hepatosplenomegaly was followed by death at 18 months of age in this child with a similarly affected sibling. Post-mortem liver shows a diffuse infiltration of the liver by plate cells of comparable size to hepatocytes.

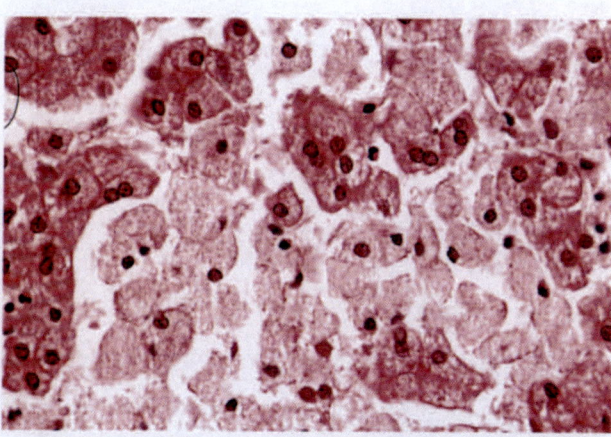

Figure 9.4 Niemann-Pick disease. Same case as Figure 9.3. Higher magnification shows that the abnormal pale cells have a granular, finely vacuolated, cytoplasm. Although most affected cells have small histiocyte nuclei, a few are probably altered hepatocytes.

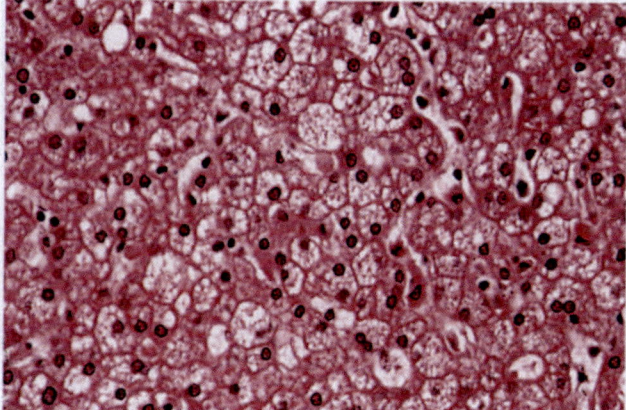

Figure 9.5 Hurler's syndrome. Severely retarded child, with a similarly affected elder sibling, showed a progressive deterioration and died aged 13 years. Post-mortem liver shows a uniform fine vacuolation of hepatocytes which is in no way specific. In this case there was no associated fibrosis.

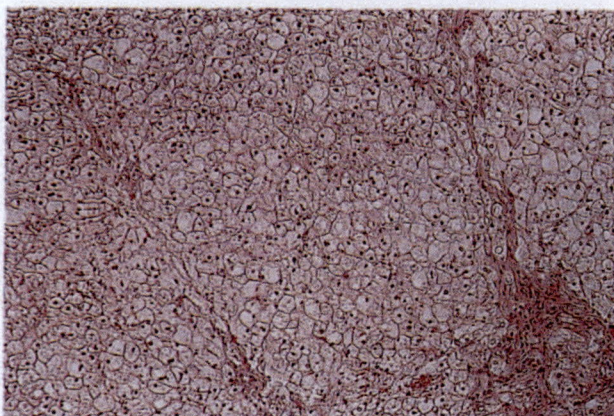

Figure 9.6 Glycogen storage disease, Type III. A 6-month-old infant who presented with hepatomegaly. Biopsy shows the classical empty plant-like pale hepatocytes with obliteration of sinusoids. Note also the thin fibrous spurs radiating from portal tracts.

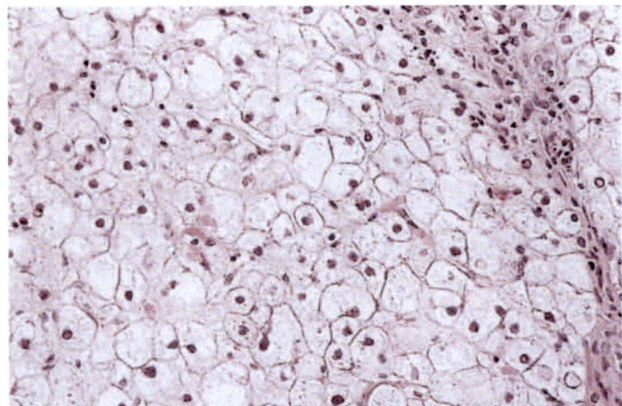

Figure 9.7 Glycogen storage disease, Type III. Same case as Figure 9.5. Higher magnification shows that there is some variation in hepatocyte size. There are a few vacuolated nuclei adjacent to the portal tract on the right of the field.

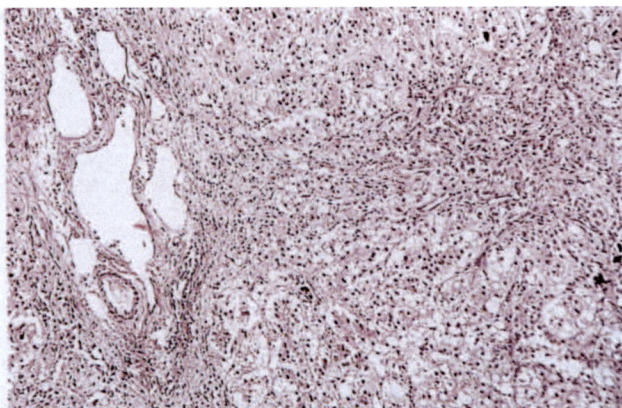

Figure 9.8 Galactosaemia. A 3–week–old infant presented with jaundice. Laparotomy and exploration of biliary tree revealed no abnormality. Liver biopsy taken at that time shows generalized pallor of liver cells due to the presence of fat droplets and considerable architectural disturbance in the form of pericellular fibrosis extending into the parenchyma from the portal tract on the right (galactosaemia was proved biochemically).

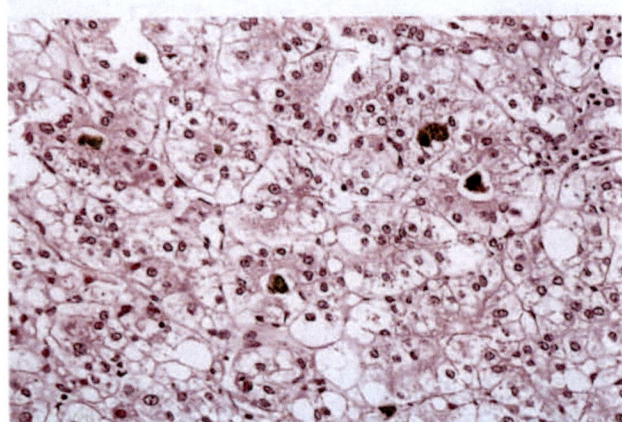

Figure 9.9 Galactosaemia. Same case as Figure 9.8. Higher magnification shows the distinctive mixture of 'rosettes' of liver cells, each with a bile plug at its centre, and multiple fat droplets.
The author is deeply indebted to Dr F J Paradinas who kindly provided the slides from which Figures 9.8 and 9.9 were prepared.

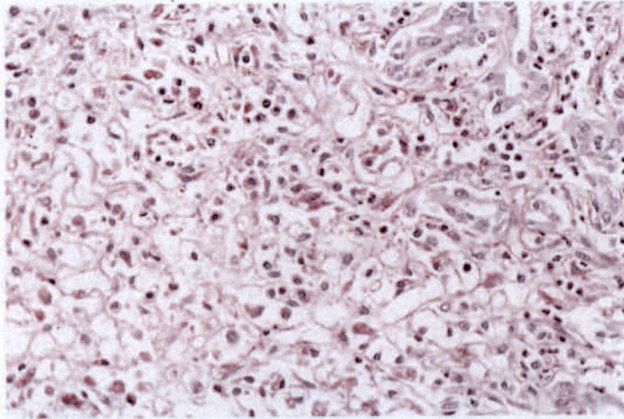

Figure 9.10 Hereditary fructose intolerance. An 18-year-old female, previously undiagnosed, was well until she was given a dextrose-based plasma expander under anaesthetic for a routine operation—she developed fulminant liver failure and died. The biopsy shows massive necrosis with a total absence of hepatocytes. Occasional phagocytes can be seen, and there is ductular proliferation (upper right). PAS after diastase.

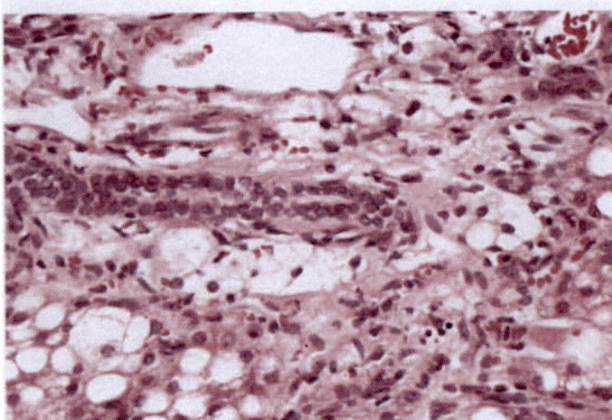

Figure 9.11 Mannosidosis. A 5-year-old child presented with hepatosplenomegaly. A small number of vacuolated foam cells, which were faintly PAS-positive, are present in portal tracts. Identical cells were also present in the lamina propria of a jejunal biopsy.

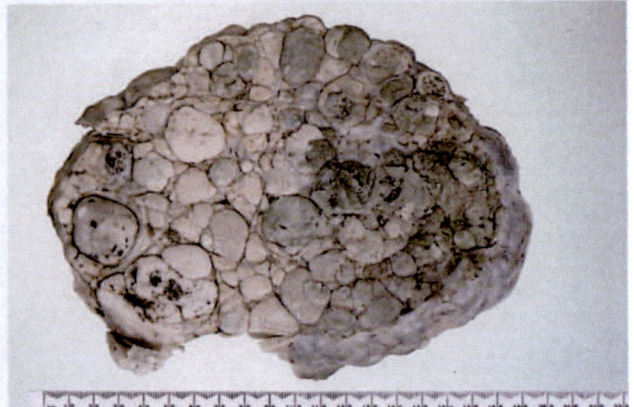

Figure 9.12 Tyrosinaemia. The liver of a 5-year-old child with an established cirrhosis, in which there are multiple foci of hepatocellular carcinoma (most of the nodules more than 1 cm in diameter represent tumour).

tyrosinosis) is associated with permanent liver damage[4]. In its acute form it may lead to death in infancy, and in its chronic form to death in the first decade. Microscopically, the changes are not specific, and are those of progressive liver injury with fibrosis and cirrhosis[18,19]. Focal lipid infiltration is common. Dysplastic nodules followed by hepatocellular carcinoma develop in up to 30% of patients who survive beyond two years of age (Figure 9.12)[19].

REFERENCES

1. Ishak, K. G. and Sharp, H. L. (1987). Metabolic errors and liver disease. In MacSween, R. N. M., Anthony, P. P. and Scheuer, P. J. (eds). Pathology of the liver. 2nd edn. pp. 99–180. Edinburgh: Churchill Livingstone
2. Filipe, M. I. and Lake, B. D. (1990). Histochemistry in Pathology. Edinburgh: Churchill Livingstone
3. Stanbury, B., Wyngarden, J. B., Fredrickson, D. S., Goldstein, J. L. and Brown, M. S. (eds.). (1983). The Metabolic Basis of Inherited Disease. 5th edn. New York: McGraw-Hill.
4. Ghishan, F. K. and Greene, H. L. (1990). Inborn errors of metabolism that lead to permanent liver injury. In Zakim, D. and Boyer, T. D. (eds). Hepatology. A textbook of liver disease. 2nd edn. pp. 1300–1348. Philadelphia: Saunders
5. James, S. P., Stomeyer, F. W. and Chang, C. (1981). Liver abnormalities in patients with Gaucher's disease. Gastroeneterology, 80, 126–133
6. Wenger, D. A., Barth, G. and Githens, J. H. (1977). Nine cases of sphingomyelin lipidosis, a new variant in Spanish American children. Juvenile variant of Niemann-Pick disease with foamy and sea-blue histiocytes. Am. J. Dis. Child., 131, 955–961
7. Portmann, B. C. (1993). Paediatric liver disease. In Wight, D. G. D. (eds). Liver, Biliary Tract and Exocrine Pancreas. 3rd edn. Vol. 11. Systemic Pathology. Symmers, W. S. C. Series ed. Edinburgh: Churchill Livingstone
8. Beaudet, A. L., Ferry, G. D., Nichols, B. L. and Rosenberg, H. S. (1977). Cholesterol ester storage disease: clinical, biochemical and pathological studies. J. Pediatr., 90, 910–914
9. Bale, P. M., Clifton-Bligh, P., Benjamin, B. N. P. and Whyte, H. M. (1971). Pathology of Tangier disease. J. Clin. Pathol., 24, 609–616
10. Kelly, T. E. (1976). The mucopolysaccharidoses and mucolipidoses. Clin. Orthop., 114, 116–136
11. Spranger, J. (1975). Mucolipidoses 1. In Bergsma, D. (eds). Disorders of Connective Tissue. New York: Stratton Intercontinental Medical Book Corporation
12. McAdams, A. J., Hug, G. and Bove, K. E. (1974). Glycogen storage disease, types I to X. Criteria for morphological diagnosis. Hum. Pathol., 5, 463–487
13. Fink, A. S., Appleman, H. D. and Thompson, N. W. (1985). Hemorrhage into a hepatic adenoma and type Ia glycogen storage disease: a case report and review of the literature. Surgery, 97, 117–124
14. Segal, S. (1983). Disorders of galactose metabolism. In Stanbury, B., Wyngarden, J. B., Fredrickson, D. S., Goldstein, J. L. and Brown, M. S. (eds). The Metabolic Basis of Inherited Disease. 5th edn. pp. 161–191. New York: McGraw-Hill
15. Monk, A. M., Mitchell, A. J. H. and Milligan, D. W. A. (1977). The diagnosis of classical galactosaemia. Arch. Dis. Child., 52, 943–946
16. Gitzelman, R., Steinmann, B. and van den Berghe, G. (1983). Essential fructosuria, hereditary fructose intolerance, and fructose 1,6-diphosphatase deficiency. In Stanbury, B., Wyngarden, J. B., Fredrickson, D. S., Goldstein, J. L. and Brown, M. S. (eds). The Metabolic Basis of Inherited Disease. 5th edn. pp. 118–140. New York: McGraw-Hill
17. Schulte, M. J. and Lenz, W. (1977). Fatal sorbitol infusion in a patient with fructose-sorbitol intolerance [letter]. Lancet, 2, 188
18. Prive, L. (1967). Pathological findings in patients with tyrosinaemia. Can. Med. Assoc. J., 97, 1054–1056
19. Dehner, L. P., Snover, D. C., Sharp, H. L., Asher, N. A., Nakhleh, R. and Day, D. L. (1989). Hereditary tyrosinaemia type I (chronic form): Pathologic findings in the liver. Hum. Pathol., 20, 149–158

The liver plays an important role in the metabolism of a great variety of ingested substances which may include both environmental toxins and drugs taken for therapeutic purposes. It is therefore uniquely susceptible to these agents and furthermore its metabolic activity may actually increase the toxicity of a whole variety of different substances. Typically drugs either cause liver cell injury, which includes both fatty change and necrosis, or cholestasis, but a number of other changes such as fibrosis, vascular injury and tumours have also been increasingly recognized.

Historically, occupational exposure to toxic chemicals was an important hazard of many industrial processes. With improvements in the working environment the emphasis has now switched to the domestic scene where there remain a few well-known toxic hazards, such as dry-cleaning fluids and 'mushrooms'. However, therapeutic agents are now the most important toxic cause of liver disease in modern practice. It has been estimated that they are responsible for some 2–5% of all cases of jaundice, whilst in the geriatric population this figure may be as high as 20%. Furthermore drugs account for as much as 25% of serious liver disease associated with acute hepatic failure.

The rôle of the pathologist is probably greater in the interpretation of drug-induced hepatic lesions than in those of other organs, such as kidney or heart, where physiological methods can provide useful parameters[1]. Drugs may be responsible for almost any type of liver disease and thus regularly mimic that due to other causes, such as viral hepatitis and biliary obstruction. It is thus essential to maintain a high index of suspicion and regard any therapeutic agent that the patient may be taking as a potential hepatotoxin even although this effect may not previously have been documented[2]. A clear clinical history is mandatory and crucial, since a diagnosis can rarely be made on morphological grounds alone[3,4]. It is, however, vital that the correct diagnosis is reached, since continued use or re-exposure to the drug in question may lead to severe or fatal liver cell necrosis or chronic liver disease.

GROUND-GLASS CELLS

Cells with a uniform finely granular eosinophilic cytoplasm, often with a peripheral clear space and a displaced nucleus, were first described in the German literature and related to induction of smooth endoplasmic reticulum (SER) by drugs such as chlorpromazine and rifampicin (Figure 10.1)[5,6]. These cells have a predilection for acinar zone 3, and are a common finding in liver biopsies with no pathological significance. Similar 'induced' ground glass cells are also quite frequently seen in cholestasis (Figure 16.3) and alcoholic injury[7]. Subsequently, similar ground glass cells were seen in carriers of hepatitis B surface antigen (Chapter 7). Rather similar cytoplasmic inclusions have also been seen as a manifestation of cyanamide toxicity[8].

PATHOGENESIS

Drugs and toxins can affect the liver in one of two ways. The effect may be predictable and dose-related or it may be unpredictable and idiosyncratic.

Predictable liver injury

This, as the term implies, is the expected outcome of exposure to these agents. The liver damage is often a zonal necrosis which follows a short latent period and is reproducible in experimental animals. The extensive animal tests on new drugs effectively detect this type of lesion and thus there are very few medicinal agents, at least in therapeutic dosage, which now belong to this group.

Predictable toxins may be able to cause liver damage directly. Substances such as tannic acid, ethionine, beryllium, white phosphorus[9] and aflatoxin are all primary cytotoxic agents of this type. They usually cause zonal necrosis, often in the periportal regions (zone 1), and interfere with the cell metabolism by a wide range of different mechanisms, although they frequently involve interference in nucleic acid or protein synthesis. More commonly, substances must first undergo metabolic transformation within the liver cell, usually by the cytochrome P450 mixed function oxidative enzyme system (MFOS) within the smooth endoplasmic reticulum (phase I reactions). The newly formed toxic metabolites, by covalent binding to the cell macromolecules, produce cytotoxic injury[10]. Although this is most often centrilobular zonal necrosis, carcinogens may be newly formed in this manner and metabolites may also be responsible for the cholestatic response to some drugs. The toxic metabolites may be further metabolized and rendered harmless as polar molecules suitable for excretion in bile or urine. As well as the initial dose of the toxin ingested, the rate of degradation of the intermediate metabolites depends on a host of other factors such as hormone balance, diet, other drugs (especially enzyme inhibitors or inducers) and the availability of glutathione for conjugation (phase II reactions).

The potential of other drugs to influence the metabolic outcome is well illustrated by experience with anti-tuberculous drugs. When isoniazid was combined with para aminosalicylic acid as the standard treatment for tuberculosis, hepatic reactions to isoniazid were uncommon, because PAS is an enzyme inhibitor. In contrast, when combined with rifampicin, an enzyme inducer, liver damage (see below) is significantly more common.

The classical liver cell poisons CCl_4 and $CHCl_3$ belong to the predictable group, as do paracetamol and C17-alkylated anabolic and contraceptive steroids. Paracetamol is of interest because in therapeutic doses it is readily conjugated to sulphate or glucuronide. In overdose, however, the liver stores of glucuronide and sulphate are rapidly depleted, allowing excess unconjugated reactive metabolites to cause liver cell injury by interaction with essential macromolecules. The reactive metabolites themselves are inactivated by conjugation with glutathione which also may, in certain circumstances, become depleted.

Unpredictable liver injury

Most therapeutic drugs cause liver damage unpredictably. The overall incidence tends to be low, the hepatic lesions are not dose-related and they occur after a relatively long and variable latent period which may be anything from weeks to years. This type of effect cannot usually be reproduced in experimental animals, and thus the causal relationship may be very difficult to prove. Furthermore, because of the low incidence of lesions (may be less than 1 in 10 000) they are usually not picked up in the preliminary therapeutic trials of a new drug.

Traditionally, unpredictable lesions were regarded as manifestations of hypersensitivity, but it seems probable that only a proportion are true examples of hypersensitivity[11]. Here the reactive metabolite may combine with the macromolecules of the cell to form a neoantigen which excites a cell-mediated or humoral response[10]. In these cases, the latent period is often constant and there are morphological features, such as tissue eosinophilia and epithelioid granulomas, as well as systemic evidence to point to a drug hypersensitivity. The drug or a metabolite may act as a hapten which, in combination with macromolecules, can lead to either humoral or cell-mediated responses.

In other examples, however, there are no ancillary features suggestive of hypersensitivity and thus the damage may be attributable to the accumulation of hepatotoxic reactive metabolites comparable to predictable lesions, but differing in that the enzyme system responsible for their synthesis is aberrant and idiosyncratic.

In unpredictable injury the picture is often morphologically more similar to viral hepatitis rather than a zonal necrosis – an observation which lends further support to the idea of immune aggression as a pathogenic mechanism.

CLASSIFICATION

The spectrum of drug injury in practice is best classified on a morphological basis (Table 10.1).

In the discussion which follows no attempt is made to provide a comprehensive list of drugs which can cause liver disease–a number of comprehensive accounts is available[12-15]. Instead, a few of the more common drugs responsible for each of the different morphological patterns is listed in each section. In addition, one representative drug from each of the main categories is considered in detail as an illustrative example.

Zonal necrosis

This is the commonest response to predictable toxins. Changes are usually detectable biochemically and visible morphologically within hours of exposure. However, since the changes are both predictable and reversible, there is not often a good indication for liver biopsy. Most of these substances, for example carbon tetrachloride, Amanita phalloides[16] and paracetamol overdose, cause centrilobular (zone 3) necrosis which is sharply demarcated from the surviving liver (Figures 10.2–10.5). Although there may be condensation of reticulin, the basic framework survives, allowing regeneration to replace the lost cells within a few days. Surviving liver cells may show small or large droplet fatty change, especially at the interface with the necrotic zone (Figure 10.2). Kupffer cells proliferate and often form prominent aggregates filled with granular yellow brown PAS-positive ceroid pigment (Figure 10.6). These persist for days or weeks after the recovery of the liver cells, and gradually migrate towards the portal areas over a time-scale of months. Even when necrosis is very severe, there is nearly always a surviving rim of liver cells in zone 1 around the portal tract (Figure 10.4). This is in contrast to the unpredictable hepatitic injury where total loss of liver cells from some lobules is well described.

Paracetamol (acetaminophen)

Paracetamol hepatotoxicity has become well known in the last 25 years or so as its popularity as a potential suicide agent has increased. Although not particularly effective in this respect (the overall mortality is only about 20%)[17] it seems unlikely that paracetamol would be approved by the Committee on Safety of Medicines if it were discovered today. Toxic effects at therapeutic dosage are uncommon but well recognized[18]. In doses in excess of 6 g, however, liver damage is predictable and due to excessive accumulation of a reactive metabolite formed by the cytochrome P450 system[19]. In England, this single agent is responsible for up to 50% of all cases of fulminant hepatic failure[20]. The morphological changes are identical to those described above[21,22]. Despite the often quite extensive centrizonal liver cell necrosis (Figure 10.4), an inflammatory response is rarely well developed and usually inconspicuous. Kupffer cells phagocytose the cell debris following the acute hepatocyte injury, often forming groups of four or five cells filled with strongly PAS positive ceroid (Figure 10.6). They may also contain iron pigment. Portal reaction is unusual. In the most severe cases there may be a little associated bile duct proliferation. Death in acute liver failure, about 4–6 days after

Table 10.1 Classification of drug-induced hepatic injury

			Examples
Acute	Cytotoxic	Zonal necrosis	Paracetamol, carbon tetrachloride
		Hepatitic reaction	Isoniazid, methyl dopa, halothane
		Fatty liver	Alcohol, glucocorticoids, sodium valproate
		Steatohepatitis	Alcohol, perhexiline maleate, amiodarone
		Inclusion bodies	Disulfiram, cyanamide
	Cholestasis	With inflammation	Chlorpromazine
		Uncomplicated	Anabolic and contraceptive steroids
	Granulomas		Isoniazid, phenylbutazone
Chronic	Chronic hepatitis		Methyldopa
	Fibrosis and cirrhosis		Methotrexate, hypervitaminosis A
	Vascular injury*	Peliosis hepatitis	Anabolic steroids
		Veno-occlusive disease	Pyrrolizidine alkaloids, azathioprine
		Budd-Chiari syndrome	Contraceptive steroids
	Neoplasia†	Adenoma	Anabolic steroids
		Hepatocellular carcinoma	Aflatoxin
		Cholangiocarcinoma	Thorotrast
		Angiosarcoma	Vinyl chloride, thorotrast

* see Chapter 18
† see Chapters 22–24 for further discussion

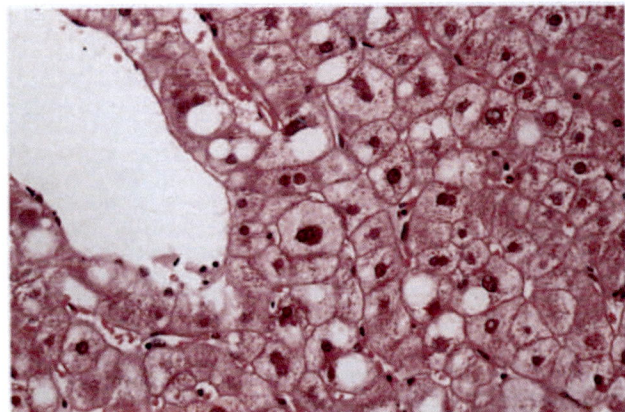

Figure 10.1 Ground glass cells, drug-induced. A number of hepatocytes are enlarged with pale uniform cytoplasm, but note that this is less homogeneous and less eosinophilic than is seen in HBsAg carriers (Chapter 7).

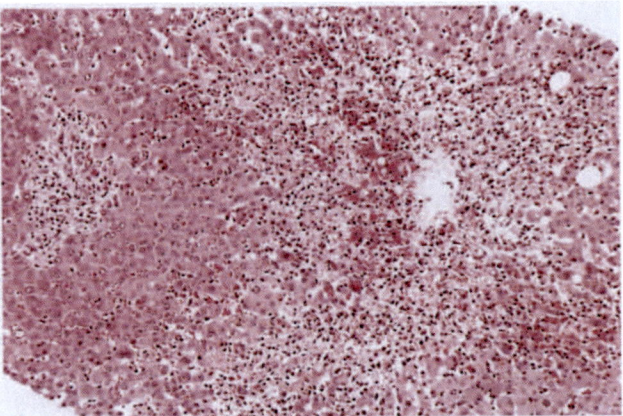

Figure 10.2 Carbon tetrachloride injury. An 18-year-old male presented in acute liver failure following inhalation of carbon tetrachloride fumes. Biopsy shows clearly demarcated centrilobular liver cell necrosis. Periportal liver cells are showing regenerative activity in the form of twinning of liver cell plates. There are a few fat droplets at the interface between necrotic and surviving hepatocytes. This patient died soon after biopsy.

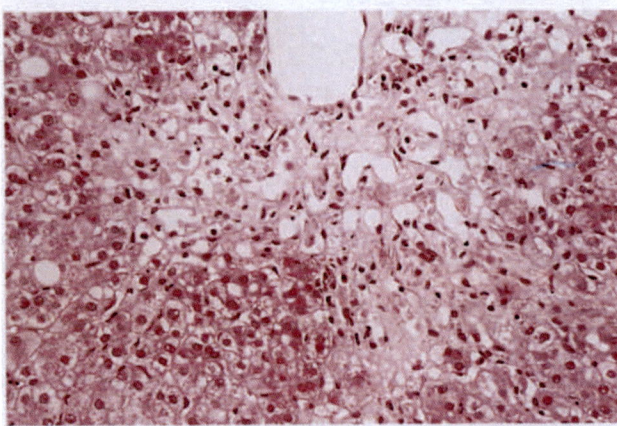

Figure 10.3 Carbon tetrachloride injury. A 34-year-old male was presented with jaundice after cleaning a carpet with carbon tetrachloride. Biopsy shows sharply demarcated centrilobular liver cell dropout, representing both less severe injury and a later stage than Figure 10.2. This patient made a complete recovery.

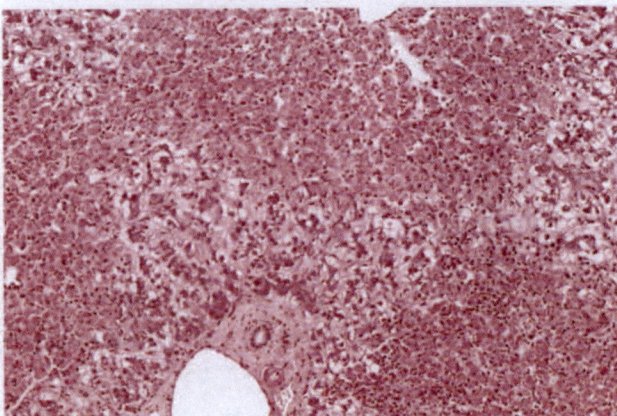

Figure 10.4 Paracetamol injury. A four-year-old child developed acute jaundice 2 days after accidental ingestion of paracetamol. Note the acute coagulative necrosis of hepatocytes in acinar zones 2 and 3, closely resembling ischaemic necrosis (Chapter 18). There is also ballooning of the surviving hepatocytes. The injury is comparable to that seen in Figure 10.2, although the changes are both more acute and more severe.

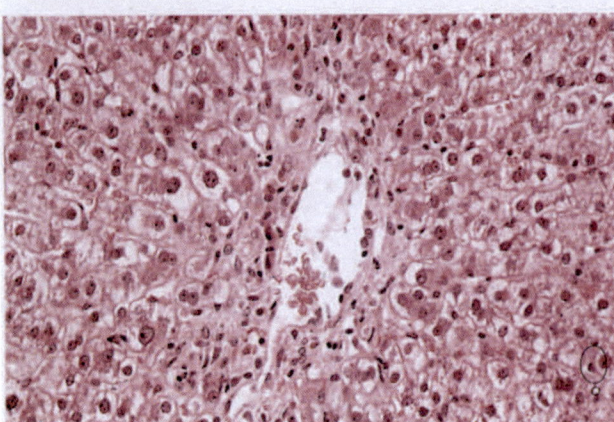

Figure 10.5 Paracetamol injury. Another case of acute onset of jaundice 2 days after the ingestion of paracetamol in a suicide attempt. Biopsy at 4 days shows a small area of hepatocyte dropout immediately adjacent to the terminal venule. The remaining liver cells are unaffected and appear normal. The changes are much less severe than those in Figure 10.4, and are very comparable to those in Figure 10.3. This patient made a full recovery.

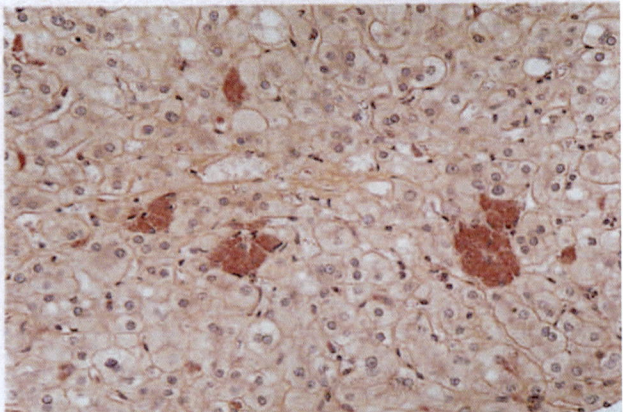

Figure 10.6 Paracetamol injury. A similar case to that shown in Figure 10.5, biopsied 6 days after drug ingestion, showing that prominent PAS-positive ceroid-filled Kupffer cells are the only remaining sign of acute liver injury. Note also the evidence of liver cell regeneration in the form of twinning of liver cell plates. PAS diastase.

ingestion, is the rule if more than about 50% of the liver cells are destroyed[21]. If the patient survives the acute phase there is complete recovery. Although there may be some persistent fibrosis initially, by a year after exposure this has usually resolved. There is no evidence that paracetamol is an initiator of chronic active hepatitis[23]. These complications can all be prevented if treatment with N-acetylcysteine, a sulphydryl rich compound which is able to restore the hepatocyte levels of glutathione which are necessary for the phase II conjugation, is instituted within 10–20 hours of ingestion[24].

The main condition likely to be confused with this type of necrosis is hypoxic liver injury which also is associated with sharply circumscribed foci of necrosis at the centre of the lobule. Indeed there has been a suggestion that ischaemia may play a part in the pathogenesis of paracetamol injury[17]. However, ischaemic necrosis is more likely to be associated with coagulative necrosis both of liver cells and of the supporting cells leading to persistence of necrotic ghost cells. Predictable liver cell necrosis is not likely to be confused with hepatitic injury because, apart from variable fat and/or ballooning degeneration of the liver cells adjacent to the necrosis, the surviving liver cells appear normal and there is no lobular disarray. However, the latter should not be confused with broadening of the liver cell plates due to regeneration which is, of course, regularly seen following this type of necrosis.

Zonal necrosis other than centrilobular is much less common[13]. Acinar zone 1 necrosis, as mentioned above, follows ingestion of a number of poisons, such as white phosphorus, aflatoxin and ferric sulphate (Figure 10.7). Proteus endotoxin may produce a similar picture. Midzonal necrosis is rare but has been described following beryllium and frusemide ingestion.

Hepatitic reactions

In contrast to zonal necrosis, these are usually the result of unpredictable injury. Drugs may produce a focal or spotty necrosis accompanied by lobular disarray, which is indistinguishable from viral hepatitis. When drugs do cause hepatitis, however, it is more likely to be severe and has a high mortality. Such fatal cases are comparable to fulminant viral hepatitis, and like viral hepatitis the liver may show massive necrosis with total loss of liver cells in some lobules (Figure 10.8), or even large portions of liver. Here there is no sparing of periportal liver cells, and there may be a florid reactive bile duct proliferation extending into the otherwise empty parenchyma from the portal tracts. Halothane (see below), and certain monoamine oxidase inhibitors such as iproniazid, are particularly associated with this type of reaction. Biopsy clearly plays little part in the management of these patients, since liver failure often precludes biopsy on technical grounds. Post-mortem biopsy and autopsy may, however, provide useful diagnostic information.

All forms of virus hepatitis may cause massive necrosis indistinguishable from drug hepatitis. Morphological features are unlikely to be helpful in making this distinction. Even hepatitis B is not usually detectable in sections during acute hepatitis. Thus indirect methods such as serological parameters may be necessary, and even then the evidence in favour of the drug may be no more than circumstantial.

Less severe hepatitis may likewise be indistinguishable from viral hepatitis (Figure 10.9). There may be the same lobular disarray with ballooning degeneration of some liver cells, occasional acidophil bodies, loss of other liver cells and an associated Kupffer cell reaction. Portal tracts may contain mixed inflammatory cells and show some bile duct proliferation (Figure 10.10). There may be

some spillover of chronic inflammatory cells, particularly lymphocytes, into the parenchyma as in viral hepatitis.

Apart from an appropriate history, there is a number of features which are helpful in correctly attributing a hepatitic reaction to a drug aetiology[25]. Fat in hepatocytes is unusual in viral hepatitis (with the exception of hepatitis C), but is not unusual in association with drugs (Figures 10.9–10.11). Acidophil bodies may be more numerous, more irregular in outline and more likely to retain a nuclear remnant than in viral hepatitis (Figures 10.11–10.13)[3]. Inflammation may be less than expected and necrosis disproportionately severe in relation to the patient's clinical condition and biochemical changes. Significant numbers of eosinophils within the portal infiltrate are a helpful feature when present but occur in less than 50% of cases. Accompanying granulomas in the absence of an obvious cause are also a useful pointer but they are more usually seen in the absence of a lobular hepatitis (see below). The early appearance of peripheral cholestasis and bile duct damage are also occasionally seen. Thus any additional or unusual morphological feature seen in a biopsy in which the principal change is a lobular hepatitis should make one think of a drug aetiology. The distinction is of considerable importance, since withdrawal of the drug is usually followed by recovery whilst continued use or re-exposure may precipitate massive necrosis.

All degrees of hepatocellular necrosis may be found, from the focal necrosis described above to massive necrosis. Bridging necrosis (sometimes called subacute) is thus also occasionally encountered (Figure 10.14). A great range of different drugs has been implicated in this type of injury, and it is necessary to maintain a high index of clinical suspicion that a drug might be involved in all cases of serologically negative hepatitis. It cannot be overemphasized that any drug must be considered as a potential hepatotoxin, even if not previously implicated.

Methyldopa

This is a drug which may rarely produce an acute hepatitic picture of this type. Clinically and pathologically the picture may be indistinguishable from viral hepatitis[26]. Onset is usually heralded by a typical hepatitic prodrome, occurring most often within four weeks of starting methyldopa. Histologically, too, the changes may be indistinguishable from acute viral hepatitis (Figures 10.9, 10.10 and 10.12) with the same range of severity from mild lobular hepatitis through bridging necrosis to massive necrosis. Tissue eosinophilia is uncommon. The mortality is approximately 10%. In the remaining patients, recovery is usually prompt on withdrawal of the drug.

In a small number of cases, however, methyldopa is associated with a *chronic active hepatitis*-like clinical and pathological syndrome. Histologically[27], the CAH is typical (Figure 10.15) with a portal tract-based chronic inflammatory infiltrate which includes many plasma cells as well as other mononuclear cells. This extends into the parenchyma causing piecemeal necrosis with ballooning degeneration of periportal liver cells. If the drug is not withdrawn cirrhosis may develop, as following any chronic hepatitis. However, withdrawal of the drug at any stage is usually followed by complete resolution of all activity and return of the liver to normal if there has not already been irreversible damage. There is immunological evidence that the mechanism of liver damage may be comparable to that in autoimmune chronic active hepatitis[28].

Chronic hepatitis is also well known following oxyphenisatin[29], isoniazid[30], and nitrofurantoin[31]. Perhexiline maleate[32] (now obsolete) and amiodarone are unusual since both produce an alcoholic-injury type of picture (often termed *non-alcoholic steatohepatitis*, Chapter 13)

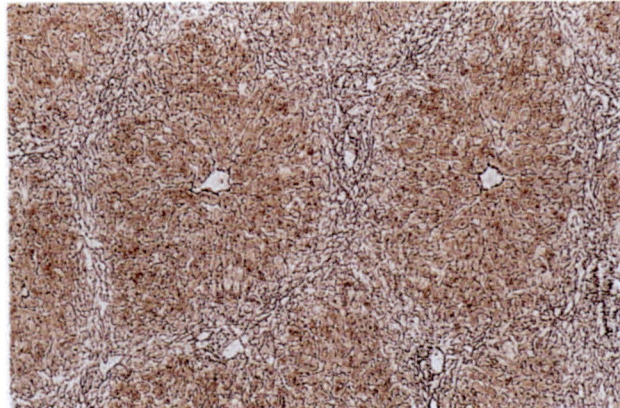

Figure 10.7 Zone 1 necrosis seen in an African child who died of liver failure, thought to be the result of ingestion of a toxin (undefined, possibly aflatoxin). Note the very striking collapse and condensation of reticulin in acinar zone 1 leading to portal to portal links, but wholly normal parenchyma in zones 2 and 3. Untoned reticulin.

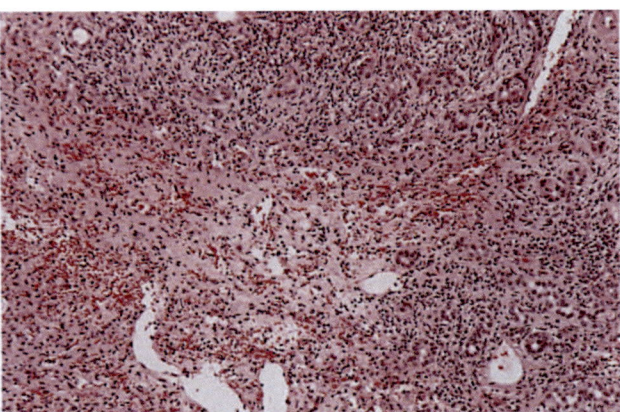

Figure 10.8 Hydralazine, fulminant hepatitis. A 50-year-old female with chronic renal failure and hypertension was treated with hydralazine. The onset of jaundice several months later was rapidly followed by acute hepatic failure. No serological evidence of viral hepatitis. Biopsy shows multilobular necrosis with a complete absence of hepatocytes. Portal tracts are expanded and inflamed with some bile duct proliferation. The patient died.

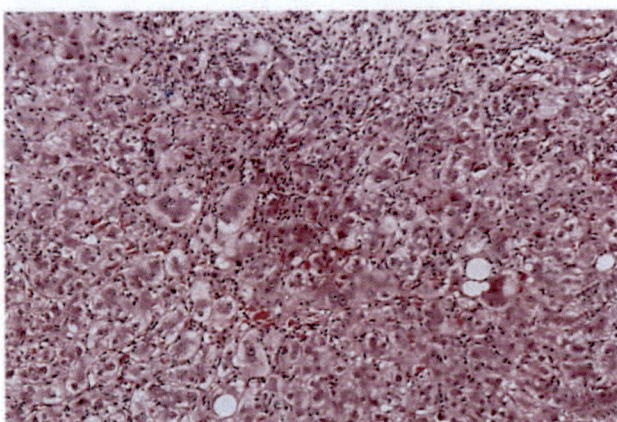

Figure 10.9 Methyldopa hepatitis. Acute onset of hepatocellular jaundice in a 59-year-old male, 3 weeks after commencing treatment with methyldopa. Biopsy shows a severe lobular hepatitis, with lobular disarray, ballooning degeneration and mononuclear cell infiltration.

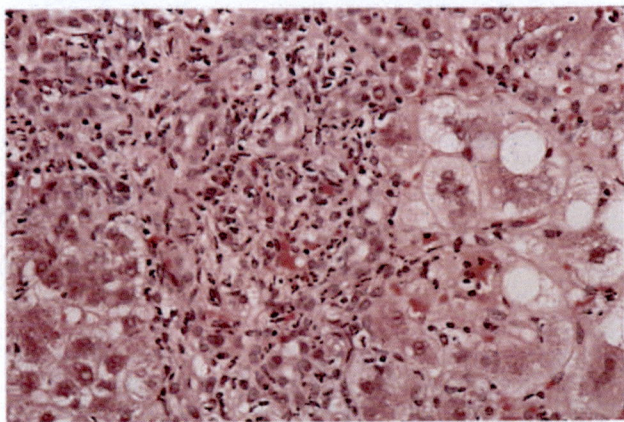

Figure 10.10 Methyldopa hepatitis. Same case as Figure 10.9. There is infiltration of this portal tract by both acute and chronic inflammatory cells. Eosinophils are not conspicuous. There is a little piecemeal necrosis at the limiting plate with several periportal hepatocytes showing ballooning degeneration.

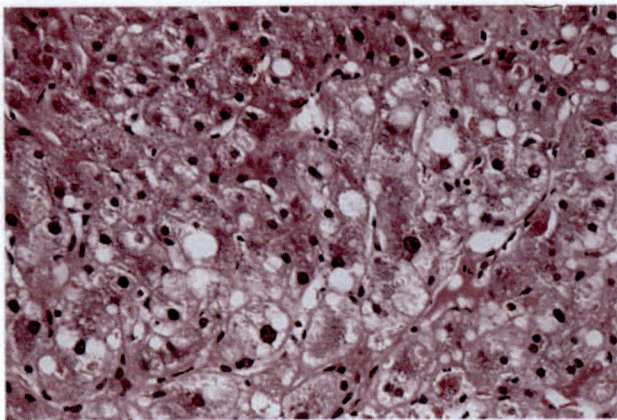

Figure 10.11 Indomethacin hepatitis. Onset of jaundice in an elderly patient taking indomethacin, biochemically hepatocellular. Biopsy shows a rather mild lobular hepatitis with some swelling of centrilobular hepatocytes. As in Figure 10.9 the only feature which is inconsistent with viral hepatitis is the rather conspicuous large droplet fatty change.

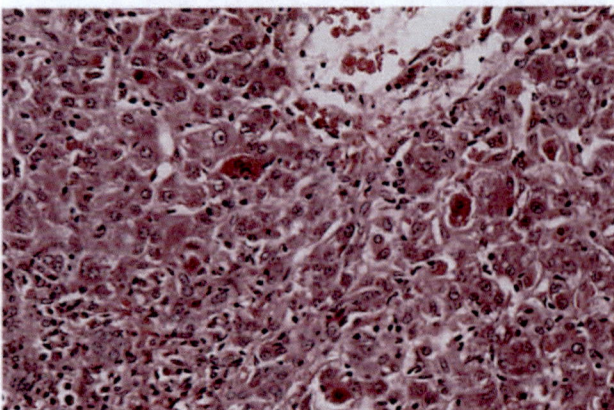

Figure 10.12 Methyldopa hepatitis. Another case showing a lobular hepatitis with numerous acidophil bodies visible in this field. They all have a somewhat irregular outline and their nuclei are retained.

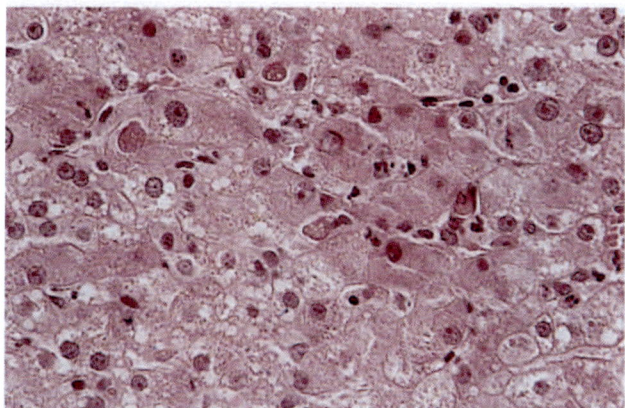

Figure 10.13 Rifampicin hepatitis. Acute onset of jaundice 7 days after starting rifampicin for suspected recurrence of tuberculosis. As in the previous case, this was biochemically hepatocellular. Biopsy shows a lobular hepatitis in which both fat and acidophil bodies are unusually prominent.

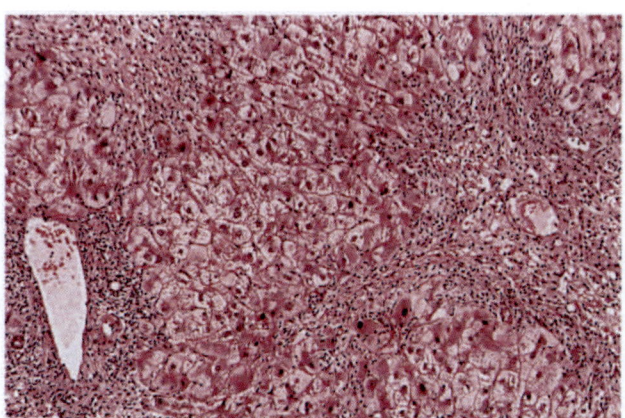

Figure 10.14 Amitryptiline hepatitis. A 56-year-old female developed an acute hepatic illness whilst taking amitryptiline. Biopsy shows hepatocyte necrosis with a distribution corresponding to acinar zone 3. There is bridging necrosis linking the terminal venule (right) with portal tract (left) and terminal venules with one another (not shown). Surviving periportal liver cells show regenerative changes. Inflammation is relatively inconspicuous. This patient recovered on withdrawal of the drug.

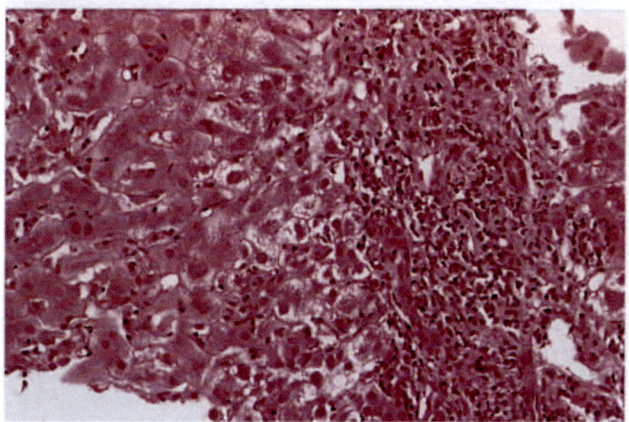

Figure 10.15 Methyldopa chronic active hepatitis. This patient continued to take methyldopa for several weeks after the onset of jaundice. Biopsy shows a predominantly periportal and portal chronic inflammation with piecemeal necrosis of a few periportal hepatocytes. Withdrawal of the drug was followed by rapid recovery without further treatment.

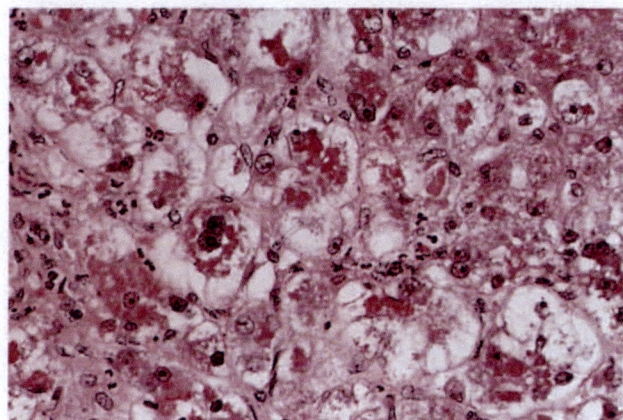

Figure 10.16 Perhexiline maleate injury. Note the striking resemblance to alcoholic hepatitis (Chapter 13) with numerous ballooned hepatocytes containing clumped eosinophilic Mallory's hyalin.

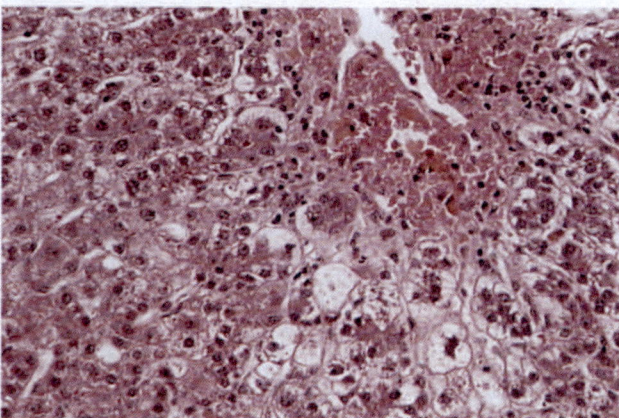

Figure 10.17 Halothane hepatitis. Acute onset of hepatocellular jaundice a few days after a second halothane anaesthetic. Biopsy shows striking sharply demarcated, centrilobular necrosis comparable to that due to chloroform. Note the ceroid-filled Kupffer cells in the necrotic zone. The remaining liver cells show active regeneration, but, inferiorly, there is also some lobular disarray with ballooning degeneration of liver cells, a hepatitic component.

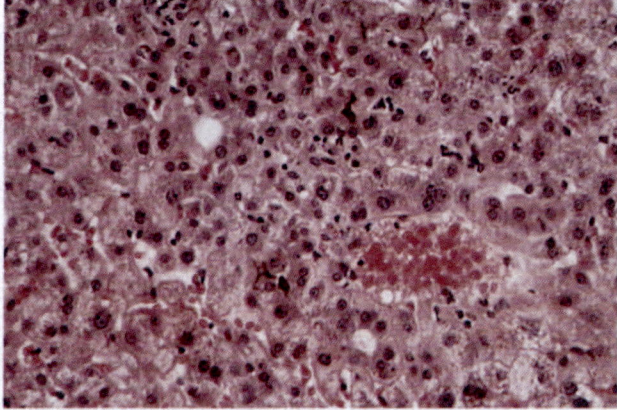

Figure 10.18 Anabolic steroids, cholestasis. Long-term treatment of aplastic anaemia with anabolic steroids. An increased dose was followed by cholestatic jaundice which had been present for several weeks at the time of biopsy. This shows a pure cholestasis together with some secondary changes such as tubule formation (below central vein) and Kupffer cell reaction, but there is no hepatocyte damage.

with numerous ballooned cells containing Mallory's hyalin (Figure 10.16)[33]. Since all of these agents may also cause acute liver injury, and since chronic hepatitis usually follows prolonged exposure, it seems reasonable to speculate that continuing subtle injury has begun long before the patient presents with chronic injury[34]. Many of these patients have the complete clinical syndrome of lupoid hepatitis with accompanying elevation of serum gamma-globulin, together with antinuclear and smooth muscle antibodies, all providing strong support for the view that chronic hepatitis has an immunological basis.

Several series have shown that drugs may make a significant contribution to the overall pool of chronic active hepatitis[30], responsible for the disease in nearly half of one series of 85 patients[35]. The most commonly implicated drug in these series has been oxyphenisatin, and indeed, this drug has now been withdrawn from the market.

Halothane

There has been considerable dispute as to whether or not halothane can be implicated as a hepatotoxin, but there is now a consensus that halothane hepatitis is a distinct although rare syndrome[36]. Early evidence was circumstantial, but more recently challenge studies have shown recurrence of fever and hepatitis after re-exposure to halothane, but not to control anaesthetic[37]. Hepatitis is more likely to follow multiple exposures, with re-exposure within four weeks of being seen in about half of all cases[38]. The mortality is greater than 50% in recognized cases, although a proportion of the milder ones may well go unrecognized. The commonest presentation is with unexplained fever in the post-operative period. Arguments still rage about whether the liver damage is a result of hepatotoxicity or whether it is immunologically mediated. In support of a hypersensitive mechanism are the finding of other stigmata, such as fever, rashes and arthralgias in a proportion of patients. Peripheral blood eosinophilia is seen in about 30%[38]. There is recent evidence that antibodies to hepatocyte neoantigens might be involved in the pathogenesis of liver injury[39].

Histologically the lesion associated with halothane is unusual in that it has some features of a hepatitis and some of a predictable type of hepatotoxicity, (Figure 10.17)[40,41]. Liver cells show lobular disarray, with swelling of some cells, lytic necrosis of others and acidophil bodies. Fat droplets may be seen but usually only in the most severe cases[42]. There is a mesenchymal reaction in portal tracts which may or may not include eosinophils but is overall less intense than in viral hepatitis. Confluent necrosis is quite common, especially in fatal cases, but in contrast to viral hepatitis it has an irregular but mainly centrilobular distribution (Figure 10.17) and rarely involves whole lobules. The areas of necrosis are very sharply demarcated from surviving parenchyma and it is this feature which resembles injury due to substances such as carbon tetrachloride.

Fatty liver

Fatty liver may be produced by a wide variety of agents, but in clinical practice alcohol is much the commonest cause (Chapter 13). Many substances which produce zonal necrosis, but especially white phosphorus and carbon tetrachloride, show large droplet fatty change in the surviving liver cells at the margin of the necrotic zone (as described above). Spotty fatty change may also be seen in association with the hepatic reaction caused by some drugs. Methotrexate and other antineoplastic agents may cause large droplet fatty change in association with

fibrosis. Glucocorticoids also cause significant macrovesicular fat. In all these cases, the fat *per se* has little clinical or functional significance other than as a cause of hepatomegaly.

In contrast, the microvesicular fatty change seen in centrilobular liver cells following intravenous tetracycline[43], like that seen in acute fatty liver of pregnancy and in Reye's syndrome (Chapter 12), appears to represent an acute form of hepatic injury. This effect is predictable and dose-related but is only seen when large doses are administered, usually by intravenous injection, and is thought to be the consequence of inhibition of hepatic triglyceride secretion. Despite the rather bland appearance, the prognosis is poor[3]. Sodium valproate may produce a rather similar picture[44].

Granulomas

Granulomas are a common response to drugs but may be difficult to distinguish from those due to other causes (see also Chapter 19). Histiocytic nodules of Kupffer cell granulomas within the parenchyma are a common response to drugs but are also seen in many other circumstances and thus have little or no diagnostic significance. True epithelioid granulomas, with or without giant cells, are found in about 5–10% of all liver biopsies in routine practice. Sarcoidosis accounts for about a third of all cases, whilst tuberculosis is the cause in less than a sixth. A presumed drug aetiology may also account for up to a third of all cases of granulomas[45]. The drugs most often incriminated include antihypertensives (including methyldopa), antibiotics (sulphonamides, isoniazid), antirheumatic agents (phenylbutazone, aspirin), but there are also many others.

There are no particular pathogenic features of drug-induced granulomas[45]. They may be found in any part of the liver, but some portal tract involvement is usual. The granulomas are non-caseating and usually discrete and surrounded by a mixed inflammatory infiltrate. The latter sometimes includes eosinophils in quite large numbers, when it is a helpful feature. Healing may leave a small collagenous scar. The granulomas may be present as an isolated finding or part of a hepatitic, cholestatic or mixed picture[34].

Cholestasis

Cholestasis may be a result of either predictable or unpredictable injury. In its purest form, the only morphological finding may be rather inconspicuous and small bile plugs in centrilobular cells, despite marked elevation of serum bilirubin levels.

This uncomplicated type of cholestasis follows ingestion of C17 alkylated anabolic steroids (Figures 10.18–10.20), oral contraceptives and oestrogens, and is largely predictable, although individual susceptibility does vary[46,47]. The cholestatic jaundice of pregnancy is of similar type and patients who develop this usually also become jaundiced if they take oral contraceptives. Inflammatory changes in these livers are minimal (Figure 10.19) and only develop if cholestasis is prolonged (the consequences of prolonged cholestasis are described in Chapter 16, and the tumours which are occasionally associated with steroid hormones in Chapter 22).

Cholestasis with inflammation is probably the commonest drug reaction seen in the liver. Here bile thrombi are much more obvious and the secondary changes may also be more marked. There is often also evidence of a mild lobular hepatitic reaction with occasional focal necroses and acidophil bodies (Figure 10.21). Binucleate liver cells and mitoses are also sometimes present. Portal tracts contain variable numbers of inflammatory cells (Figure

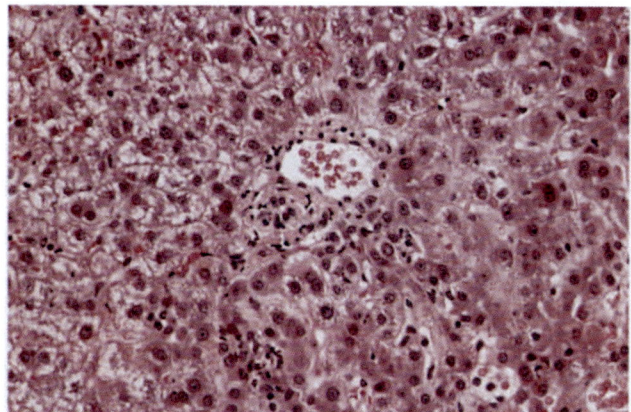

Figure 10.19 Anabolic steroids, cholestasis. Same case as Figure 10.18. The portal tract is entirely normal with no inflammatory changes. Periportal liver cells are showing some regenerative activity.

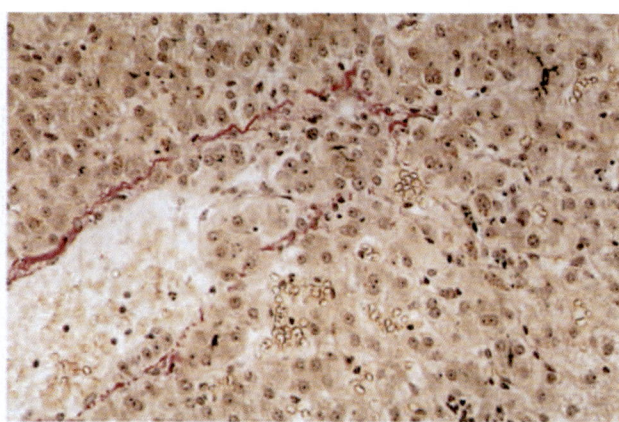

Figure 10.20 Anabolic steroid injury. Same case as Figures 10.18 and 10.19. This section shows prolapse of hepatocytes into the central vein, another type of injury attributable to long-term anabolic steroids. Peliosis hepatis (see Chapter 22) was also present elsewhere in the biopsy. Elastic van Gieson.

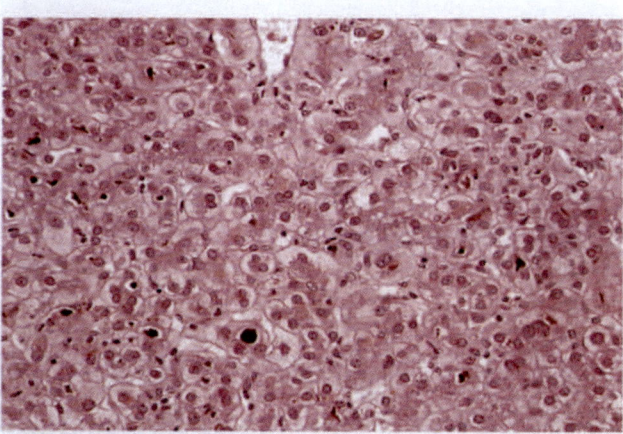

Figure 10.21 Chlorpromazine cholestasis. A patient with cholestatic jaundice attributed to chlorpromazine. Canalicular cholestasis is marked in this case and there are also a few multinucleate hepatocytes.

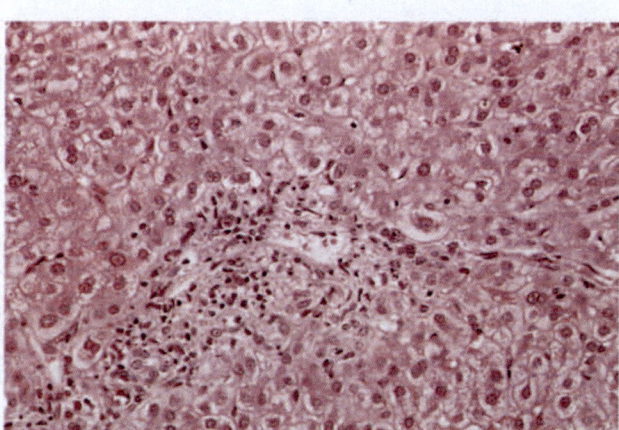

Figure 10.22 Chlorpromazine cholestasis, same case as Figure 10.21. The portal tract contains a few inflammatory cells which are mostly lymphocytes with, in this instance, very few eosinophils. Compare this with Figure 10.19.

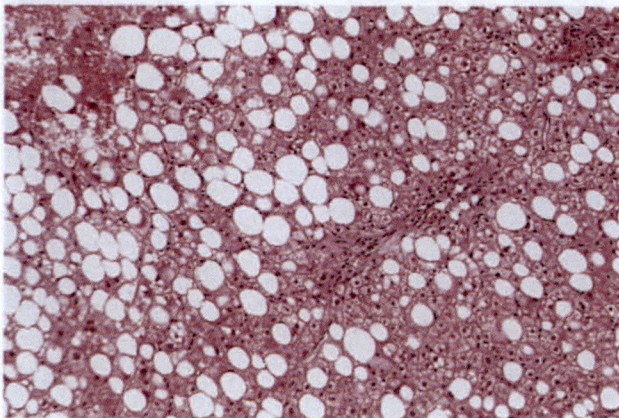

Figure 10.23 Methotrexate therapy. A 58-year-old female with severe psoriasis, treated with methotrexate for about 5 years. Biopsy shows extensive large droplet fatty change but only trivial portal fibrosis. These appearances could easily be attributable to methotrexate, but fatty change of this severity is also common in psoriatics not being treated with this drug.

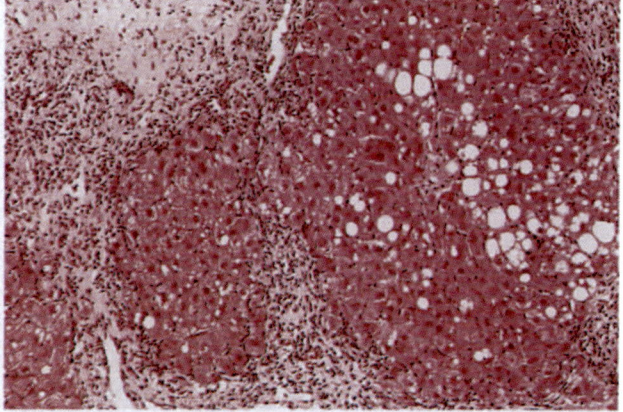

Figure 10.24 Methotrexate injury. A 33-year-old male with severe psoriasis treated with methotrexate for 18 months. Biopsy shows advanced portal fibrosis, but hitherto preservation of lobular architecture and no regeneration nodules.

10.22). Eosinophils are occasionally quite numerous, when they may be a helpful pointer, if not actual proof of aetiology. Inflammation gradually fades with the passage of time.

Chlorpromazine

This drug is the prototype for this kind of liver injury, cholestasis occurring in 0.15–1% of patients taking the drug. There is usually a latent period of some 1–5 weeks before the onset of jaundice and complete recovery after withdrawal is the rule. Inflammatory changes, leading to some expansion of the portal tracts by a mixture of cells, but mainly lymphocytes (Figure 10.22), are maximal in the first few weeks[48], even if the condition pursues a chronic course. Persistence of jaundice, as in any prolonged cholestasis, may be followed by periportal bile plugging and this is often accompanied by more marked liver cell swelling. Rarely chlorpromazine may lead to a primary biliary cirrhosis-like syndrome[13].

Drug-induced cholestasis must be distinguished from mechanical biliary obstruction. Modern investigation, such as percutaneous cholangiography, ultrasound and computerized tomography are all making the distinction easier, but liver biopsy may still be performed. Marginal bile duct proliferation is not seen in drug cholestasis and marked portal tract oedema, neutrophils in relation to bile ducts, or bile infarcts, all favour biliary obstruction. Small collections of foam cells may, however, be seen in drug cholestasis.

In practice, therefore, the clinical and histological diagnosis of drug induced cholestasis is mainly one of exclusion.

Fibrosis and cirrhosis

Alcohol is far more likely to cause fibrosis and cirrhosis than any therapeutic drug. However, both may follow any drug-induced chronic active hepatitis if the drug continues to be taken after the onset of hepatic damage.

Methotrexate

Methotrexate therapy however, may be associated with the insidious development of cirrhosis in up to 20% of patients[49]. Chronic methotrexate therapy is usually part of the long-term therapy of severe psoriasis, which itself may be associated with significant fatty change[50,51] which is at least in part due to factors such as alcohol intake and obesity. It is thus important that the liver should be biopsied prior to starting treatment. Methotrexate damage is directly related to duration of therapy and appears more likely to occur if small doses are given frequently[34]. The earliest changes noted are large droplet fatty change (Figure 10.23), followed by stellate portal tract fibrosis (Figure 10.24). Inflammatory changes are minimal and there is very poor correlation of the histological deterioration with biochemical and clinical parameters[52]. Regular biopsy is thus mandatory in the management of any patient on long-term therapy.

Cirrhosis resembling primary biliary cirrhosis is a rare complication of cholestatic jaundice of the type caused by chlorpromazine (see above), whilst drug-induced hepatic vein thrombosis or veno-occlusive disease may lead to a type of congestive or cardiac cirrhosis. Vinyl chloride and chronic arsenic ingestion both lead to a chronic non cirrhotic fibrosis of the liver[53]. Serial biopsies have shown both capsular and portal fibrosis which extends into the periportal sinusoids and may ultimately cause portal hypertension. The condition is sometimes referred to as hepatoportal sclerosis and is followed in a proportion of patients by the development of angiosar-coma (Chapter 24). *Hypervitaminosis A* can lead to similar sinusoidal fibrosis associated with increased numbers of perisinusoidal lipocytes (Ito cells)[54].

Vascular disorders (Chapter 18) and neoplasms (Chapters 22–24) are considered elsewhere.

A comprehensive tabulated list of drugs known to have caused various hepatic diseases can be found in references[12-14].

REFERENCES

1. Popper, H. (1975). The role of the human pathologist in the management of drug-induced hepatic injury. Hum. Pathol., 6, 649–651
2. Scheuer, P. J. (1988). Drugs and toxins. In Liver Biopsy Interpretation. 4th edn. pp. 99–112. London: Baillière Tindall
3. Rubin, E. (1980). Iatrogenic hepatic injury. Hum. Pathol., 11, 312–331
4. Black, M. M. (1992). Investigations of liver disease and drug toxicity. Curr. Opin. Gastroenterol., 8, 439–448
5. Gudat, F., Bianchi, L., Sonnabend, W., Thiel, G., Aenishaenslin, W. and Staider, G. A. (1975). Pattern of core and surface expression in liver tissue reflects state of specific immune response in hepatitis B. Lab. Invest., 32, 1–9.
6. Popper, H. (1975). The ground glass hepatocyte as a diagnostic hint. Hum. Pathol., 6, 517–520.
7. Thomsen, P., Poulsen, H. and Petersen, P. (1976). Different types of ground glass hepatocytes in human liver biopsies: morphology, occurrence and diagnostic significance. Scand. J. Gastroenterol., 11, 113–119
8. Vazquez, J. J., Guillen, F. J., Zozaya, J. and Lahoz, M. (1983). Cyanamide-induced liver injury. A predictable lesion. Liver, 3, 225–230
9. Salfelder, K., Doehnert, H. R., Doehnert, G., Sauerteg, K., Deliscano, T. R. and Fabrega, S. E. (1972). Fatal phosphorus poisoning. A study of forty-five autopsy cases. Beitr. Pathol., 147, 321–340
10. Tredger, J. M. and Davis, M. (1991). Drug metabolism and hepatotoxicity. Gut, Supplement, S34–S39
11. Pohl, L. (1990). Drug-induced allergic hepatitis. Semin. Liver Dis., 10, 305–315
12. Ludwig, J. and Axelsen, R. (1983). Drug effects on the liver. An updated tabular compilation of drugs and drug-related hepatic disease. Dig. Dis. Sci., 28, 651–666
13. Zimmerman, H. J. and Ishak, K. G. (1987). Hepatic injury due to drugs and toxins. In MacSween, R. N. M., Anthony, P. P. and Scheuer, P. J. (eds). Pathology of the Liver. 2nd edn. pp. 503–573. Edinburgh: Churchill Livingstone
14. Stricker, B. H. and Spoelstra, P. (1985). Drug-induced Hepatic Injury. Amsterdam: Elsevier
15. Bass, N. M. and Ockner, R. K. (1990). Drug-induced liver disease. In Zakim, D. and Boyer, T. D. (eds). Hepatology. A textbook of liver disease. 2nd edition edn. pp. 754–791. Philadelphia: Saunders
16. Wepler, W. and Opitz, K. (1972). Histological changes in the liver biopsy in Amanita phalloides intoxication. Hum. Pathol., 3, 249–254
17. Clark, R., Thompson, R. P. H., Borirakchanyavat, V., Widdop, B., Davidson, A. R., Goulding, R. and Williams, R. (1973). Hepatic damage and death from overdose of paracetamol. Lancet, 1, 66–70
18. Boukowsky, H. L., Mudge, G. H. and McMurty, R. J. (1978). Chronic hepatic inflammation and fibrosis due to low doses of paracetamol. Lancet, 1, 1016–1018
19. Black, M. (1980). Acetaminophen toxicity. Gastroenterology, 78, 382–392
20. O'Grady, J. G., Alexander, G. J. M., Hayllar, K. M. and Williams, R. (1989). Early indicators of prognosis in fulminant hepatic failure. Gastroenterology, 97, 439–445
21. Portmann, B., Talbot, I. C., Day, D. W., Davidson, A. R., Murray-Lyon, I. M. and Williams, R. (1975). Histopathological changes in the liver following paracetamol overdose: correlation with clinical and biochemical parameters. J. Pathol., 117, 169–181
22. Zimmerman, H. J. (1981). Effects of aspirin and acetaminophen in the liver. Arch. Intern. Med., 141, 333–342
23. Neuberger, J., Davis, M. and Williams, R. (1980). Long-term ingestion of paracetamol and liver disease. J. R. Soc. Med., 73, 701
24. Smilkstein, M. J., Knapp, G. L., Fulig, K. W. and Rumack, B. H. (1988). Efficacy of oral N-acetylcysteine in the treatment of acetaminophen overdose. Analysis of the national multicenter study (1976–1985). N. Engl. J. Med., 319, 1557–1562

25. Bianchi, L., De Groote, J., Desmet, V., Gedigk, P., Korb, G., Popper, H., Poulsen, H., Scheuer, P. J., Schmid, M., Thaler, H. and Wepler, W. (1974). Guidelines for diagnosis of therapeutic drug-induced liver injury in liver biopsies. Review by an international group. Lancet, 1, 854–857

26. Rodman, J. S., Deutsch, D. J. and Gutman, S. I. (1976). Methyldopa hepatitis. A report of six cases and review of the literature. Am. J. Med., 60, 941–948

27. Toghill, P. J., Smith, P. G., Benton, P., Brown, R. C. and Matthew, H. L. (1974). Methyldopa liver damage. Br. Med. J., 3, 545–548

28. Neuberger, J., Kenna, J. G., Nouri Aria, K. and Williams, R. (1985). Antibody mediated hepatocyte injury in methyl dopa induced hepatotoxicity. Gut, 26, 1233–1239

29. Reynolds, T. B., Peters, R. L. and Yamada, S. (1971). Chronic active and lupoid hepatitis caused by a laxative, oxyphenisatin. N. Engl. J. Med., 285, 813–820

30. Maddrey, W. C. and Boitnott, J. K. (1977). Drug-induced chronic liver disease. Gastroenterology, 72, 1348–1353

31. Sharp, J. R., Ishak, K. G. and Zimmerman, H. J. (1980). Chronic active hepatitis and severe hepatic necrosis associated with Nitrofurantoin. Ann. Intern. Med., 92, 14–19

32. Pessayre, D., Bichara, M., Feldmann, G., Degott, C., Potet, F. and Benhamou, J.-P. (1979). Perhexiline maleate-induced cirrhosis. Gastroenterology, 76, 170–177

33. Simon, J. B., Manley, P. N., Brien, J. F. and Armstrong, P. W. (1984). Amiodarone hepatotoxicity simulating alcoholic liver disease. N. Engl. J. Med., 311, 167–172

34. Zimmerman, H. J. (1979). Drug-induced chronic hepatic disease. Med. Clin. N. Am., 63, 567–582

35. Dietrichson, O. (1975). Chronic active hepatitis. Aetiological considerations based on clinical and serologic studies. Scand. J. Gastroenterol., 10, 617–624

36. Dienstag, J. L. (1980). Halothane hepatitis: allergy or idiosyncracy. N. Engl. J. Med., 303, 102–104

37. Wright, R., Eade, O. E., Chisholm, M., Hawksley, M., Lloyd, B., Moles, T. M., Edwards, J. C. and Gardner, M. J. (1975). Controlled prospective study of the effect on liver function of multiple exposures to halothane. Lancet, 1, 817–820

38. Walton, B., Simpson, B. R., Strumin, L., Doniach, D., Perrin, J. and Appleyard, A. J. (1976). Unexplained hepatitis following halothane. Br. Med. J., 1, 1171–1176

39. Kenna, J. G., Neuberger, J. and Williams, R. (1988). Evidence for expression in human liver of halothane-induced neoantigens recognized by antibodies in sera from patients with halothane hepatitis. Hepatology, 8, 1635–1641

40. Peters, R. L., Edmondson, H. A., Reynolds, T. B., Meister, J. C. and Curphey, T. J. (1969). Hepatic necrosis associated with halothane anaesthesia. Am. J. Med., 47, 748–764

41. Benjamin, S. B., Goodman, Z. D., Ishak, K. G., Zimmerman, H. J. and Irey, N. S. (1985). The morphologic spectrum of halothan-induced hepatic injury: analysis of 77 cases. Hepatology, 5, 1163–1171

42. Wills, E. J. (1978). A morphological study of unexplained hepatitis following halothane anaesthesia. Am. J. Pathol., 9I, 11–32

43. Peters, R. L., Edmondson, H. A., Mikkelsen, W. P. and Tatter, D. (1967). Tetracycline-induced fatty liver in non-pregnant patients. Am. J. Surg., 113, 622–632

44. Zimmerman, H. J. and Ishak, K. G. (1982). Valproate induced hepatic injury: analysis of 23 fatal cases. Hepatology, 2, 591–597

45. McMaster, K. R. and Hennigar, G. R. (1981). Drug induced granulomatous hepatitis. Lab. Invest., 44, 61–73

46. Westaby, D., Ogle, S. J., Paradinas, F. J., Randell, J. B. and Murray-Lyon, I. M. (1977). Liver damage from long-term methyltestosterone. Lancet, 2, 261–263

47. Paradinas, F. J., Bull, T. B., Westaby, D. and Murray-Lyon, I. M. (1977). Hyperplasia and prolapse of hepatocytes into hepatic veins during long-term methyl testosterone therapy: possible relationships of these changes to the development of peliosis hepatis and liver tumours. Histopathology, 1, 225–246

48. Regal, R. E., Billi, J. E. and Glazer, H. M. (1987). Phenothiazine-induced cholestatic jaundice. Clin Pharm, 6, 787–794

49. Dahl, M. G. C., Gregory, M. M. and Scheuer, P. J. (1971). Liver damage due to methotrexate in patients with psoriasis. Br. Med. J., 1, 625–630

50. Nyfors, A. (1976). Liver biopsies from psoriatics related to methotrexate therapy. 1. Findings in 123 consecutive non-methotrezate treated patients. Acta Pathol. Microbiol. Scand. [A], 84, 253–261

51. Nyfors, A. and H., P. (1976). Liver biopsies from psoriatics related to methotrexate therapy. 2. Findings before and after methotrexate therapy in 88 patients. A blind study. Acta Pathol. Microbiol. Scand. [A], 84, 262–270

52. Nyfors, A. (1977). Liver biopsies from patients related to methotrexate therapy 3. Findings in post-methotrexate liver biopsies from 160 psoriatics. Acta Pathol. Microbiol. Scand. [A], 85, 511–518

53. Thomas, L. B., Popper, H., Berk, P. D., Selikoff, I. and Falk, H. (1975). Vinyl chloride induced liver disease. From idiopathic portal hypertension (Banti's syndrome) to angiosarcomas. N. Engl. J. Med., 292, 17–22

54. Forouhar, F., Nadel, M. S. and Gondos, B. (1984). Hepatic pathology in vitamin A toxicity. Ann Clin Lab Sci, 14, 304–310

Cirrhosis

11

There has been controversy over the precise definition of cirrhosis but there now seems to be general agreement[1] that it is characterized by diffuse, that is to say involving the whole liver although not necessarily equally, fibrosis with the normal lobular architecture converted into structurally abnormal nodules. Although earlier definitions included a statement about necrosis, this has now generally been dropped since, even when an important pathogenetic factor, there is frequently little or no evidence of liver cell necrosis in established cirrhosis. In many ways, cirrhosis can be regarded as the end-stage response of the liver to a wide variety of different insults and an important feature of the diagnosis is that it is generally regarded as irreversible and inevitably fatal. (Wilson's disease under effective treatment may be an important exception to this rule, see Chapter 15) Thus it is important that diagnosis should be accurate.

Diffuseness can of course only be inferred from blind needle biopsy and it is most important that the interpretation should be made in context with the clinical and biochemical findings. These too, however, may be very unreliable[2] in inactive cirrhosis. Additional information about the macroscopic appearance of the liver gleaned at laparotomy or laparoscopy should thus always be taken into consideration. Figure 22.4 gives an example of the importance of this kind of correlation. Although the surgical wedge biopsy taken at laparotomy is wholly abnormal and apparently cirrhotic, the surgeon was able to report that this was an isolated nodule in an otherwise normal liver with a smooth surface. This is thus an example of focal nodular hyperplasia (Chapter 22). Conversely, diffuse nodularity without fibrosis, as in nodular regenerative hyperplasia (Chapter 22), is not cirrhosis. Finally, there is a number of conditions which are not considered to be cirrhotic because, although there may be both diffuse fibrosis and parenchymal nodularity, the basic lobular architecture is preserved within the nodules (Table 11.1). Congenital hepatic fibrosis and the earlier phases of primary biliary 'cirrhosis' are two examples of this phenomenon.

Cirrhotic nodules lack normal lobular organization and are surrounded by fibrous bands of variable thickness

Table 11.1 Conditions which may be confused with cirrhosis morphologically

Precirrhotic conditions
Biliary cirrhosis (early)
Venous outflow obstruction
Alcoholic hepatitis
Chronic active hepatitis
Sarcoidosis fibrosis

Fibrosis which is not normally cirrhotic
Ductal plate malformations
Radiation fibrosis
Schistosomiasis
Gaucher's disease

Focal conditions
Partial nodular transformation
Focal nodular hyperplasia
Cystic fibrosis

Miscellaneous
Severe hepatocellular necrosis with bridging

(Figures 11.2 and 11.3). The liver cell plates may be of normal single cell thickness, particularly if they are derived from dissection of pre-existing lobules by passive septa. More commonly they display some evidence of regeneration in the form of large cells, often multinucleate or polyploid, with twinning of liver cell plates. This can best be recognized by the position of the nuclei on the sinusoidal surface. Larger nodules may show evidence of uneven growth with foci of actively growing cells compressing their neighbours. Nodules may or may not contain internal vessels. When these are present they may be structurally abnormal, for example portal tracts may be abnormally small, or they may have an abnormal relationship to one another. There is often an excess of efferent veins. These vessels may be pre-existing or newly formed or modified.

There are two main clinical consequences of cirrhosis, the effects of portal hypertension and of liver cell failure. Although both are often in operation, terminal patients usually present with one or the other in the first instance.

PORTAL HYPERTENSION

Portal hypertension is usually considered to be due to a post-sinusoidal compression of hepatic vein tributaries by nodules; however, since there is almost no pressure drop from the hepatic sinusoid to the vena cava[3], a sinusoidal block is probably equally as important. This is due partly to a reduction in the vascular bed by fibrosis and partly to perisinusoidal fibrosis. Added to these are the effects of arteriovenous anastomoses within the septa, which bring arterial pressure to bear on the portal vein, and of portal fibrosis. Paradoxically the splenomegaly, which is one of the consequences of portal hypertension, may aggravate it by increasing splenic blood flow. The important clinical consequence of portal hypertension is the development of extrahepatic portal–systemic shunts. The latter may contribute to the increased susceptibility to infection of patients with cirrhosis.

The distended thin-walled veins in the submucosa of the lower oesophagus are easily traumatized by food passing down the oesophagus and once bleeding has started it may be difficult or impossible to stop. Hence variceal haemorrhage is a common cause of death in cirrhosis. Portal hypertension may also occur in any form of portal fibrosis without cirrhosis.

LIVER CELL FAILURE

Liver cell failure, manifest as jaundice, portal systemic encephalopathy and bleeding diathesis, may be a consequence of continuing liver cell necrosis as in acute alcoholic injury superimposed upon the cirrhosis. However, independently of liver cell integrity, intrahepatic portal systemic shunts and reduced efficiency of the intrahepatic microcirculation caused by new perisinusoidal basement membrane formation and fibrosis will deprive the body of liver cell function. These haemodynamic changes may thus contribute to liver cell failure. They may also permit endotoxins and other substances normally filtered out by the liver to gain access to the systemic circulation and perhaps contribute to the increased tendency to infection, leucocytosis, cardiovascular changes

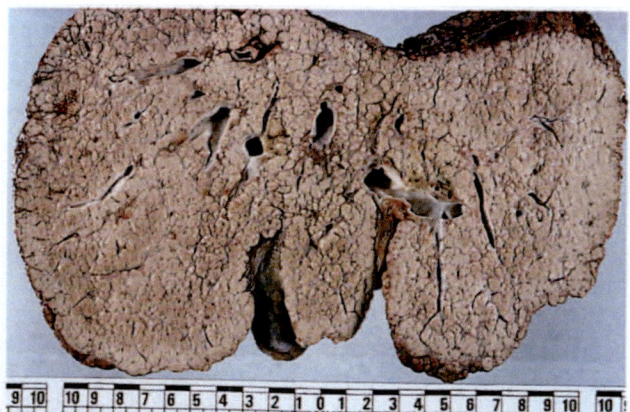

Figure 11.1 Micronodular cirrhosis. A 51-year-old male with known alcoholic liver disease died of gastrointestinal haemorrhage due to bleeding from oesophageal varices. The liver weighed 1440 g and section shows a typical micronodular cut surface with uniform nodules all about 0.3 cm in diameter.

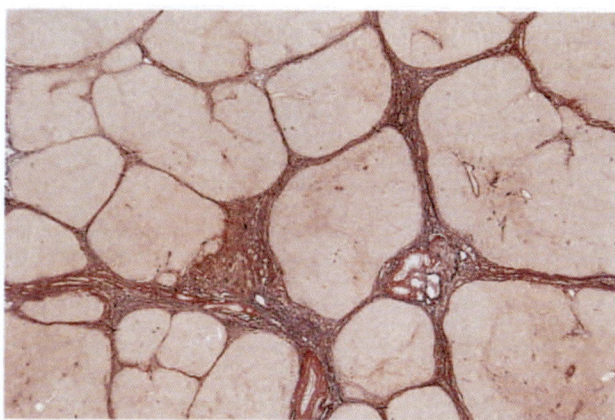

Figure 11.2 Micronodular cirrhosis. A 25-year-old female with micronodular cirrhosis following chronic active hepatitis. The liver was removed at transplantation and shows very uniform nodules all near to lobular size and most without vessels. The septa are thin. Elastic van Gieson.

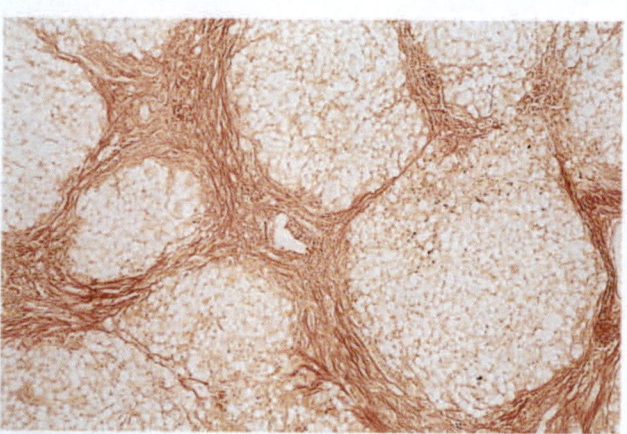

Figure 11.3 Micronodular cirrhosis, alcoholic. A 68-year-old male with long history of alcoholism died with progressive hepatic failure. Section shows typical alcoholic cirrhosis in which all the nodules are of lobular size or less and devoid of vascular structures because pre-existing portal tracts, and terminal hepatic venules have been linked by fibrous septa. Note also marked diffuse fatty change. Elastic van Gieson.

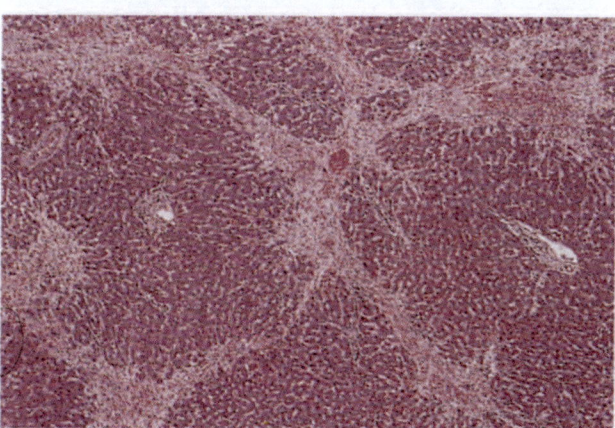

Figure 11.4 Cardiac fibrosis/cirrhosis. A 71-year-old male with long standing chronic lung disease and congestive heart failure (same case as Figure 18.17). The section has an overall resemblance to Figure 11.4, but here the lobules are outlined by central to central fibrous septa with portal tracts at the centre of the nodules.

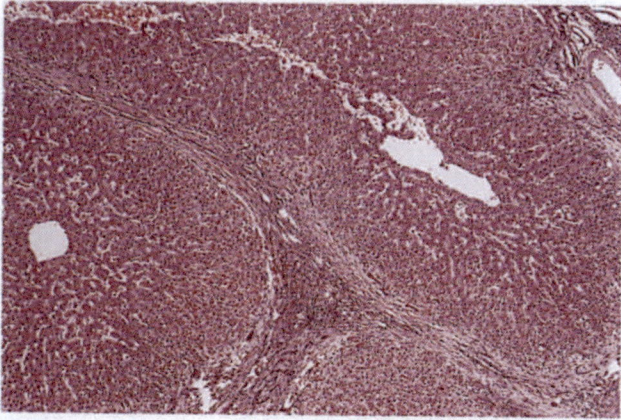

Figure 11.5 Biliary fibrosis/cirrhosis. A 44-year-old female with recurrent biliary strictures following surgery to the biliary tract eventually developed a nodular liver with portal hypertension. The section shows biliary fibrosis with septa linking adjacent portal tracts. Note, however, that the lobular architecture is preserved with normal terminal hepatic venules.

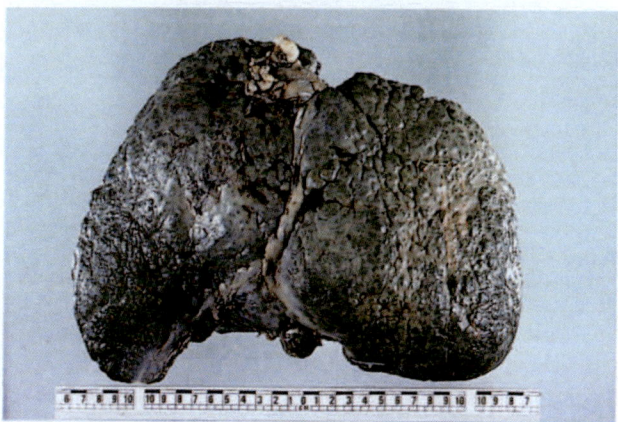

Figure 11.6 Primary biliary cirrhosis. A 56-year-old male with a 4-year history of PBC. The liver is characteristically very dark green and micronodular. Biliary obstruction causes an identical picture.

and renal effects of liver failure. Finally, both the portal hypertension, by increasing lymph flow, and liver cell failure, through hypoalbuminaemia, contribute to ascites.

CLASSIFICATION

Although many pathologists still use the traditional terms, such as portal cirrhosis and post-necrotic cirrhosis, these are misleading and should no longer be used. Two methods of classification are currently in use: morphological and aetiological, both of which are complementary to one another. Neither is ideal. For example, the disease in an individual patient may change from one morphological category to another and the cause of many cases of cirrhosis remains undetermined.

Morphological classification

Morphological classification on the basis of nodular size, although now well established, is of somewhat limited value. The same morphological pattern can be produced by a variety of causal agents and a single agent can produce a variety of morphological patterns. Nevertheless, it may be of epidemiological value and may reflect aetiology and stage of evolution and prognosis to some extent. A practical point of not inconsiderable importance is that a diagnosis of micronodular cirrhosis by needle biopsy can almost always be made confidently, whereas that of macronodular cirrhosis is often by implication only.

Micronodular cirrhosis (monolobular, portal, Laennec's)

This is defined as cirrhosis in which virtually all the nodules are less than 0.3 cm in diameter, and thus correspond roughly in size to a pre-existing lobule which measures 0.1–0.2 cm in diameter. There is often a striking uniformity of nodular size and septa tend to be slender (Figures 11.1 and 11.2). The liver as a whole may be of normal size but is frequently enlarged. The micronodular pattern is usual but not invariable in cirrhosis due to alcohol, biliary obstruction, haemochromatosis and Indian childhood cirrhosis. The colour of the liver or of the biopsy may give a clue to the aetiology. Alcoholic injury is frequently associated with fatty infiltration which may cause considerable hepatic enlargement and impart a pale yellow colour to the biopsy which will float in fixative. In biliary obstruction, the liver is usually dark green in colour, whilst in haemochromatosis it is dark brown.

Microscopically the nodules are usually devoid of vascular structures, especially in the alcoholic where they are generally considered to arise by a process of dissection of pre-existing lobules (Figure 11.3). In this group typically there is fibrosis around the terminal venule communicating with that in the expanding portal tracts so that sublobular nodules of parenchyma are surrounded and separated by irregular portal-central bridges[4]. All major vessels are then peripheral to these nodules. In other cases, however, portal tracts (especially in the cirrhosis following venous outflow obstruction (Figure 11.4), or terminal venules (for example in biliary obstruction or haemochromatosis (Figure 11.5), may be found within nodules.

Macronodular cirrhosis (multilobular, post-necrotic)

Here the nodules are generally greater than 0.3 cm in diameter and often reach 3 cm or more. Any liver with a significant proportion of larger nodules should probably be put into this group. The mixed category sometimes used serves only to bring the morphological classification further into disrepute, since if criteria were to be strictly applied, virtually all livers would be classified as mixed. Macroscopically, macronodular livers may be of normal size but are frequently reduced sometimes to as little as 700–800 g.

Two subcategories can be recognized[1]. In one, the macronodules are divided by slender, sometimes incomplete and blind-ending septa which tend to link portal tracts (Figures 11.7 and 11.8). This is known as incomplete septal cirrhosis and the nodularity is not always apparent macroscopically (Figure 11.7). This type may cause considerable problems of diagnosis by biopsy. It seems to be a particularly common type in the tropical and subtropical areas of the world and is especially associated with hepatitis B.

The other subcategory contains the traditional 'hobnail' liver with large macronodules often separated by broad septa (Figures 11.9–11.11). The latter may contain several adjacent portal tracts, often best recognized by elastic stains, and are thus assumed to have been formed by a process of collapse (hence the old term post-necrotic cirrhosis (Figure 11.12). This collapse is not necessarily part of the original process but may be secondary. Only in primary collapse will there be preservation of normal relationships between portal tract and portal tract, and with efferent veins (Figure 11.12). The left lobe seems particularly susceptible to primary collapse and is often very small (Figure 11.11).

As already stated, larger nodules may have residual or newly grown vascular structures. These frequently show an excess of efferent veins and normal relationships are not seen. Portal tracts when present are often abnormally small.

There is a tendency for micronodular livers to become macronodular with the passage of time. This is particularly true if the primary cause can be withdrawn, for example, if the alcoholic stops drinking. In micronodular cirrhosis the balance is in favour of liver cell destruction rather than regeneration at a lobular level; whereas in macronodular cirrhosis, although there is some regeneration as shown by the presence of large nodules, the overall reduction in size may largely be attributable to secondary collapse not necessarily caused by the original agent. Carcinoma less commonly complicates micronodular cirrhosis than macronodular, although haemochromatosis – which is usually micronodular – is an exception to this rule since it probably has the highest incidence of malignant transformation of any cirrhosis in the UK. In both situations it may merely be a reflection of longer survival (see Chapter 23).

Pathogenesis

Necrosis

All types of cirrhosis are often assumed to follow necrosis of liver cells. In some cases this is frank and obvious, as following viral hepatitis or alcoholic injury. In other cases it may be low grade injury, as in certain metabolic disorders[5]. However, it seems probable that a single episode of necrosis alone is insufficient to cause cirrhosis, as follow-up studies of patients surviving fulminant viral hepatitis[6] have shown that restitution to normal is the rule. Thus there must be sustained injury to liver cells. This may be due to continued presence of the cause, as in metabolic or enzymic abnormalities, or continued exposure to alcohol in the alcoholic. In addition to the primary cause Popper[5] has identified three additional or secondary factors which may operate, to which a fourth and fifth should probably be added.

(1) *Immunological hepatocellular injury.* This is now well established as playing a major role in the pathogenesis of the chronic hepatitis and cirrhosis following hepatitis

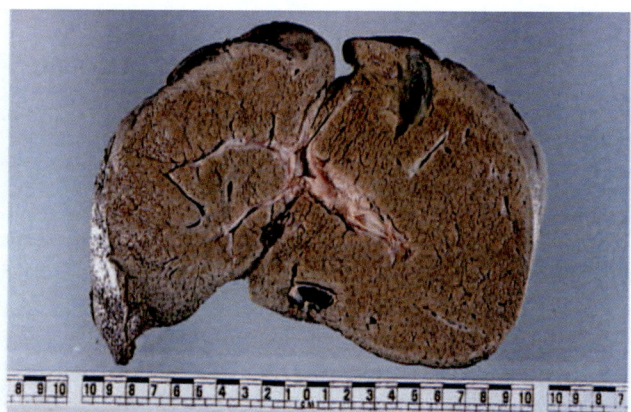

Figure 11.7 Incomplete septal cirrhosis. A 34-year-old male who presented with portal hypertension. The liver, which weighed 1450 g, had a smooth capsular surface but the cut surface is faintly nodular.

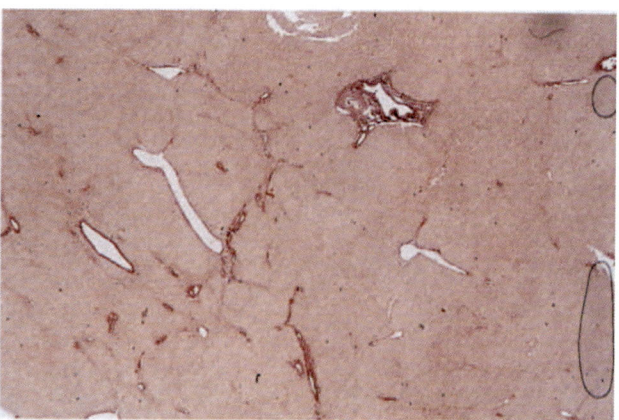

Figure 11.8 Incomplete septal cirrhosis. Same case as Figure 11.7. The section shows that although the relationships of central veins and portal tracts are abnormal, septa are thin and poorly developed in this part of the liver. Elsewhere fibrosis was more marked. Elastic van Gieson.

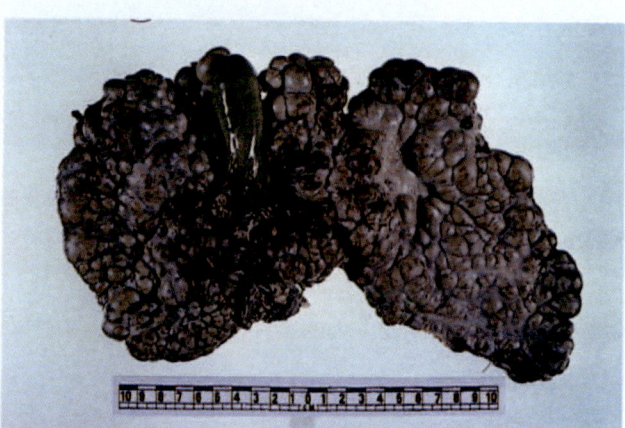

Figure 11.9 Macronodular cirrhosis (idiopathic). A 25year-old male with insidious onset of portal hypertension with oesophageal varices. The liver was excised at transplantation and weighed 1195 g. It has a typical 'hob-nail' external surface. On section, the nodules measured up to 3 cm in diameter.

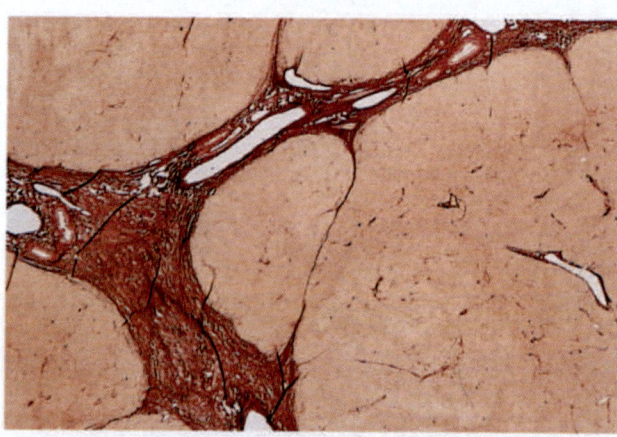

Figure 11.10 Macronodular cirrhosis. Same case as Figure 11.9. Note the large nodules with internal vessels and thin septa. This photograph is at the same magnification as Figure 11.2. Elastic van Gieson.

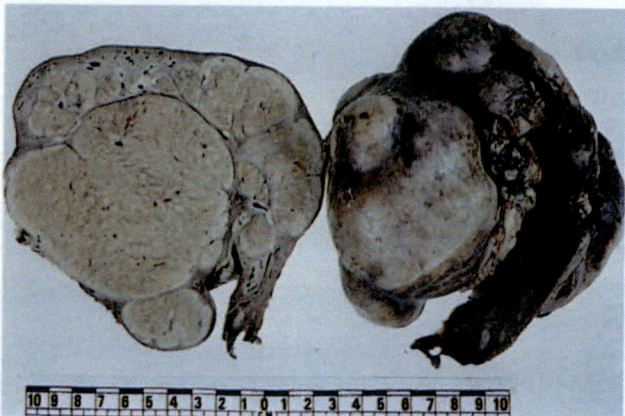

Figure 11.11 Macronodular cirrhosis (idiopathic). A 29-year-old female with portal hypertension and oesophageal varices. The excised liver weighed 750 g and was cut coronally, both halves being photographed together. The cut surface shows that the right lobe consists of a small number of very large nodules whilst the left lobe (lower right on each slice) has collapsed completely. This is the classic picture of 'post-necrotic scarring'.

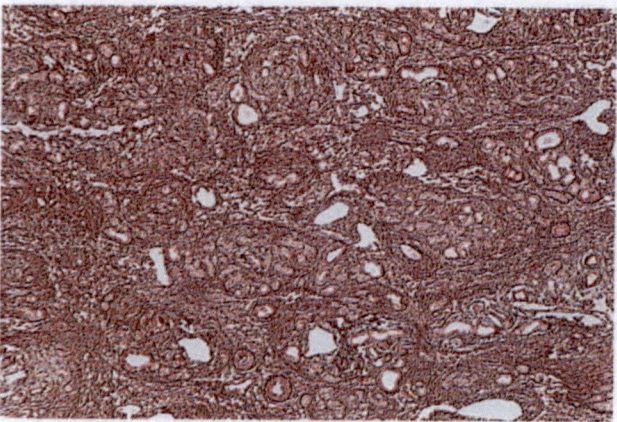

Figure 11.12 Macronodular cirrhosis, primary collapse. Same case as Figure 11.11. This section from the left lobe shows complete disappearance of hepatocytes with collapse of the lobular architecture. Nevertheless normal relationships between central veins and portal tracts are preserved, thus the collapse was probably part of the primary attack upon the liver. Reticulin, neutral red.

B infection. Contrary to previous teaching, it is the mild or inapparent case which is more likely to be followed by chronic disease. The liver damage is thought to be antibody-mediated by an autoimmune mechanism following failure of elimination of the virus. There is good correlation between the morphological features of chronic hepatitis, especially piecemeal necrosis, in these cases and clinical signs of decompensation. Drugs such as oxyphenisatin and methyldopa may operate in a very similar manner and indeed the chronic hepatitis may clear when the drug is withdrawn. Autoimmune chronic hepatitis has a similar mechanism, with an immunological attack being mounted against a self-protein. The mere presence of chronic hepatitis therefore does not indicate a particular aetiological diagnosis.

(2) *Anoxic injury.* This may be caused by the abnormal vascular communication already described and by encirclement of liver cells by fibrosis. The consequence may be collapse and cell loss impossible to distinguish from that due to other causes, and is thought to be a major cause of secondary collapse. This should not be confused with the hypovolaemic necrosis seen commonly as a terminal event following gastrointestinal haemorrhage. This is an acute coagulative necrosis often with a pseudolobular distribution in the centre of nodules (Figure 18.8).

(3) *Bile injury.* This may be part of the primary cause or secondary to obstruction of canaliculi within nodules, and most often at the point of entry into the septa. Bile retention leads to feathery degeneration and necrosis in the usual way.

(4) *Copper accumulation.* In primary biliary cirrhosis, as in any prolonged cholestasis, there is a secondary failure of excretion of copper in the bile and this may itself be responsible for tissue damage (see Chapter 17).

(5) *Portal blood deprivation.* Deprivation of hepatotrophic factors in portal blood, particularly insulin, is the main cause of liver atrophy in Eck's fistula, and in Starzl's portal diversion experiments[7]. This is also the main explanation for the atrophy of liver cells that occurs in a Zahn's infarct, which is due to occlusion of a portal vein branch (Chapter 10). A similar explanation can account for the nodularity reported in portacaval diversion in rats[8] and which is seen in *nodular regenerative hyperplasia*, where there is atrophy of cells in zone 3 and reactive hyperplasia of those in zone 1[9]. It seems very probable that the late development of nodularity in biliary cirrhosis, occurring after portal fibrosis is well-established, is primarily due to this mechanism (Chapter 17).

Inflammation
Injury or death of liver cells is followed by inflammation. Lymphocytes and plasma cells usually predominate, but eosinophils and neutrophils are occasionally seen, the latter particularly in association with proliferating bile ductules and cells containing hyalin. Parenchymal inflammation is a good guide to activity and speed of progression of the disease, and is particularly associated in this context with piecemeal necrosis (Figure 11.13). Inflammation confined to septa is of much lesser significance.

Fibrosis
Following isolated liver cell injury, normal total liver cell mass is rapidly achieved through the organ's capacity for regeneration. If, however, regeneration occurs in a liver whose architecture has been disturbed by diffuse fibrosis,

then it is likely to be nodular, especially if the agent concerned has also damaged the basic acinar framework[10]. The key to cirrhosis is thus fibrosis, which may have many causes and almost certainly occurs by way of more than one pathogenetic route. Most fibrosis is comparable to that in wound repair, namely it follows inflammation, itself caused by a variety of stimuli. The inflammatory cells are then responsible for secretion of a variety of cytokines, including various interleukins, transforming growth factor β and platelet derived growth factor, all of which stimulate fibrosis[11,12]. It seems probable that the main source of new collagen within the parenchyma is the sinusoidal lipocyte (Ito cell)[13,14]. In conditions where there is little evidence of liver cell necrosis or of inflammation, such as haemochromatosis, iron-laden hepatocytes may directly stimulate cytokine release[15].

The more rapid development of true cirrhosis, in both biliary obstruction and iron overload, in childhood than in adults may be a reflection of the increased capacity for growth and regeneration of the child's liver.

Aetiological classification

Table 11.2 lists various types of cirrhosis, grouped by possible mechanism of fibrosis. It is clear that some conditions may have more than one mechanism. For example, as already discussed above, the sustained injury to liver cells in chronic hepatitis B infection may well have a strong or even dominant immunological component.

Table 11.2 Aetiological classification of cirrhosis*

Initiating factor	Examples
Hypoxia	Cardiac Budd-Chiari syndrome Veno-occlusive disease
Drugs & Toxins	Alcohol Methyl Dopa
Infective	Hepatitis B Hepatitis D Hepatitis C
Immunological	Autoimmune chronic hepatitis
Metabolic	Wilson's disease Haemochromatosis α_1-Antitrypsin deficiency Tyrosinaemia Glycogen storage disease Galactosaemia
Cholestasis	Primary biliary cirrhosis Primary sclerosing cholangitis Secondary biliary cirrhosis
Miscellaneous	Cryptogenic Indian childhood cirrhosis

* Based on Wight, D. G. D. (1993). Introduction, reactions of the liver to injury. In Wight, D. G. D. (ed.). *Liver, Biliary Tract and Endocrine Pancreas.* Vol. 11. Systemic Pathology. Symmers, W. S. C., series ed. 3rd edn. Edinburgh: Church Livingstone

DIAGNOSIS OF CIRRHOSIS BY BIOPSY

Although diagnosis can usually be confidently made on surgical wedge biopsies, these can be misleading as subcapsular fibrosis is sometimes an isolated finding[16]. However if the biopsy is sufficiently large it will be seen that only in cirrhosis do the changes extend into the deeper part of the liver. Needle biopsies may pose considerably more problems. Many of these have been resolved by the appearance of needles with a cutting

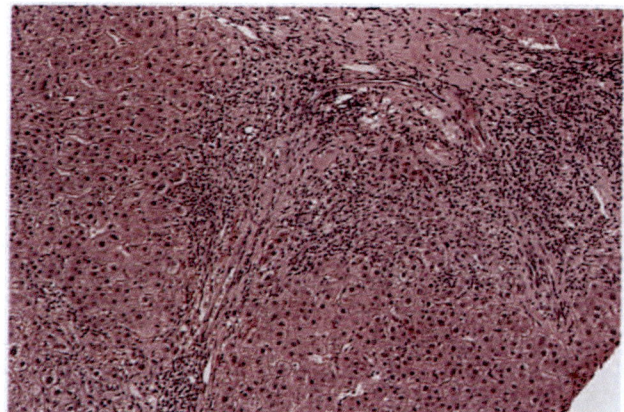

Figure 11.13 Active macronodular cirrhosis. A 54-year-old female patient with chronic active hepatitis which has progressed to cirrhosis. Section shows continuing 'activity' with piecemeal necrosis at the periphery of the nodules as well as chronic inflammatory cell infiltration of the septa.

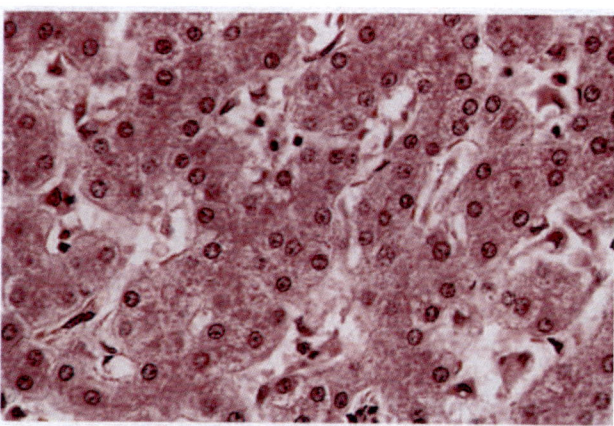

Figure 11.14 Macronodular cirrhosis. This section shows a focus of regenerative activity with twinning of liver cell plates. Note that in many cases the hepatocyte nuclei are adjacent to the sinusoidal edge of the cell.

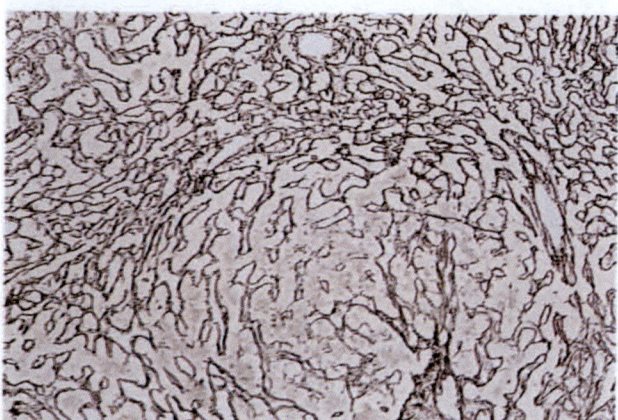

Figure 11.15 Macronodular cirrhosis. This section provides evidence of differential growth rates within a single nodule. The focus of twin cell plates (below centre) is apparently causing compression of the adjacent thin plates. Reticulin.

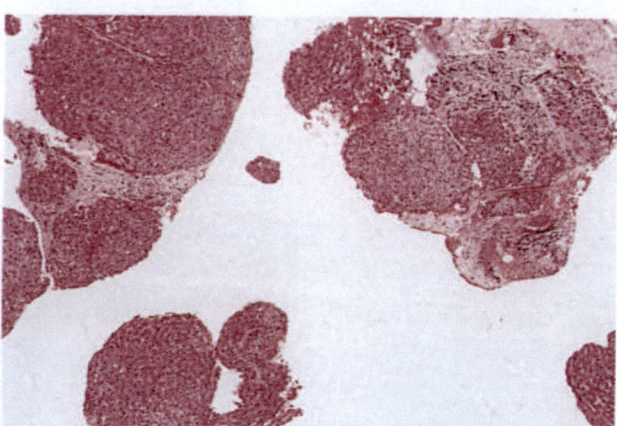

Figure 11.16 Macronodular cirrhosis. This aspiration biopsy has fragmented, providing strong suspicion of cirrhosis, although the liver tissue itself contains little direct evidence of cirrhosis other than the rounded contour of the fragments.

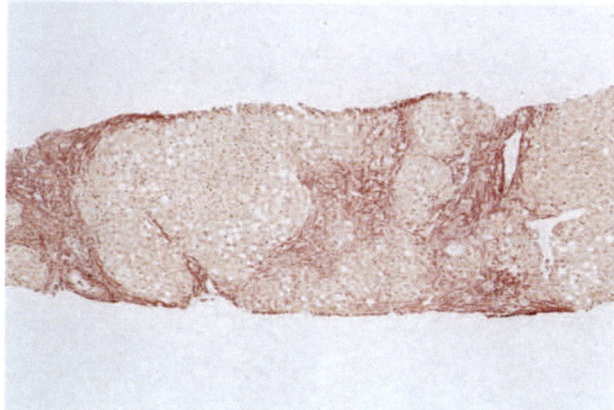

Figure 11.17 Macronodular cirrhosis. Same patient as Figure 11.16. A subsequent biopsy performed by the same operator but with a needle with a cutting action. The biopsy now includes septa as well as parenchyma and its cirrhotic nature can be confirmed. Elastic van Gieson.

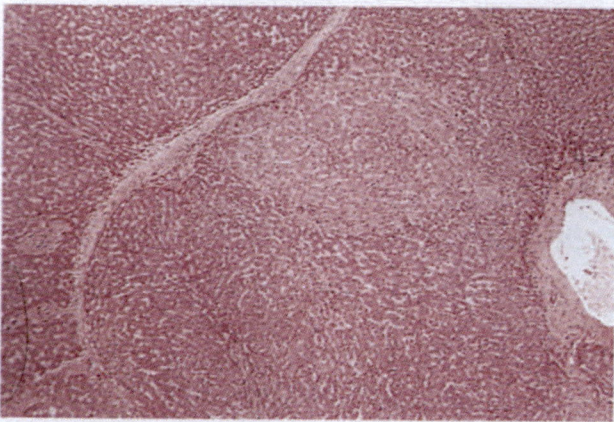

Figure 11.18 Incomplete septal cirrhosis. Same case as Figure 11.7 and 11.8. Note the long, thin, curved septum traversing the field and an abnormal lobular architecture.

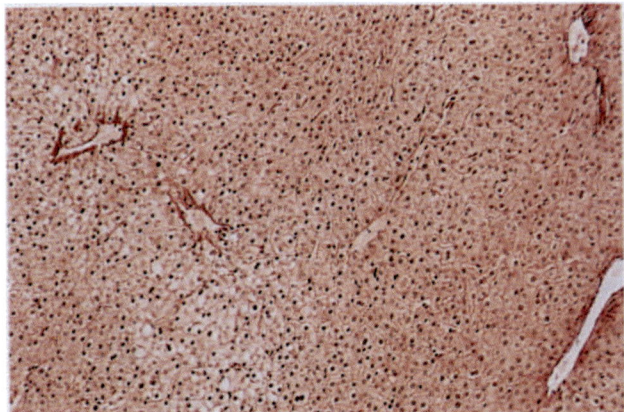

Figure 11.19 Macronodular cirrhosis. Same case as Figure 11.9 and 11.10. Section from within a nodule showing a great excess of terminal hepatic venules. Elastic van Gieson.

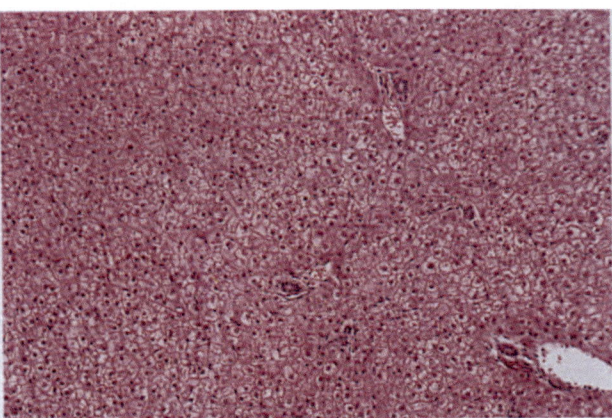

Figure 11.20 Macronodular cirrhosis. Same case as Figure 11.9, 11.10 and 11.19. Another section shows abnormal lobular architecture with several very small portal tracts, consisting only of a small bile duct.

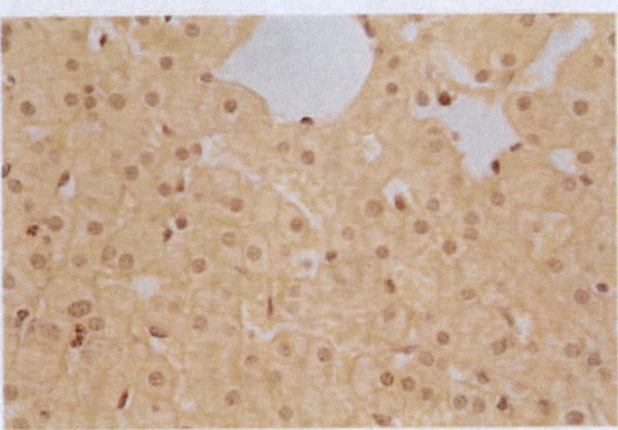

Figure 11.21 Macronodular cirrhosis. A 40-year-old patient with a macronodular cirrhosis following chronic active hepatitis. Note the complete absence of lipofuscin around this efferent vein. PAS diastase, ponceau S counterstain.

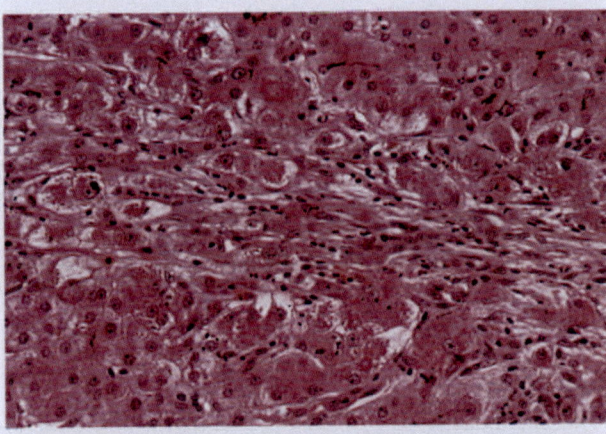

Figure 11.22 Cirrhosis, hyalin and peripheral cholestasis. Abundant hyalin can be seen in hepatocytes adjacent to the horizontal septum and bile plugs are visible, particularly at the top of the field.

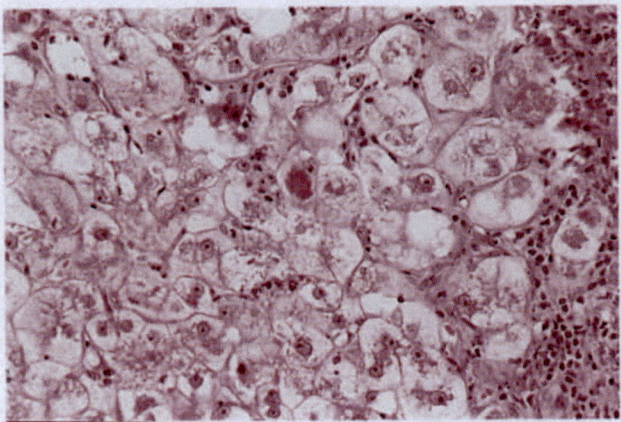

Figure 11.23 Active cirrhosis, hyalin. Hyalin and ballooning near the periphery of a cirrhotic nodule. Note also the chronic inflammatory cell infiltrate and piecemeal necrosis at the right margin.

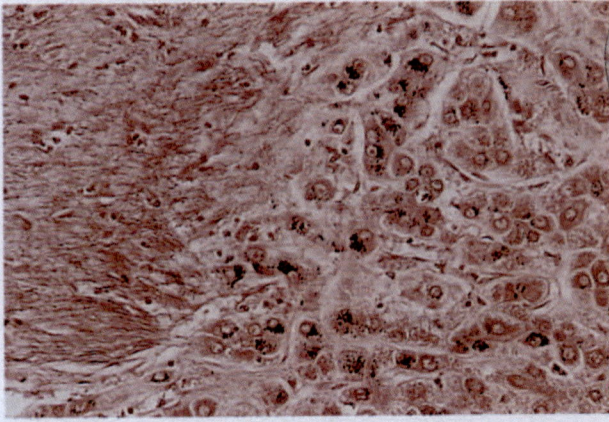

Figure 11.24 Cirrhosis, copper-associated protein. Black granules of copper-associated protein in peripheral hepatocytes. Orcein.

action, such as the Trucut®, since, unlike the aspiration needles of Menghini type, these are not deflected by connective tissue, and fragmentation is uncommon. Nevertheless, modern versions of the latter are also highly successful and they have the advantage that it is often possible to produce a much larger specimen than the Trucut®.

The main problems in diagnosis are two-fold. Firstly, is the liver cirrhotic, and, if so, what is the aetiology? Conditions which may be confused with cirrhosis are those conditions which cause fibrosis alone but which do not usually go on to a true cirrhosis (Table 11.1), or in which cirrhosis has not yet developed. It is clearly most important that cirrhosis should not be over-diagnosed because of the therapeutic and prognostic implications of this diagnosis. The diagnosis of micronodular cirrhosis is usually straightforward but a confident diagnosis of macronodular cirrhosis may be much more difficult. Helpful points include the following:

(1)   The presence of several nodules clearly surrounded by connective tissue septa. A single apparent nodule may merely represent tangential cutting of a promontory of parenchyma in a liver which is merely fibrotic.

(2)   Regenerative activity in the form of variation in liver cell size with twinning of liver cell plates (Figure 11.14) and evidence of differential growth and compression of other liver cells (Figure 11.15). Evidence of liver cell dysplasia (Chapter 23).

(3)   Fragmentation of the biopsy, especially if performed by an experienced operator (Figures 11.16 and 11.17). Connective tissue or reticulin stains may demonstrate fibrous tissue partly or wholly encircling the fragments.

(4)   Septa traversing the specimen especially if linking central and portal canals or if bent or zigzag and associated with abnormal lobular architecture (Figure 11.18).

(5)   Abnormal lobular architecture with excessive efferent veins (Figure 11.19), efferent veins in contact with septa, abnormal spacing of vessels, abnormal portal tracts (Figure 11.20), scanty or absent lipofuscin around efferent vessels in an adult (Figure 11.21).

These features may enable a fairly confident diagnosis of macronodular cirrhosis even in the complete absence of fibrous tissue.

COMPLICATIONS AND SECONDARY PHENOMENA

These are changes which may be seen in cirrhosis of any cause and thus do not give any clues to the aetiology.

(1)   Cholestasis. The presence of bile thrombi, particularly at the periphery of nodules, is common and probably due to fibrosis and distortion of the canaliculi at the point of entry into the septa (Figure 11.22). Cholestasis may also be due to drug therapy (for example, methyltestosterone to control itching), or to biliary obstruction by gallstones which are more common in cirrhosis.

(2)   Bile duct proliferation is common in any liver injury[17], and *per se* bears little relationship to the cause; it is often accompanied by a little inflammatory cell infiltration which may include neutrophils.

(3)   Mallory's hyalin (Figures 11.22 and 11.23) is commonly found in liver cells at the periphery of nodules in conditions as diverse as biliary obstruction, Wilson's disease, Indian childhood cirrhosis and α_1-antitrypsin deficiency. Similarly, copper accumulation, shown by orcein positivity (Figure 11.24), is a common sequel to biliary obstruction.

(4)   Iron accumulation may be a complication of portacaval anastomosis but is sometimes seen in cirrhosis of any cause, probably as a result of spontaneous shunting.

Finally, having taken all these secondary phenomena into consideration, it may be possible to detect certain additional morphological features and patterns which point to a particular aetiology. These are discussed individually in the appropriate chapter but can be summarized as follows:

(1)   Abundant fat, focal necroses with neutrophils and pericellular fibrosis all suggest alcoholic aetiology (Chapter 13). Similar changes may be seen in certain metabolic disorders of childhood, e.g. tyrosinosis, in a quite different clinical setting (Chapter 9).

(2)   Large amounts of iron in parenchymal cells, septa and phagocytes suggest haemochromatosis (Chapter 14).

(3)   Large amounts of peripheral copper-associated protein, combined often with abundant hyalin, suggest primary biliary cirrhosis and should prompt a search for other features of the disease, such as the characteristic bile ductules (Chapter 17). However, copper-associated protein is also found in biliary obstruction (Chapter 16), some phases of Wilson's disease (Chapter 15), Indian childhood cirrhosis and primary sclerosing cholangitis.

(4)   PAS-positive diastase-resistant globules point to α_1-antitrypsin deficiency (Chapter 8).

(5)   The architecture of the nodules may be very helpful (see above), particularly in alcoholic cirrhosis, biliary and cardiac fibrosis.

In a significant number of cases no cause for cirrhosis can be discovered by morphological examination.

REFERENCES

1.   Anthony, P., Ishak, K. G., Nayak, N. C., Poulsen, H. E., Scheuer, P. J. and Sobin, L. H. (1978). The morphology of cirrhosis. J. Clin. Pathol., 31, 395–414

2.   Carlisle, R., Galambos, J. T. and Warren, W. D. (1979). Relationship between conventional liver tests, quantitative function tests and histopathology in cirrhosis. Dig. Dis. Sci., 24, 358–362

3.   Laut, W. W. (1977). Hepatic vasculature – a conceptual review. Gastroenterol., 73, 1163–1169

4.   Friedman, S. L., Millward-Sadler, G. H. and Arthur, M. J. P. (1992). Liver fibrosis and cirrhosis. In Millward-Sadler, G. H., Wright, R. and Arthur, M. J. P. (eds). Wright's Liver and Biliary Disease. 3rd edn. pp. 821–881. London: W B Saunders

5.   Popper, H. (1977). Pathological aspects of cirrhosis. Am. J. Pathol., 87, 228–264

6.   Karvountzis, G. G., Redeker, A. G. and Peters, R. L. (1974). Long-term follow-up studies of patients surviving fulminant viral hepatitis. Gastroenterol., 67, 870–877

7.   Starzl, T. E. and Terblanche, J. (1979). Hepatotrophic substances. In Popper, H. and Schaffner, F. (eds). Progress in Liver Diseases. VI. pp. 135–151. New York: Grune and Stratton

8.   Weinbren, K. and Washington, S. L. A. (1976). Hyperplastic nodules after portacaval anastomosis in rats. Nature (London), 264, 440

9.   Wanless, I. R. (1990). Micronodular transformation (nodular regenerative hyperplasia) of the liver: a report of 64 cases among 2,500 autopsies and a new classification of benign hepatocellular nodules. Hepatology, 11, 787–797

10. Wight, D. G. D. (1993). Introduction, reactions of the liver to injury. In Wight, D. G. D. (ed). Liver, Biliary Tract and Exocrine Pancreas. Vol. 11. Systemic Pathology. Symmers, W. S. C. Series ed. 3rd edn. Edinburgh: Churchill Livingstone

11. Bissell, D. M. and Roll, J. (1990). Connective tissue metabolism and hepatic fibrosis. In Zakim, D. and Boyer, T. D. (eds). Hepatology. A textbook of liver disease. 2nd edition edn. pp. 424–444. Philadelphia: Saunders

12. Andus, T., Bauer, J. and Gerok, W. (1991). Effects of cytokines on the liver. Hepatology, 13, 364–375

13. Gressner, A. M. and Bachem, M. G. (1990). Cellular sources of non-collagenous matrix proteins: rvle of fat-storing cells in fibrogenesis. Semin. Liver Dis., 10, 30–46

14. Bissell, D. M., Friedman, S. L., Maher, J. J. and Roll, F. J. (1990). Connective tissue biology and hepatic fibrosis: report of a conference. Hepatology, 11, 488–498

15. Bacon, B. R. and Britton, R. S. (1990). The pathology of hepatic iron overload: a free radical mediated process? Hepatology, 11, 127–137

16. Petrelli, M. and Scheuer, P. J. (1967). Variation in subcapsular liver structure and its significance in the interpretation of wedge biopsies. J. Clin. Pathol., 20, 743–748

17. Masuko, K., Rubin, E. and Popper, H. (1964). Proliferation of bile ducts in cirrhosis. Arch. Pathol., 78, 421–431

Fatty Liver

12

Fatty change or steatosis in the liver is an extremely common finding, both in biopsies and at post-mortem. The fat is predominantly triacylglycerol (triglyceride) and may occur in the form of small droplets (microvesicular) or a single large vacuole which displaces the nucleus to one side of the cell (macrovesicular). Liver cell involvement may be focal, diffuse or zonal. Minor changes are frequently insignificant and cannot be attributed to any particular cause. The normal liver contains only about 5% of fat by weight, but in severe fatty change this may rise to 50% or more. Fatty change *per se* causes no consistent biochemical abnormality and is usually asymptomatic, although a few patients may recognize some fullness or tenderness over the liver[1]. In general, fatty liver is not regarded as a precirrhotic or prefibrotic condition, although some aetiological agents such as alcohol may cause both fatty change and cirrhosis. Fatty liver has been regarded as a cause of sudden death[2], although this is not a view which has general acceptance.

The pathogenesis of fatty change is complex. Fat which enters the liver cell is derived partly by transfer from fat stores and partly as chylomicra following absorption by the gut; there it is converted to triacylglycerol. Within the liver cells there is new synthesis of cholesterol and fatty acid and of phospholipid, the last necessary for micellar dispersal of the fat within the cell. Some fatty acid is also oxidized as an energy source. Finally, all three lipids in varying proportion are exported from the cell attached to a carrier apoprotein, also synthesized in the liver, as lipoproteins. Thus fat accumulation in the liver cell may occur by any one or more of four different mechanisms; namely increased entry, increased synthesis, diminished utilization or diminished removal. There is rarely a single explanation for fatty change in any individual condition; much more frequently several, or indeed all, of the above mechanisms may operate to a greater or lesser extent.

The causes of fatty liver are shown in Table 12.1. In developed countries fatty liver is most often due to obesity, diabetes mellitus, alcoholic liver disease, intestinal disease and, especially at post-mortem, debilitating diseases such as malignancy, or infections and cardiac failure. It can also increasingly be attributed to drugs, of which corticosteroids are probably the most common offenders. In underdeveloped countries, malnutrition is the commonest cause of fatty liver.

Whatever the cause of the fatty change, both fat cysts (Figure 12.1) and lipogranulomas (Figure 12.2) are occasional secondary phenomena especially when fat is abundant. Fat cysts result from the coalescence of several fat droplets to form a single larger globule. This often results in the extracellular leakage of fat which stimulates a mesenchymal reaction–a lipogranuloma. Most lipogranulomas consist of a few macrophages and other mononuclear cells grouped around a fat droplet[3]. There is occasionally also giant cell formation. Healing may be followed by the appearance of a small stellate scar[3].

The presence of fat is usually assumed by its morphology, since routine paraffin processing removes all lipids, leaving the characteristic circular empty spaces. Usually its recognition in this manner poses no problems. However, the microvesicular fat encountered in conditions such as acute fatty liver of pregnancy and in Reye's syndrome (q.v.) may be overlooked by anyone unfamiliar

Table 12.1 Causes of fatty change

Macrovesicular fat

Drugs and Toxins
Alcohol
Corticosteroids
Bleomycin
Methotrexate
Warfarin

Inherited metabolic diseases (Chapter 9)
Galactosaemia
Hereditary fructose intolerance
Tyrosinaemia
Wilson's disease
Glycogen storage disease (Type 1)
Homocystinuria
Refsum's disease
Schwachman's syndrome
Abetalipoproteinaemia
Familial hepatosteatosis

Acquired metabolic diseases
Diabetes mellitus
Obesity
Jejuno-ileal bypass
Starvation, protein-calorie malnutrition
Total parenteral nutrition
Inflammatory bowel disease
Cachexia and severe anaemia
Hyperlipidaemia

Microvesicular fat

Acute fatty liver of pregnancy
Reye's syndrome
Salicylate toxicity
Sodium valproate toxicity
Tetracycline
Aflatoxins
Alcoholic foamy degeneration
Miscellaneous inherited diseases

with the conditions. To confirm the presence of fat it is necessary to apply fat stains to frozen sections. Frozen sections should certainly be cut if either of the latter conditions are suspected clinically[4]. A useful clue to the presence of large quantities of fat is a biopsy which floats in its fixative. Macroscopically, in autopsy specimens for example, fat imparts a yellowish-brown colour to the cut surface of the liver which is also often manifestly greasy. The colour is due to excess carotenes and other lipochromes.

Although liver biopsy is the most reliable method for establishing the diagnosis of fatty liver, a number of non-invasive techniques such as computerized tomography and nuclear magnetic resonance are increasingly reliable at detecting total quantities of lipid[5,6]. They do not, however, give any guide to distribution or to other changes such as inflammation and fibrosis.

NON-ALCOHOLIC STEATOHEPATITIS (NASH)

It is now recognized that the full histological spectrum of alcoholic hepatitis, in particular ballooning of hepatocytes with Mallory's hyalin and pericellular fibrosis (see Chapter 13), may be seen in a wide range of conditions which are associated with fatty change (Table 12.2)[7]. Whilst some cases due to drugs such as amiodarone and perhexilene maleate may be associated with abundant Mallory body formation[6], two recent studies concluded that it was impossible to distinguish between NASH and alcoholic injury on morphological grounds alone[8,9]. It is important that the pathologist should recognize that these other conditions exist, and thus the diagnosis of alcoholic liver disease must not be made in the absence of a full clinical history.

Table 12.2 Causes of non-alcoholic steatohepatitis

Diabetes mellitus
Morbid obesity
Jejuno-ileal bypass
Intestinal resection
Total parenteral nutrition
Drugs   glucocorticoids
amiodarone
perhexilene maleate
nifedipine

LARGE DROPLET FAT (MACROVESICULAR STEATOSIS)

The commonest causes of macrovesicular fat are alcohol ingestion (considered separately in Chapter 13), cachexia and diabetes mellitus.

Diabetes mellitus

Fatty liver occurs in over 50% of patients with late-onset (Type II) diabetes mellitus[10] where it may merely be a manifestation of obesity and thus shows the same variability of amount and distribution. However, focal large droplet fatty change is the most common pattern. Glycogen vacuolation of nuclei, particularly of liver cells in the immediate periportal region (Figure 12.3), is an extremely common finding and the combination of this with the fat is characteristic but not diagnostic of diabetes. Similar changes may not only be found in presymptomatic Wilson's disease, seen in quite a different clinical setting, but also in other much less specific conditions, such as acute and chronic infections[11]. Fat is much less commonly seen in the livers of juvenile diabetics.

Rarely, obese diabetics may develop NASH in the absence of exposure to alcohol, which may be associated with cirrhosis[12,13]. This, however, is exceptional and cirrhosis in diabetics is regarded as more likely to be genuinely alcoholic or due to viral hepatitis.

Malnutrition and kwashiorkor

Kwashiorkor is attributable to severe protein malnutrition in the presence of adequate total calorie intake in the form of carbohydrate and/or lipid[14]. It is widely prevalent in parts of Africa and India and is seen particularly in children who would otherwise be growing rapidly. Affected children show peripheral oedema, skin and hair changes, and a striking potbelly due to massive hepatic enlargement. Fat accumulation is due to a combination of increased mobilization of fat from stores and a failure of synthesis of carrier apoprotein.

The liver is large, yellow and greasy, and at its most advanced, the cut surface may even resemble adipose tissue (Figure 12.4). Microscopically the large droplet fat is predominantly in acinar zone 1 before becoming diffuse in more advanced cases. Here, too, the quantity of fat may be so extreme as to resemble adipose tissue. Inflammatory changes or cholestasis are rare. Slight portal fibrosis may be seen, but progression to cirrhosis, contrary to previous beliefs, does not occur[15]. If the child survives, recovery is complete. In total starvation, in which there is calorie as well as protein malnutrition, fatty change is inconspicuous[14].

Toxic liver injury, terminal fatty change

Here fatty change either has no particular distribution or may represent a sublethal liver cell injury and has a similar distribution to any accompanying necrosis. Thus in cardiac failure or following ingestion of halogenated hydrocarbons there may be a zone of fatty change adjacent to the central liver cell loss (Figure 12.5). Fatty change accompanying some forms of acute gastroenteritis and lymphoma deposits may predominantly affect acinar zone 1 (Figure 12.6). Fatty change is also one of the commonest hepatic manifestations of inflammatory bowel disease (Chapter 20). The fat seen in some cases of Wilson's disease is rather characteristically distributed around the periphery of the liver cell cytoplasm.

Jejuno-ileal bypass

Following its introduction in 1963 as a treatment for massive obesity, several thousand bypass operations were performed. In the majority of patients there was a rapid initial weight loss accompanied by an increase in the hepatic lipid. Weight loss and hepatic changes then seem to stabilize. However, a proportion of patients developed progressive liver disease. One to two per cent developed jaundice and died of liver failure – usually less than 6 months after surgery. The mechanism of these acute deaths is quite unknown and many occurred despite reversal of the shunt. Apart from the increased fat (Figure 12.7), all series[16,17] showed a percentage of cases with portal tract changes and centrilobular pericellular fibrosis (Figure 12.8). Even more significant has been the appearance of florid NASH, with portal to central septa and, in about 3%, nodule formation and cirrhosis, the last occasionally with astonishing speed[18]. There was very poor correlation between any of these changes and biochemical results and thus some authors[19,20] felt that regular biopsy should be a mandatory part of follow-up in these cases.

It is tempting to speculate that the fibrosis and cirrhosis are the consequence of malnutrition. However, it has been shown in experimental animals[21] that whilst bypass alone may be fatal, bypass plus resection of the redundant bowel is followed by survival and adaptation. Alternative hypotheses include the effects of bacterial action leading to formation of toxic products and the synthesis of toxic lithocholate in the large bowel. Thus the balance of evidence would seem to point to a metabolic rather than a nutritional cause but, as yet, the problem remains unresolved. Because of the significant risk of serious problems the procedure has now been almost completely abandoned.

Obesity

Some degree of fatty change is almost invariable in severe or what in recent years has come to be called 'morbid' obesity[22]. This is defined as twice ideal weight or 100 lb (45.3 kg) greater than ideal weight. The fat may be focal, zonal – when it is usually centrilobular – or diffuse. It is usually large droplet, but there is no consistent relationship between distribution or quantity of fat and the size of the patient. Its main cause is generally considered to be an increased transport of fat to the liver as a result of over-nutrition and increased synthesis by the liver[23]. Very similar changes occur in the hyperlipoproteinaemia syndromes.

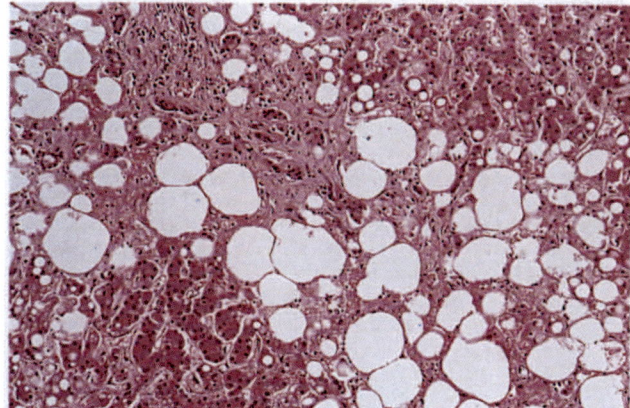

Figure 12.1 Fat cysts. Severe periportal fatty change from a case of Weber-Christian disease showing coalescence of fat droplets to form fat cysts.

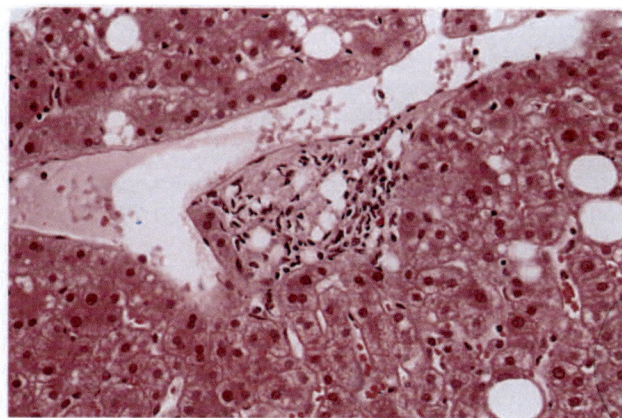

Figure 12.2 Lipogranuloma composed of lymphocytes and macrophages surrounding several fat droplets and situated next to a central vein.

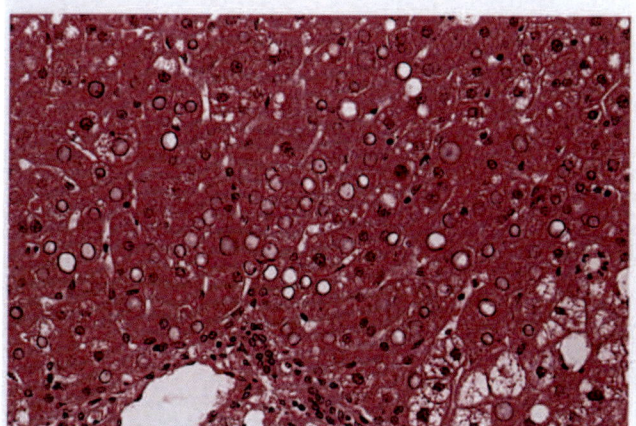

Figure 12.3 Fat, massive obesity. Grossly obese patient showing widespread large droplet fatty change with, in addition, slight centrilobular sclerosis. Elastic van Gieson.

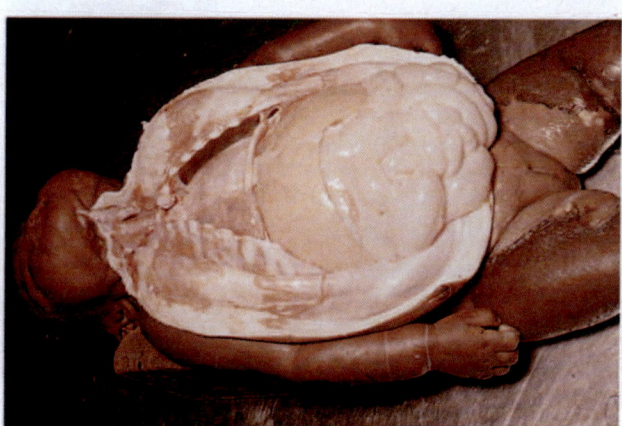

Figure 12.4 Kwashiorkor. An African child who died of malnutrition, showing that the liver resembles adipose tissue.

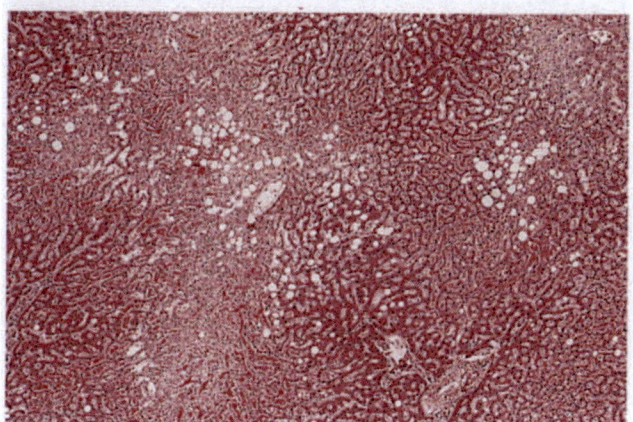

Figure 12.5 Fat, chronic passive congestion. Classic nutmeg liver at post-mortem showing fatty change at the interface between the centrilobular congestion and surviving healthy cells.

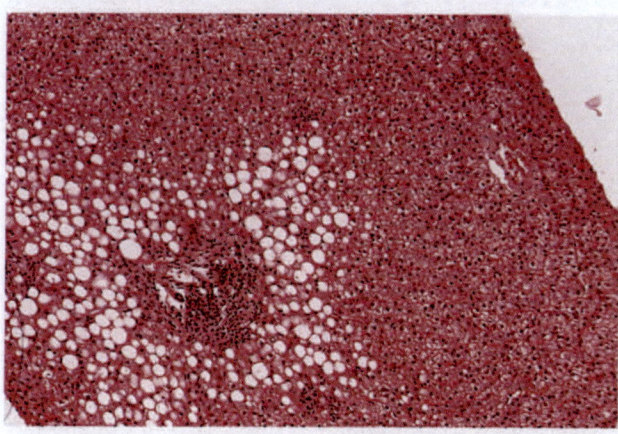

Figure 12.6 Periportal fat. A 6-month-old infant with acute gastroenteritis. Biopsy shows striking periportal distribution of fat.

A number of large studies have demonstrated that, in addition to the fat, a few patients show some structural abnormalities in their livers[17,19,23]. Ten to twenty per cent of patients show minor degrees of portal chronic inflammation and fibrosis, often with minor bile duct proliferation. More significantly, up to 9% show some evidence of NASH (Figure 12.9) with or without focal accumulation of inflammatory cells. The changes are not thought to be progressive in the majority of cases[7,24].

Total parenteral nutrition

Fatty change occurs in some patients receiving total parenteral nutrition (TPN)14 when it is generally also accompanied by significant canalicular cholestasis. Although generally mild and reversible, after prolonged therapy some patients develop cirrhosis[25].

FINE DROPLET FAT (MICROVESICULAR STEATOSIS)

The main conditions associated with microvesicular fat are shown in Table 12.1. In most cases, careful attention to the clinical history combined with the histological findings will lead to the correct diagnosis. Only two conditions will be considered in detail.

Acute fatty liver of pregnancy (AFL)

This was the first condition with this pattern of fat accumulation to be described[26]. It typically afflicts primigravidae in the last few weeks of pregnancy[27], with an overall prevalence of 1 in 14 000 pregnancies[28]. There may or may not be associated pre-eclampsia. The onset can be sudden or may follow a short prodrome, followed by vomiting and the onset of jaundice and coma[29]. Clinically it is indistinguishable from severe acute viral hepatitis, which is much more common and accounts for 40% of all causes of jaundice in pregnancy[30], and may have a similar biochemical profile, although hypoglycaemia is also common in AFL. The mortality for both mother and baby is very high–probably exceeding 80% if not diagnosed early. However, the condition may well be more common than previously recognized and thus, by inclusion of milder variants, the true mortality is probably much lower[31]. Prompt intervention by Caesarean section leads to immediate recovery of the mother – and resolution of the histological changes – and may also save the infant[32]. The total course of the illness is less than 2 weeks and if recovery occurs it is complete. Liver biopsy is the mainstay of diagnosis.

Macroscopically the liver is usually reduced in size and is pale in colour. Microscopically the appearances are wholly distinctive (Figures 12.10 and 12.11). The liver cells, with the exception of a narrow rim of periportal cells, are diffusely abnormal with pale cytoplasm filled with fine vacuoles. There is no displacement of the nucleus and anyone unaware of this condition might easily overlook their nature, unless a frozen section is stained for fat with Oil-red-O. Inflammatory changes are usually minor and confined to portal tracts. The pathogenesis remains quite unknown.

Reye's syndrome

Since it was first described in 1963[33] over 800 cases of Reye's syndrome have been reported. It is a condition of world-wide distribution, mainly affects children, is characterized by rapid onset of convulsions and coma, and is often fatal. At necropsy there is a characteristic microvesicular fatty infiltration of the liver, kidneys and other viscera[34]. Clinically there is usually a history of a mild prodromal illness which is often recovering when there is a sudden deterioration, frequently heralded by vomiting and followed by a progressive loss of consciousness. Jaundice is unusual. The mortality is about 40% in cases diagnosed during life, but others are only diagnosed at necropsy. If recovery occurs, it is complete[35].

The pathogenesis is quite unknown, but epidemiological and experimental studies suggest an unusual interaction between infective agents, particularly varicella virus and influenza B, and environmental factors such as aspirin[36]. Ultrastructurally there are distinctive changes, particularly in the mitochondria[37]. These have been linked to reduced activity of the mitochondrial urea-cycle enzymes in an attempt to explain the encephalopathy. However, it has yet to be established that they are not merely secondary changes.

Microscopically the liver shows a diffuse fatty change which is mainly microvesicular. The liver cell nucleus remains undisplaced at the centre of the cell and the cytoplasm is filled by numerous small vacuoles (Figure 12.12). These tend to be smaller at the centre of the lobule than at the periphery and without a fat stain on a frozen section may not be recognized as fat[4]. There may be some periportal liver cell necrosis and/or glycogen loss. Inflammatory changes are usually confined to the portal tracts. Liver structure and ultrastructure return to normal within 2 months of clinical recovery.

FOCAL FATTY CHANGE

Brower[38] described a series of cases of localized nodules of fatty change found incidentally at post-mortem. The authors felt that it is probably more common than generally realized and pointed out that the lesions might be confused with space occupying lesions such as tumour or abscess. In a number of reported cases the fat has been accompanied by other conditions such as cirrhosis or focal nodular hyperplasia, but in over 40 cases the surrounding liver was normal or nearly so[39].

Macroscopically, they are usually subcapsular in location, up to 4 cm in diameter, with a yellowish cut surface and often a scalloped border. Histologically, they show diffuse or even zonal large droplet fatty change. The remaining liver may show much milder fatty change and they may be the consequence of local ischaemia superimposed upon conditions regularly producing fatty change.

DIFFERENTIAL DIAGNOSIS OF FATTY CHANGE

Minor degrees of fatty change rarely have an attributable cause. Evidence of alcoholic liver disease should always be sought. but it is important to appreciate that other conditions such as diabetes mellitus, drugs such as corticosteroids or perhexilene maleate and even otherwise uncomplicated obesity, are occasionally associated with very similar changes. Hyperlipoproteinaemia and drugs should always be considered as possible causes. The rare conditions, Reye's syndrome and fatty liver of pregnancy, usually have a typical clinical setting, but when they are suspected, some or all of the biopsy should be retained for frozen section and fat stains. Similarly in certain metabolic disorders, fat may be a helpful diagnostic clue, for example in galactosaemia, but is rarely a dominant feature histologically.

REFERENCES

1. Leevy, C. M. (1962). Fatty liver: a study of 270 patients with biopsy-proven fatty liver and a review of the literature. Medicine (Baltimore), 41, 249–276
2. Randall, B. (1980). Fatty liver and sudden death. A review. Hum. Pathol., 11, 147–151

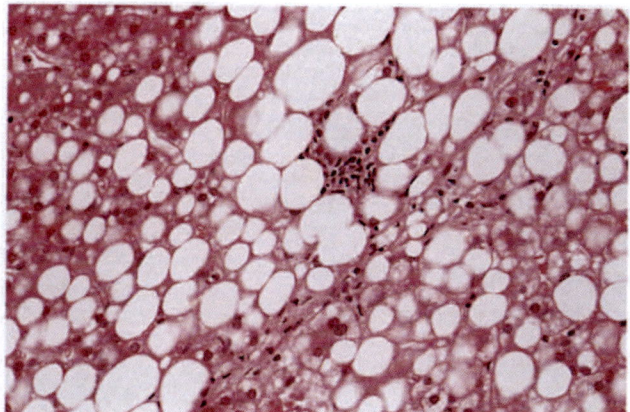

Figure 12.7 Fat, massive obesity. Biopsy taken 2 years after jejuno-ileal bypass operation. Severe fatty change persists with scattered inflammatory foci composed predominantly of lymphocytes.

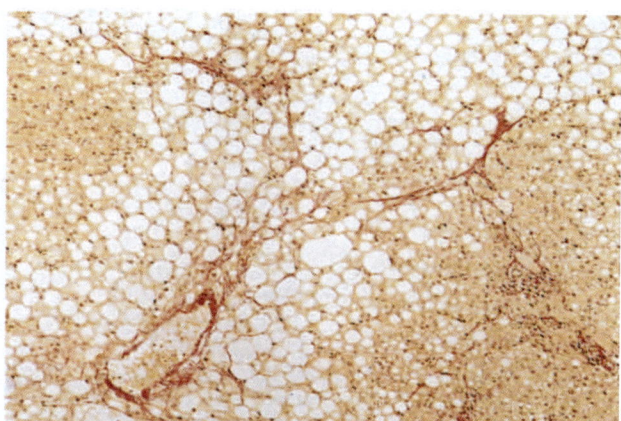

Figure 12.8 Fat, massive obesity. Same biopsy as Figure 12.7 showing some progression of the architectural disturbance seen prior to bypass. Slender fibrous septa now link central veins and portal tracts. Elastic van Gieson.

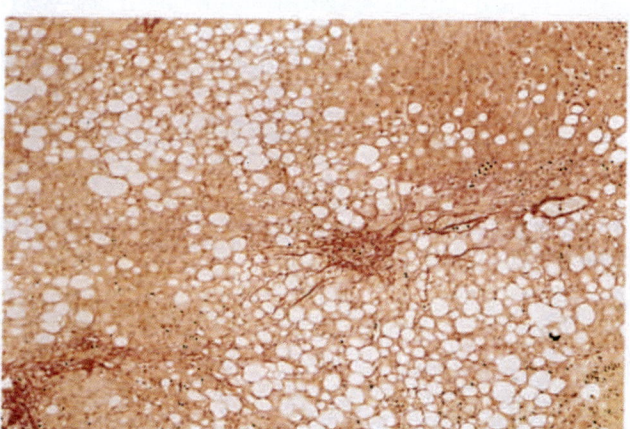

Figure 12.9 Fat, massive obesity. The same grossly obese patient as shown in Figures 12.7 and 12.8 whose liver prior to bypass shows widespread large droplet fatty change with, in addition, slight centrilobular sclerosis–a manifestation of non–alcoholic steatohepatitis.

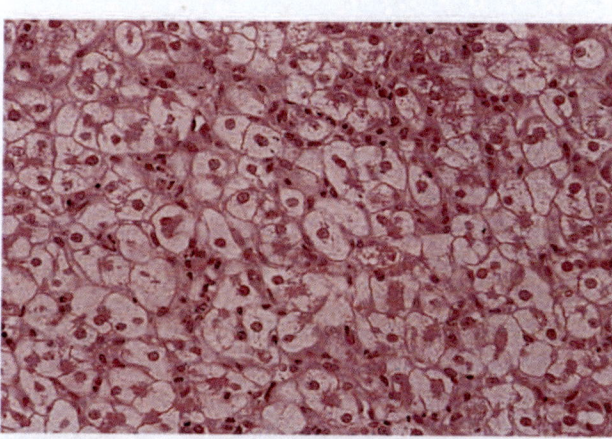

Figure 12.10 Acute fatty liver of pregnancy. Severe pre-eclamptic toxaemia in last trimester of first pregnancy, followed by ante-partum haemorrhage and a stillborn infant. Acute onset of jaundice at time of delivery. Biopsy shows marked pallor of hepatocyte cytoplasm with fine peripheral vacuolation.

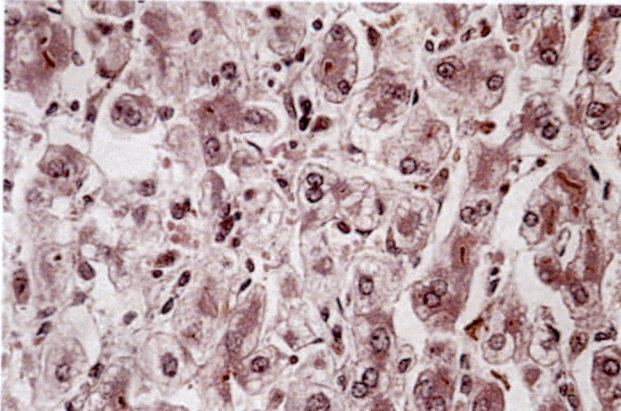

Figure 12.11 Acute fatty liver of pregnancy. A different case with a similar history, although this patient died a few days after the onset of jaundice. Sections show similar peripheral pallor which is now much more obviously vacuolated. Cholestasis, which was mainly centrilobular, is also quite prominent.

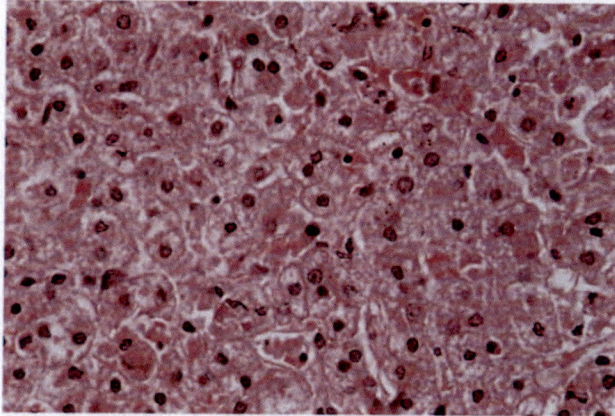

Figure 12.12 Reye's syndrome. A 16-month-old child developed encephalopathy and died after an indeterminate febrile illness. At post-mortem the liver was slightly enlarged and pale. Sections show a uniform fine vacuolation of hepatocytes, without displacement of the nucleus, which could easily be overlooked. Fat stains were strongly positive.

3. Christoffersen, P., Braendstrup, O., Juhl, E. and Poulsen, P. (1971). Lipogranulomas in human liver biopsies with fatty change. Acta Pathol. Microbiol. Scand, 79A, 150–158

4. Wigger, H. J. (1977). Frozen section of the liver in diagnosis of Reye's syndrome. Am. J. Surg. Pathol., 1, 271–274

5. Levenson, H., Greensite, F., Hoefs, J. et al. (1991). Fatty infiltration of the liver: quantification with phase contrast MR imaging at 1.5t versus biopsy. AJR, 156, 307–312

6. Burt, A. D. and MacSween, R. N. M. (1993). Fat, alcohol, iron. In Wight, D. G. D. (ed). Liver, Biliary Tract and Exocrine Pancreas. Vol.11. Systemic Pathology. Symmers, W. S. C., series ed. 3rd edn. Edinburgh: Churchill Livingstone

7. Lee, R. G. (1989). Nonalcoholic steatohepatitis: a study of 49 patients. Hum. Pathol., 20, 594–598

8. Itoh, S., Youngel, T. and Kawagoe, K. (1987). Comparison between non-alcoholic steatohepatitis and alcoholic hepatitis. Am. J. Gastroenterol., 82, 650–654

9. Diehl, A. M., Goodman, Z. and Ishak, K. G. (1988). Alcohol-like liver disease in non-alcoholics. A clinical and histologic comparison with alcohol-induced liver injury. Gastroenterology, 95, 1056–1062

10. Stone, B. G. and Van Thiel, D. H. (1985). Diabetes mellitus and the liver. Semin. Liver Dis., 5, 8–28

11. Creuzfeldt, W., Frerichs, H. and Sickinger, K. (1970). Liver diseases and diabetes mellitus. In Popper, H. and Schaffner, F. (eds). Progress in Liver Diseases. III. pp. 371–401. New York: Grune and Stratton

12. Thaler, H. (1975). The relationship of steatosis to cirrhosis. Clin. Gastroenterol., 4, 273–280

13. Falchuk, K. R., Fiske, S., Trey, C., Haggett, R. and Federman, M. (1980). Pericentral hepatic fibrosis in diabetes mellitus. Gastroenterology, 78, 535–541

14. Quigley, E. M. and Zetterman, R. K. (1988). Hepatobiliary complications of malabsorption and malnutrition. Semin. Liver Dis., 8, 218–228

15. Cook, G. C. and Hutt, M. S. R. (1967). The liver after kwashiorkor. Br. Med. J., 2, 454–457

16. Peters, R. L. (1977). Patterns of hepatic morphology in jejunoileal bypass patients. Am. J. Clin. Nutr., 30, 53–57

17. Marrubio, A. T., Rucker, R. D., Schneider, P. D., Hastmann, J. P., Varco, R. L. and Buchwald, H. (1979). Liver in morbid obesity and following bypass surgery. Surg. Clin. N. A., 59, 1079–1093

18. Spellberg, M. A. and Bermundez, F. (1977). Rapid development of micronodular cirrhosis following small bowel bypass for obesity. Am. J. Gastroenterol., 68, 354–358

19. Galambos, J. T. and Wills, C. E. (1978). Relationship between 505 paired liver tests and biopsies in 242 obese patients. Gastroenterology, 74, 1191–1195

20. Hocking, M. P., Duerson, M. C., Alexander, R. W. and Woodward, E. R. (1981). Late hepatic histopathology after jejunoileal bypass for morbid obesity. Relation of abnormalities on biopsy and clinical course. Am. J. Surg., 141, 159–163

21. Nayak, N. C. (1987). Nutritional liver disease. In MacSween, R. N. M., Anthony, P. P. and Scheuer, P. J. (eds). Pathology of the liver. 3rd edn. pp. 265–280. Edinburgh: Churchill Livingstone

22. Falloon, W. W. (1988). Hepatobiliary effects of obesity and weight-reducing surgery. Semin. Liver Dis., 8, 229–236

23. Nasrallah, S. M., Willis, C. E. and Galambos, J. T. (1981). Hepatic morphology in obesity. Dig. Dis. Sci., 26, 325–327

24. Powell, E. E., Cooksley, W. G. E., Hanson, R., Searle, J., Halliday, J. W. and Powell, L. W. (1990). The natural history of non-alcoholic steatohepatitis: a follow-up study of forty-two patients for up to 21 years. Hepatology, 11, 74–80

25. Craig, R. M., Neumann, T., Jeejeebhoy, K. N. and Yokoo, H. (1980). Severe hepatocellular reaction resembling alcoholic hepatitis with cirrhosis after massive small bowel resection and prolonged total parenteral nutrition. Gastroenterology, 79, 131–137

26. Sheehan, H. L. (1940). Pathology of acute yellow atrophy and delayed chloroform poisoning. J. Obstet. Gynaecol. Br. Emp., 47, 49–62

27. Rolfes, D. B. and Ishak, K. G. (1985). Acute fatty liver of pregnancy: a clinicopathological study of 35 cases. Hepatology, 5, 1149–1158

28. Pockros, P. J., Peters, R. L. and Reynolds, T. B. (1984). Idiopathic fatty liver of pregnancy: findings in ten cases. Medicine (Baltimore), 63, 1–11

29. Sherlock, S. (1983). Acute fatty liver of pregnancy and the microvesicular fat diseases. Gut, 24, 265–269

30. Hemmerli, U. P. (1966). Jaundice during pregnancy with special emphasis on recurrent jaundice during pregnancy and its differential diagnosis. Acta Med. Scand., 179 [suppl 444], 1–111

31. Riely, C. A., Latham, P. S., Romero, R. and Duffy, T. P. (1987). Acute fatty liver of pregnancy: a reassessment based on observations in nine patients. Ann. Intern. Med., 106, 703–706

32. Ebert, E. C., Sun, E. A., Wright, S. A., Decker, J. P., Librizzi, R. J., Bolognese, R. J. and Lipshutz, W. H. (1984). Does early diagnosis and delivery in acute fatty liver of pregnancy lead to improvement in maternal and infant survival? Dig. Dis. Sci., 29, 453–455

33. Reye, R. D. K., Morgan, G. and Baral, J. (1963). Encephalopathy and fatty degeneration of the viscera. Lancet, 2, 749–752

34. Kimura, S., Kobayashi, T., Tanaka, Y. and Sasaki, Y. (1991). Liver histopathology in clinical Reye syndrome. Brain Dev., 13, 95–100

35. Crocker, J. F. S. and Bagnell, P. C. (1981). Reye's syndrome: a clinical review. Can. Med. Assn. J., 124, 375–382

36. Forsyth, B. W., Horwitz, R. I. and Acampora, D. (1989). New epidemiological evidence confirming that bias does not explain the aspirin/Reye's syndrome association. JAMA, 261, 2517–2524

37. Iancu, T. C., Mason, W. H. and Neustein, H. B. (1977). Ultrastructural abnormalities of liver cells in Reye's syndrome. Hum. Pathol., 8, 421–443

38. Brower, M. K., Austin, G. E. and Lewin, K. J. (1980). Focal fatty change of the liver. A hitherto poorly recognized entity. Gastroenterology, 78, 247–252

39. Grove, A., Vyberg, B. and Vyberg, M. (1991). Focal fatty change of the liver. A review and a case associated with continuous ambulatory peritoneal dialysis. Virch. Arch. [A], 419, 69–75

For many years it was thought that liver disease in the alcoholic was due primarily to nutritional factors and that alcohol was not a hepatotoxin[1]. On the basis of animal experiments it was assumed that fatty liver alone could then lead on to fibrosis and eventually to cirrhosis. With the recognition of alcoholic hepatitis as a clinical and pathological entity, this then was regarded as an essential step in the progression to cirrhosis. Support for this view seemed to be provided by experimental studies in alcoholic and non-alcoholic human volunteers[2] and in a new animal model in baboons[2,3]. However, the rôle of malnutrition as a cofactor cannot be totally excluded[4].

The recognition of alcoholic liver disease is ultimately a tissue diagnosis, given that the morphological changes in the liver cannot be predicted on the basis of clinical or biochemical assessment. Furthermore, it is essential to exclude other forms of liver disease in chronic alcoholics; in one study, 15% of patients with a high alcohol intake were found on biopsy to have coincidental non-alcoholic liver disease[5]. The morphological spectrum of changes attributable to alcohol has been well documented[6–9].

FATTY LIVER

Fatty liver, the first recognizable lesion of alcoholic liver disease, is found in the majority of alcoholics and appears to be directly related to alcohol consumption. Clinically it is often silent despite marked hepatomegaly, although biochemically it may be accompanied by minor elevations of the serum transaminases.

There is great variation in the number of cells affected, ranging from occasional randomly distributed droplets to massive involvement, but there is a distinct tendency for fat to be preferentially located in central and mid-zones (Figure 13.1)[6]. It is predominantly macrovesicular and is fully reversible. Thus absence of fat in an alcoholic may be attributable to recent abstinence, for example on hospitalization. The basic architecture at this stage is unremarkable, although lipogranulomas are quite common in alcoholic fatty liver, as in that due to any other cause (see Chapter 12), and these may heal with a small scar. Giant mitochondria, up to 20μ in diameter (Figure 13.2), may also be seen at this stage. Whilst they are not specific for alcohol, they do at least provide a pointer to an alcoholic aetiology[10], and may correlate with recent alcohol intake.

Rarely fatty change in the alcoholic may be complicated by acute cholestasis[11] in the absence of biliary obstruction. Biopsy in these cases reveals cholestasis which is mainly centrilobular, but not necessarily any alcoholic hepatitis (Figure 13.3). In the more severe cases there may also be evidence of microscopic cholangitis, in the form of neutrophilic infiltration of portal tracts both within and between bile ducts[12]. This reaction may be seen in severe cholestasis from any cause (see Chapter 16) and does not necessarily imply either ascending cholangitis or biliary obstruction. The fat in these cases may be microvesicular in type, and has been called alcoholic foamy degeneration[13].

ALCOHOLIC HEPATITIS

Unlike fatty liver, there is no clear dose relationship between alcohol consumption and alcoholic hepatitis.

However, the majority of patients will have been drinking heavily for at least 5 years, with a total daily intake of at least 80 g ($\cong$ one bottle of wine) per day[14]. Similarly there is not always good correlation between the clinical picture and microscopic findings. At its most severe, alcoholic hepatitis can present with ascites, and progress to death from acute liver failure. More usually it causes varying combinations of malaise, fever, anorexia, abdominal pain or hepatic tenderness. There is often an associated neutrophil leucocytosis and a mild elevation of serum enzymes. A significant number of patients with microscopic hepatitis, however, are totally free of symptoms.

Microscopically, hepatitis may be seen with or without concomitant fatty change. Liver cell damage is focal and usually consists of swollen or ballooned hepatocytes which often, but not invariably, contain clumped eosinophilic refractile masses of Mallory's hyalin (or Mallory bodies). Intimately related to these degenerate cells are aggregates of neutrophil polymorphs which are usually most numerous in those cases where hyalin is most plentiful (Figures 13.4 and 13.5). Pericellular fibrosis is highly characteristic and thin perisinusoidal collagen fibres characteristically enclose single cells and small groups of cells, giving rise to a latticework or 'chicken-wire' appearance (Figure 13.6). In the non-cirrhotic liver these lesions are always predominantly centrilobular[15]. Ultrastructurally hyalin has been shown to be filamentous[16] and there is some evidence that it is related to the intermediate filaments and that its accumulation is due to a failure of the microtubular system of the cell[17]. Hyalin is also seen in a variety of other conditions, such as primary biliary cirrhosis, biliary obstruction, α_1-antitrypsin deficiency, Wilson's disease and Indian childhood cirrhosis, in all of which it is found at the periphery of nodules. In most of these there is also evidence of accumulation of copper and copper metallothionein, as shown by positive staining with rubeanic acid and orcein, and thus copper may be the main cause of damage to the microtubular system. There is even evidence of increased copper in alcoholic liver disease[18]. Recent immunological studies have shown that, whatever its origin, all hyalin contains a common antigenic determinant[19].

The extent of the hepatitic lesion varies widely. Minimal involvement is often patchy but the fully developed lesion affects every lobule and may be associated with confluent areas of liver cell loss. This may progress to involve much of zone 3 of Rappaport's acinus, leading to central to central, and central to portal, bridging necrosis, the first step in the genesis of cirrhosis (Figure 13.10). At this stage, hepatitic lesions with hyalin may be seen at the periphery of the lobule. Conversely, proliferating bile ductules are frequently seen now near to central veins (Figure 13.8). This may also occur in association with the central fibrosis seen in venous outflow obstruction (Chapter 18) and in both situations can be confusing and create the impression that the lesion is portal[15].

Other features are relatively uncommon and in no way specific for alcohol[16]. These include acidophil bodies, 'induced' hepatocytes (Chapter 16), giant mitochondria (Figure 13.2) and oxyphil granular hepatocytes[20] (which like oxyphil cells in the thyroid and other organs are rich in mitochondria).

In a few cases the hepatitic process is more severe and

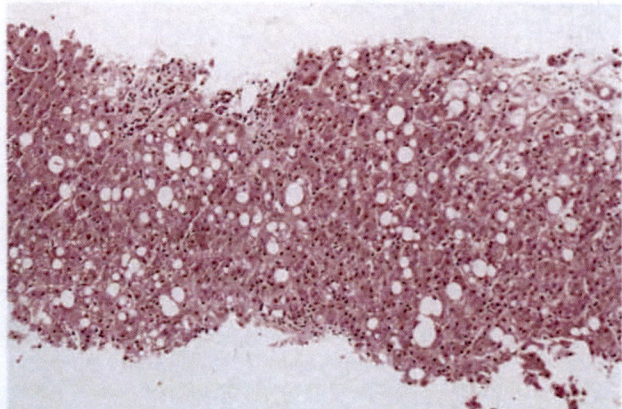

Figure 13.1 Alcoholic fatty liver. A 44-year-old female who presented with hepatomegaly. Biopsy shows large droplet fatty change of moderate degree, but no hepatitis or architectural disturbance.

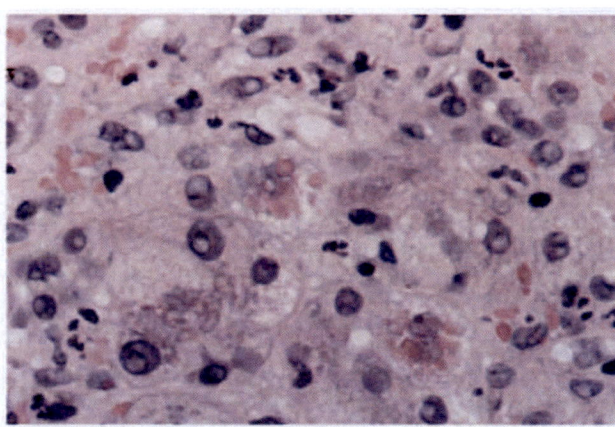

Figure 13.2 Acute alcoholic liver disease. Several hepatocytes contain groups of eosinophilic giant mitochondria.

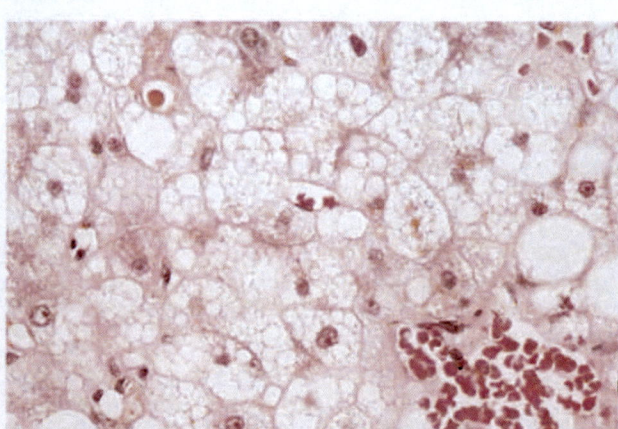

Figure 13.3 Acute alcoholic cholestasis, fatty liver. A 27-year-old male who presented with a 3-week history of progressive obstructive jaundice. Percutaneous transhepatic cholangiography failed to show dilated intrahepatic bile ducts. The biopsy shows bile canaliculi distended by bile plugs (upper left) and a uniform microvesicular fatty change, but no hepatitis. A central vein is seen lower right.

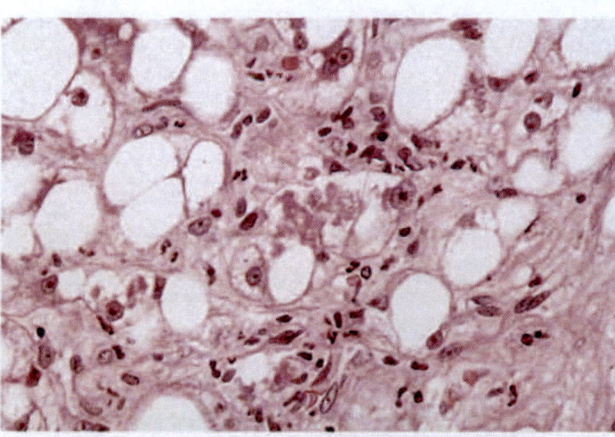

Figure 13.4 Alcoholic hepatitis. A 51-year-old female alcoholic with typical hepatitis. This biopsy shows, at the centre of the field, a ballooned hepatocyte with clumped eosinophilic hyalin surrounded by rarefied cytoplasm. Note the adjacent neutrophil polymorphs and widespread fatty change.

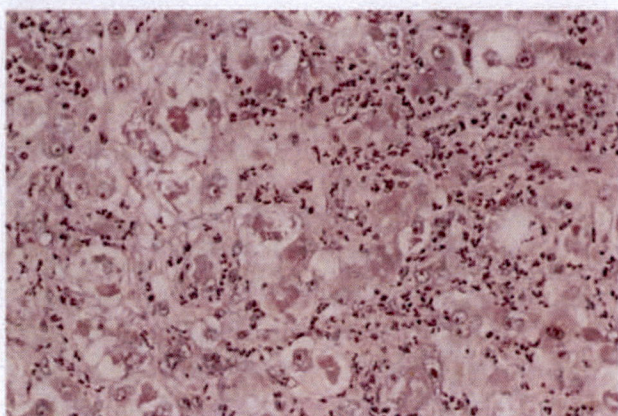

Figure 13.5 Alcoholic hepatitis. Another clinically typical case of hepatitis in a 71-year-old female alcoholic. The biopsy shows numerous degenerate hyalin-containing liver cells, many surrounded by a collar of neutrophils.

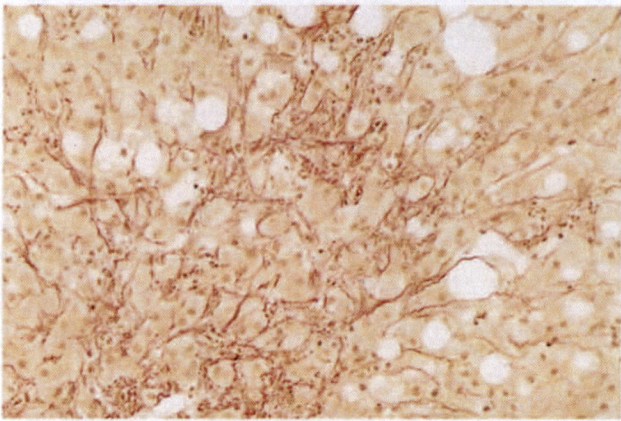

Figure 13.6 Alcoholic hepatitis. A connective tissue stain shows the remarkable pericellular fibrosis that is present, but barely detectable with the H & E. Note that this commences in the centre of the lobule (central vein bottom centre). Elastic van Gieson.

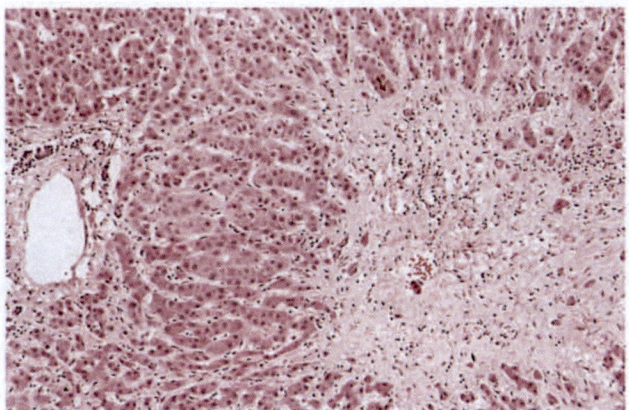

Figure 13.7 Alcoholic hepatitis, sclerosing hyaline necrosis. A 48-year-old male alcoholic who presented with acute onset of ascites which progressed to liver failure and death. The post-mortem liver shows a very sharply defined area of centrilobular fibrosis. The adjacent liver shows little evidence of fat or continuing hepatitis, probably because of the enforced abstinence during a 2-week period of hospitalization. Note the bile plug (top centre).

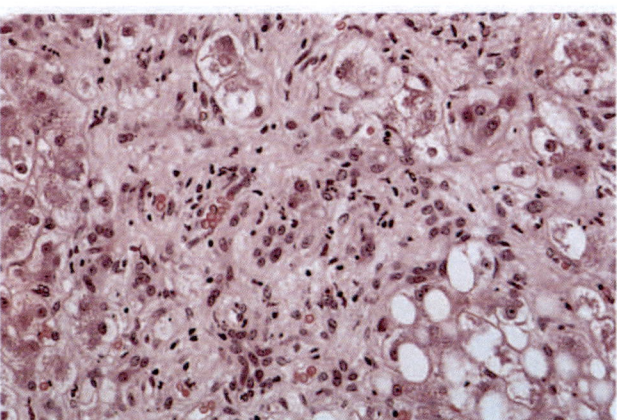

Figure 13.8 Alcoholic hepatitis, sclerosing hyaline necrosis. Same case as Figure 13.4. The section shows the centre of a lobule in which the central vein has been obliterated and replaced by fibrous tissue containing capillaries and a few bile ductules (see centre), thus simulating a portal tract. Note the ballooned hyalin containing hepatocytes in the adjacent parenchyma (top).

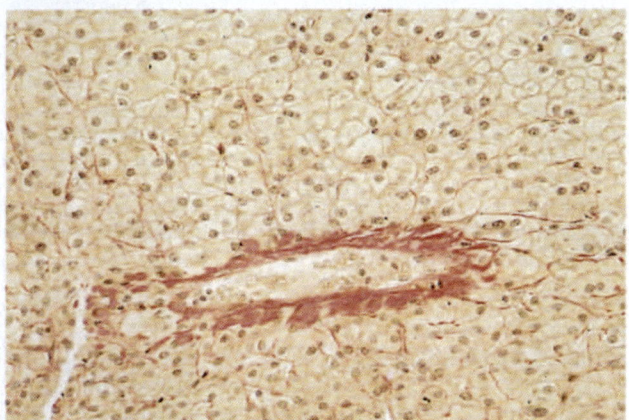

Figure 13.9 Perivenular sclerosis. A 57-year-old female alcoholic whose biopsy showed no other abnormality than this fibrous thickening of the adventitia of the central vein. Elastic van Gieson.

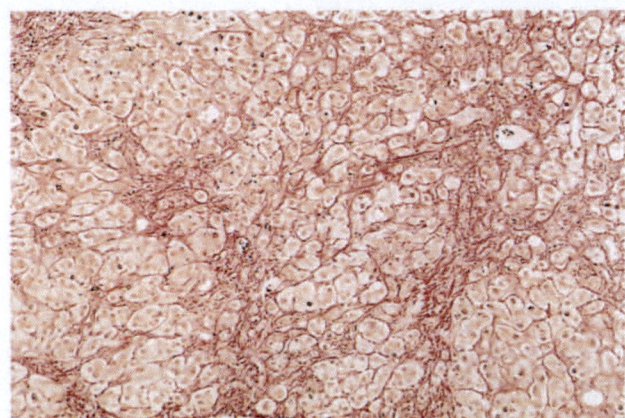

Figure 13.10 Alcoholic fibrosis. A 43-year-old female alcoholic with known liver disease, biopsied to assess prognosis. The section shows that the parenchyma is being completely broken up by thin pericellular fibrous septa, now linking central veins and portal tracts. This advanced fibrosis is theoretically reversible since there are not yet any regeneration nodules. Elastic van Gieson.

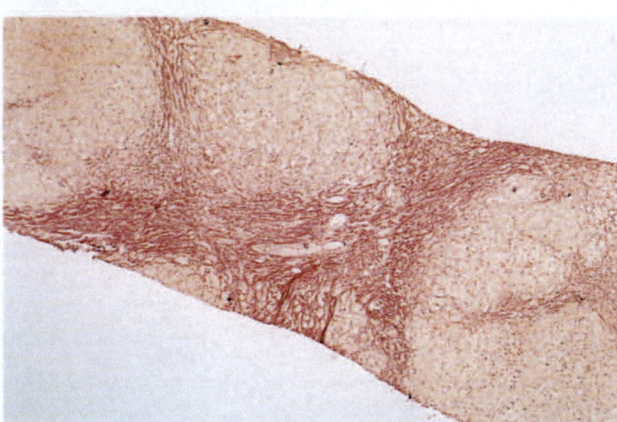

Figure 13.11 Micronodular cirrhosis. Same patient as Figure 13.1, biopsied exactly 3 years later. There has been remarkable progression from a liver which then showed only fatty change to the fully developed cirrhosis now seen. Note that the nodules are roughly of lobular size and contain no vessels, which are confined to the septa. Elastic van Gieson.

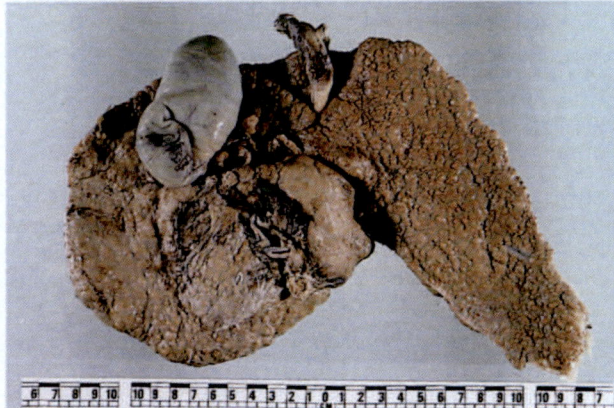

Figure 13.12 Micronodular cirrhosis. A 55-year-old male alcoholic known to have cirrhosis for several years, treated by transplantation. The excised liver weighed 1560 g and shows a typical micronodular surface. There was very little fat present histologically and this would account for the rather low weight. Hyalin was abundant.

results in marked centrilobular necrosis, termed *sclerosing hyaline necrosis* by Edmondson et al.[21]. The lesion appears as an irregular, relatively acellular. confluent, homogeneous area, often very sharply demarcated from the adjacent parenchyma (Figures 13.7 and 13.8)[6]. Thin-walled vessels tend to replace hepatic veins and there may also be inflammatory cells, bile ductules and pigmented macrophages. The surrounding liver shows continuing hepatitis. Clinically, patients tend to have an enlarged tender liver, high serum enzymes and portal hypertension[22]. The mortality is significant, as is the risk of progression to cirrhosis.

Although, as already stated, alcoholic hepatitis has generally been regarded as an essential step in the development of cirrhosis in alcoholic liver disease, recent animal experiments have now cast some doubt upon this thesis[23]. Eighteen baboons were fed alcohol for up to 6 years alongside pair-fed control animals. All animals developed fat and fibrosis, but the lesion of alcoholic hepatitis with hyalin and neutrophils was never seen. Instead, fibrosis proceeding to septum formation was mostly associated with large droplet fatty change. The distribution of the fibrosis was nevertheless very similar to that in the human condition and thus it is tempting to speculate that creeping fibrosis of this sort may also play a role in man, with hepatitis being relegated to a supplementary or incidental role[23]. This may also help to explain the occasional association of alcoholic type fibrosis in other conditions such as obesity and in association with jejuno-ileal bypass (see below and Chapter 12). The possible role of immunological factors in the pathogenesis of liver damage has also been the subject of continuing interest[24,25].

Differential diagnosis

The distinctive centrilobular necrosis with hyalin, neutrophil polymorph infiltrate and pericellular fibrosis is much more often attributable to alcohol than other aetiologies. However, non-alcoholic steatohepatitis (NASH) is infrequently seen in otherwise uncomplicated obesity[26], after jejuno-ileal bypass[26], in diabetes[27] and following treatment with drugs such as perhexilene maleate[28] and amiodarone. It is important to recognize the existence of these other causes if for no other reason than to avoid labelling such patients as alcoholics.

The centrilobular scarring associated with venous outflow obstruction is not accompanied by a hepatitic lesion and there will usually be other evidence of congestion.

Perivenular sclerosis

A few patients show a characteristic thickening of the wall of the central vein due to the deposition of a collar of collagen in the adventitial layer (Figure 13.9)[29]. This is found in up to 40% of chronic alcoholics but not in controls or moderate drinkers, and there is some evidence that its presence may identify those susceptible to the subsequent development of cirrhosis[30], although others feel that pericellular fibrosis is the true marker of progression[31].

CIRRHOSIS

Remarkable regression of alcoholic hepatitis and fibrosis is possible in patients who are able to abstain from alcohol[25], but regression becomes impossible when significant nodular regeneration has commenced. In its early stages alcoholic cirrhosis is characteristically micronodular, many of the nodules being of sublobular size in the range 1–2 mm in diameter. Initially they lack any vascular structures because they arise through a process of dissection of the lobules by fibrous septa (Figures 13.10 and 13.11), but may show continuing fat and alcoholic hepatitis, the latter tending now to be maximal at the periphery of nodules. Septa contain a variable mixture of neutrophils and chronic inflammatory cells as well as bile ductules.

With the passage of time, especially if the patient ceases to drink, regeneration may be more vigorous and larger nodules appear, leading eventually to the end-stage macronodular cirrhosis, now indistinguishable from that due to a variety of other causes (Figure 13.12). The risk of hepatocellular carcinoma (Chapter 23) is then significantly increased[32].

MISCELLANEOUS CHANGES
Alcohol-induced chronic active hepatitis

Chronic active hepatitis (CAH) which is indistinguishable from autoimmune CAH (Chapter 7) may sometimes be seen in alcoholic patients[33]. Strict criteria must be applied to exclude other causes, especially hepatitis C, but there appears to be a residue of cases directly attributable to alcohol, and the condition resolves on alcohol withdrawal. It appears to be more common in the Far East[33], where it may be found in up to 16% of chronic alcoholics.

Portal fibrosis

As explained above, although the advanced lesion of alcoholic fibrosis may appear to be portal, it is always centrilobular. However, true portal fibrosis is quite common in the liver of male chronic alcoholics[34]. Other causes for this can usually be found—the commonest being chronic pancreatitis complicated by episodes of cholangitis.

Iron accumulation

Iron accumulation occurs in up to 50% of alcoholic livers. It is found, in the non-cirrhotic liver, in hepatocytes at the periphery of lobules and probably related to the type of alcoholic beverage consumed, some having a fairly high iron content. In other cases the iron accumulation may be the consequence of cirrhosis, possibly due to the physiological effects of portacaval shunting[35]. In both sets of circumstances the quantity of iron accumulated is usually only slight and does not approach the levels seen in haemochromatosis (Chapter 14).

Others

PAS-positive diastase resistant inclusions of α_1-anti-trypsin are also quite commonly observed within liver cells in alcoholic cirrhosis. These do not appear to be in any way related to α_1-anti-trypsin deficiency since the phenotype is usually Pi M[36]. Alcohol exacerbates the cutaneous and hepatic manifestations of porphyria cutanea tarda (see Chapter 21).

Pathogenesis of alcoholic liver disease

The pathogenesis of fatty change is complex but can be explained on a biochemical basis[9]. The genesis of the other changes is less clearly understood. Alcohol itself may not be directly hepatotoxic[37]. Much accumulated data suggests that metabolites, particularly acetaldehyde, are responsible for most of the liver injury[38]. The mainly perivenular distribution of the changes may be due to the zonal distribution of the ethanol-metabolizing enzymes, combined with reduced oxygen tension.

REFERENCES

1. Best, C. H., Hartroft, W. S., Lucas, C. C. and Ridout, J. H. (1949). Liver damage produced by feeding alcohol or sugar and its prevention by choline. Br. Med. J., 2, 1001–1006
2. Rubin, E. and Lieber, C. S. (1974). Fatty liver, alcoholic hepatitis and cirrhosis produced by alcohol in primates. N. Engl. J. Med., 290, 128–135
3. Lieber, C. S. (1990). Mechanism of ethanol-induced hepatic injury. Pharmacol. Ther., 46, 1–41
4. Rothschild, M. A., Oratz, M. and Schreiber, S. S. (1989). Alcohol-induced liver disease: does nutrition play a role? Alcohol Health Res. World, 13, 229–331
5. Levin, D. M., Baker, A. L., Riddell, R. H., Rochman, H. and Boyer, J. L. (1979). Nonalcoholic liver disease. Overlooked causes of liver injury in patients with heavy alcohol consumption. Am. J. Med., 66, 429–434
6. Review by an International Group. (1981). Alcoholic liver disease: morphological manifestations. Lancet, i, 707–711
7. Popper, H., Thung, S. N. and Gerber, M. A. (1981). Pathology of alcoholic liver diseases. Semin. Liver Dis., 1, 203–216
8. MacSween, R. N. M. and Burt, A. D. (1986). Histologic spectrum of alcoholic liver disease. Semin. Liver Dis., 6, 221–232
9. Burt, A. D. and MacSween, R. N. M. (1993). Fat, alcohol, iron. In Wight, D. G. D. (ed). Liver, Biliary Tract and Exocrine Pancreas. Vol.11. Systemic Pathology. Symmers, W. S. C., series ed. 3rd edn. Edinburgh: Churchill Livingstone
10. Bruguera, M., Bertman, A., Bombi, J. A. and Rodes, J. (1977). Giant mitochondria in hepatocytes. A diagnostic hint for alcoholic liver disease. Gastroenterology, 73, 1383–1387
11. Morgan, M. Y., Sherlock, S. and Scheuer, P. J. (1978). Acute cholestasis, hepatic failure and fatty liver in the alcoholic. Scand. J. Gastroenterol., 13, 299–303
12. Afshani, P., Littenberg, G. D., Wollman, J. and Kaplowitz, N. (1978). Significance of microscopic cholangitis in alcoholic liver disease. Gastroenterology, 75, 1045–1050
13. Uchida, T., Kao, H., Quispe Sjögren, M. and Peters, R. L. (1983). Alcoholic foamy degeneration – a pattern of acute alcoholic injury of the liver. Gastroenterology, 84, 683–692
14. Galambos, J. T. (1972). Natural history of alcoholic hepatitis. III. Histological changes. Gastroenterology, 63, 1026–1035
15. Gerber, M. A. and Popper, H. (1972). Relation between central canals and portal tracts in alcoholic hepatitis. A contribution to the pathogenesis of cirrhosis in alcoholics. Hum. Pathol., 3, 199–207
16. Yokoo, H., Minick, O. T., Batti, F. and Kent, G. (1972). Morphological variants of alcoholic hyalin. Am. J. Pathol., 69, 25–40
17. French, S. W., Sim, J. S., Franks, K. E., Burbige, E. J., Denton, T. and Caldwell, M. G. (1977). Alcoholic hepatitis. In Fisher, M. M. and Rankin, J. G. (eds). Alcohol and the Liver. New York: Plenum
18. Berresford, P. A., Sunter, J. P., Harrison, V. and Lesna, M. (1980). Histological demonstration and frequency of intra-hepatocytic copper in patients suffering from alcoholic liver disease. Histopathology, 4, 637–643
19. Fleming, K. A., Morton, J. A., Carbatis, C., Burns, J., Canning, S. and McGee, J. O. (1981). Mallory bodies in alcoholic and non-alcoholic liver disease contain a common antigenic determinant. Gut, 22, 341–344
20. Gerber, M. A. and Thung, S. N. (1981). Hepatic oncocytes. Incidence, staining characteristics, and ultrastructural features. Am. J. Clin. Pathol., 75, 498–503
21. Edmondson, H. A., Peters, R. L., Reynolds, T. B. and Kuzma, O. T. (1963). Sclerosing hyaline necrosis in the liver of the chronic alcoholic. A recognizable syndrome. Ann. Intern. Med., 59, 646–673
22. Karasawa, T. and Chedid, A. (1976). Sclerosing hyaline necrosis in non-cirrhotic chronic alcoholic hepatitis. Am. J. Clin. Pathol., 66, 802–809
23. Popper, H. and Lieber, C. S. (1980). Histogenesis of alcoholic fibrosis and cirrhosis in the baboon. Am. J. Pathol., 98, 695–716
24. French, S. W., Burbige, E. J., Tarder, G., Bourke, E., Harkin, C. G. and Denton, T. (1979). Lymphocyte sequestration by the liver in alcoholic hepatitis. Arch. Pathol. Lab. Med., 103, 146–152
25. Perperas, A., Tsantoulas, D., Portmann, B., Eddleston, A. L. W. F. and Williams, R. (1981). Autoimmunity to a liver membrane lipoprotein and liver damage in alcoholic liver disease. Gut, 22, 149–152
26. Marrubio, A. T., Buchwald, H., Schwartz, M. Z. and Varco, R. (1976). Hepatic lesions of central pericellular fibrosis in morbid obesity and after jejuno-ileal bypass. Am. J. Clin. Pathol., 66, 684–691
27. Falchuk, K. R., Fiske, S., Trey, C., Haggett, R. and Federman, M. (1980). Pericentral hepatic fibrosis in diabetes mellitus. Gastroenterology, 78, 535–541
28. Pessayre, D., Bichara, M., Feldmann, G., Degott, C., Potet, F. and Benhamou, J.-P. (1979). Perhexiline maleate-induced cirrhosis. Gastroenterology, 76, 170–177
29. Van Waes, L. and Lieber, C. S. (1977). Early perivenular sclerosis in alcoholic fatty liver: an index of progressive liver injury. Gastroenterology, 73, 646–650
30. Worner, T. M. and Lieber, C. S. (1985). Perivenular fibrosis as a precursor lesion of cirrhosis. JAMA, 254, 627–630
31. Nasrallah, S. M., Nassar, V. H. and Galambos, J. T. (1980). Importance of terminal hepatic venule thickening. Arch. Pathol. Lab. Med., 104, 84–86
32. Bassendine, M. F. (1986). Alcohol–a major risk factor for hepatocellular carcinoma. J. Hepatol., 2, 513–519
33. Takase, S., Takada, N., Enomoto, N., Yasuhara, M. and Takada, A. (1991). Different types of chronic hepatitis in alcoholic patients: does chronic hepatitis induced by alcohol exist? Hepatology, 13, 876–881
34. Morgan, M. Y., Sherlock, S. and Scheuer, P. J. (1978). Portal fibrosis in the liver of alcoholic patients. Gut, 19, 1015–1021
35. Kent, G. and Popper, H. (1968). Liver biopsy in diagnosis of haemochromatosis. Am. J. Med., 44, 837–841
36. Pariente, E.-A., Degott, C., Mastin, J., Feldmann, G., Potet, F. and Benhamou, J.-P. (1981). Hepatocytic PAS-positive diastase resistant inclusions in the absence of al-anti-trypsin deficiency – high prevalence in alcoholic cirrhosis. Am. J. Clin. Pathol., 76, 299–302
37. Derr, R. F., Porta, E. A., Larkin, E. C. and Rao, G. A. (1990). Is ethanol per se hepatotoxic? J. Hepatol., 10, 381–386
38. Tsukamoto, H., Gaal, K. and French, S. W. (1990). Insights into the pathogenesis of alcoholic liver necrosis and fibrosis: Status report. 12, 599–608

Haemochromatosis and Iron Storage Disorders

14

The total body iron in an adult man is between 4 and 5 g. Approximately two-thirds of this is contained in circulating haemoglobin and. to a much lesser extent, the myoglobin and iron containing enzymes, such as mitochondrial cytochromes. The remainder, approximately 1.5 g, is stored in the liver, which is also the site of synthesis of the main protein involved in iron transport, apotransferrin. In physiological quantities, iron is principally in the form of ferritin, a complex molecule composed of a shell of protein with a core containing micellar ionic iron, dispersed through the cytoplasm and not normally visible by light microscopy. As the quantity of iron increases, ferritin molecules aggregate together and become incorporated into lysosomes. These eventually will become visible as golden-brown granules of haemosiderin, often grouped in the pericanalicular portion of the liver cell. The iron is now demonstrable histochemically by Perl's Prussian blue reaction which stains iron bright blue (care must be exercised with acid fixatives such as Zenker's, which may render a proportion of the tissue iron unstainable). In contrast to copper-staining in Wilson's disease, there is a good correlation between the amount of iron as assessed on an arbitrary four-point scale and total hepatic iron as measured chemically[1,2]. Most storage iron is found in parenchymal cells, and is derived from transferrin and from free haemoglobin. Kupffer cell iron is largely derived from the breakdown of red cells and is usually rapidly returned to the bone marrow.

A typical mixed diet contains 12 to 20 mg iron, from which approximately 10% is absorbed. Total body iron is thought to form a labile pool[3], with free exchange between the blood and synthetic, mainly haemopoietic, sites and storage sites such as mucosal cell and liver. Iron is readily taken up by the mucosal cell, particularly in the form of haem iron, and then either transferred into the circulation when needed or retained in the cell and thus shed into the intestinal lumen. Iron is transported in the blood as transferrin, which is normally relatively unsaturated. Active erythropoiesis leads to active removal of iron from the plasma; levels are then restored by movement of iron from storage sites such as the mucosal cell or the liver. Ferritin is also normally present in the circulation in small quantities and may reflect total body iron stores[4]. Serum iron, iron-binding capacity (IBC) and serum ferritin are important screening tests, since normal values in all three effectively exclude iron overload states[5].

IRON OVERLOAD

There is some confusion over the use of the terms haemosiderosis and haemochromatosis. Haemosiderosis, or siderosis, denotes an increased quantity of tissue iron without reference to its site or cause, and usually by implication an absence of tissue damage. Haemochromatosis, on the other hand, implies associated tissue damage as well as iron overload. Whatever the reason for the accumulation of iron, the liability to tissue damage is the same, although there is some evidence that reticuloendothelial iron is less harmful than parenchymal iron (see below). When the unqualified term haemochromatosis is used, it usually refers to the genetic disease idiopathic haemochromatosis.

Despite the appearance of imaging techniques such as nuclear magnetic resonance[6] which are effective quantitatively, liver biopsy is the method of choice in the diagnosis of iron overload states[2,7,8]. Both the cellular distribution of iron and the extent of tissue damage can only be assessed by direct hepatic morphology. Various semiquantitative scoring systems have been devised for the assessment of iron load, based upon histochemical stains such as Perl's Prussian blue[9]. That proposed by Sciot and colleagues is particularly useful and defines five grades from 0 (no iron) to IV (massive deposition)[10]. Quantitation can also be performed reliably by image analysis[11].

HAEMOSIDEROSIS

Small quantities of iron are occasionally seen in otherwise normal liver biopsies (Figure 14.1). Parenchymal iron is usually found in periportal liver cells and may be traced to an increase of iron intake or absorption but frequently has no obvious cause. Early presymptomatic primary haemochromatosis can never be excluded purely on morphological grounds.

In contrast, iron in reticuloendothelial cells, the Kupffer cells, is derived principally from senescent red cells, with a small contribution from necrotic liver cells and from iron in the blood not attached to transferrin. Stainable iron in Kupffer cells accumulates, therefore, most often in patients with acute haemolytic anaemia. Occasionally the iron-containing cells can be quite conspicuous (Figure 14.2), but more often they remain small and evenly spaced throughout the liver parenchyma requiring an iron stain for easy recognition. Iron may also accumulate in Kupffer cells after release from parenchymal cells in any hepatitic process (Figure 2.17) and in parenteral iron therapy. Finally, iron may accumulate because of a failure of re-utilization of iron. This is an important cause of anaemia in various chronic inflammatory states, such as rheumatoid arthritis and in malignancies. If reticuloendothelial iron accumulation is long-standing, some at least of the iron will be transferred to parenchymal cells.

PRIMARY OR IDIOPATHIC HAEMOCHROMATOSIS (IHC)

This is a metabolic disorder associated with an increased absorption of iron from a normal diet and is inherited as an autosomal recessive, closely associated with the major histocompatibility complex antigen HLA A3. The gene is thus thought to be near to the A locus on the short arm of chromosome 6, but the precise locus, and the nature of the genetic product are not yet known. The gene frequency is thought to be 1:20, giving a heterozygote frequency of 1:10 and a homozygote frequency of 1:400[12]. Clinical disease is less frequent than expected, mainly because some individuals may compensate in other ways for the increased iron absorption. This applies especially to women of child-bearing age whose menstrual blood loss may prevent the positive iron balance until after the menopause.

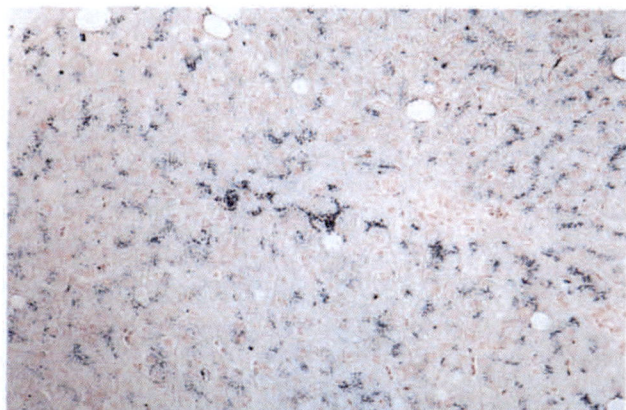

Figure 14.1 Haemosiderosis. An alcoholic patient who presented with hepatomegaly. Biopsy shows minor fatty change but no alcoholic hepatitis or cirrhosis. There is a moderate increase in iron in parenchymal cells, slightly more marked in the periportal region (centre of field), which was attributed to high iron content of the port and wine that the patient consumed. Perl's Prussian blue.

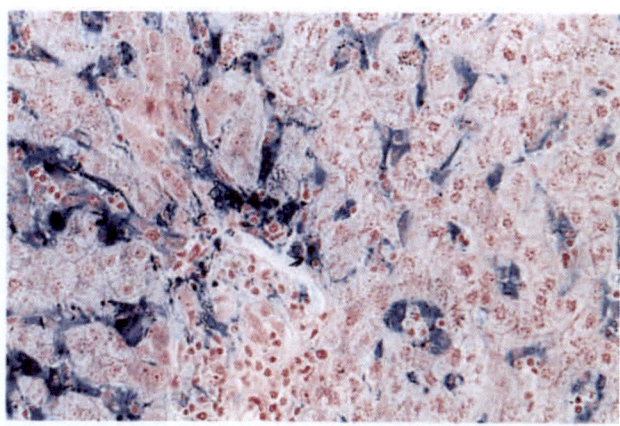

Figure 14.2 Reticuloendothelial siderosis. A 30-year-old female patient with a severe haemolytic anaemia which required multiple transfusions. The liver was biopsied at the time of splenectomy and shows massive accumulation of iron in Kupffer cells but little or no parenchymal iron. There is no architectural disturbance. Perl's Prussian blue.

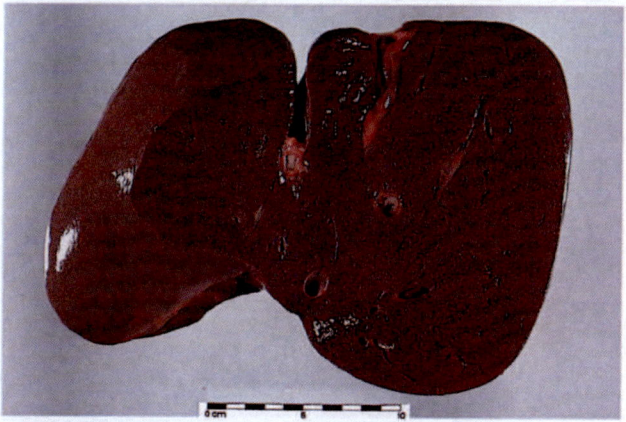

Figure 14.3 Primary haemochromatosis. The diagnosis in this case was an incidental finding at post-mortem in a 57-year-old man who died of cardiac disease. The liver is of normal size and is deep brown in colour. The capsular surface is only faintly nodular and the cut surface has a 'nutmeg' pattern without nodules.

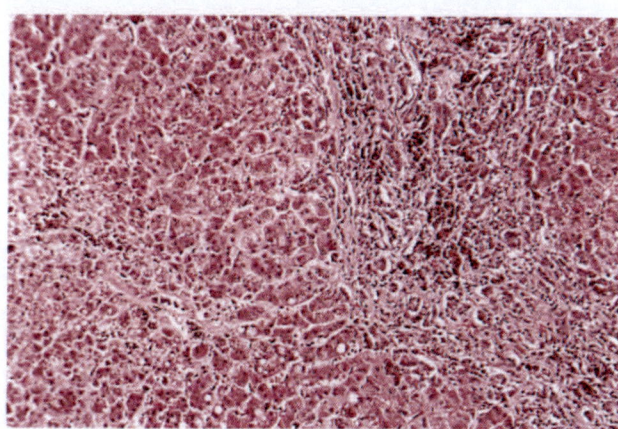

Figure 14.4 Primary haemochromatosis. Same case as Figure 14.3. The whole section has a brown hue due to iron accumulation in both parenchymal cells and portal tract phagocytes. The portal tract is expanded and fibrotic but the hepatocytes are undamaged.

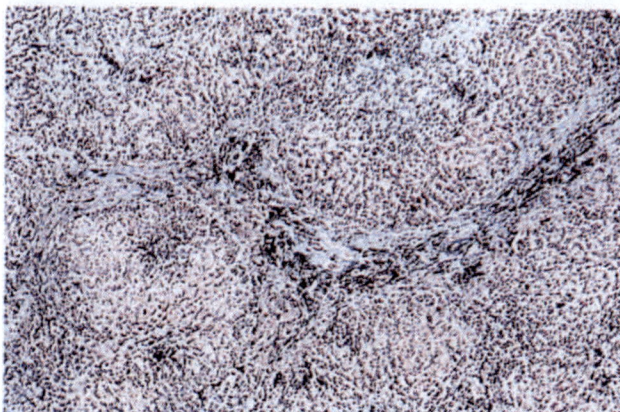

Figure 14.5 Primary haemochromatosis. Same case as Figures 14.3 and 14.4. This section more clearly demonstrates the extent of the iron accumulation and the nature of the architectural disturbance. It can be seen that the portal tract running across the centre of the field has a 'holly-leaf' outline due to fibrosis which is tending to link with neighbouring portal tracts. The parenchymal architecture is still undisturbed. Perl's Prussian blue.

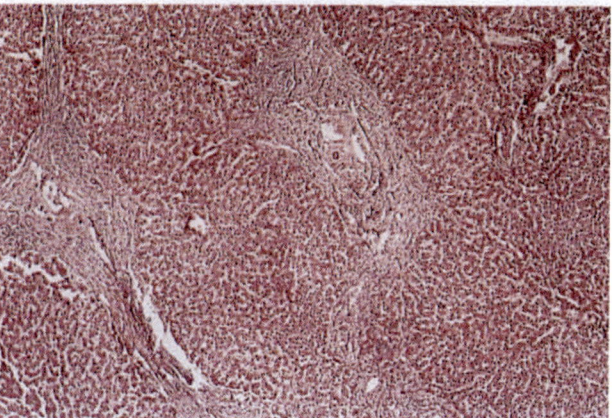

Figure 14.6 Primary haemochromatosis. Another case in which the biopsy is very similar to Figures 14.4 and 14.5 with portal tract fibrosis and preservation of lobular architecture in the presence of massive parenchymal iron deposition.

The metabolic abnormality is not yet clearly defined, but the available evidence suggests that iron absorption is excessive and inappropriate as a result of increased iron transfer across the intestinal epithelial cell. Clinical presentation usually occurs in the 40–60 year age group and the disease is ten times as frequent in men as women, possibly for the reasons given above, that women are protected to some extent from iron accumulation by menstrual blood loss and pregnancies. Total body iron stores may be 20–50 times normal and the liver iron may be as high as 40–50 g. In the established disease, when the capacity of the liver iron stores is exceeded, iron also accumulates in other parenchymal organs, particularly the endocrine glands, heart muscle and joints where it may cause diabetes mellitus, cardiac failure or arthropathy. Although iron also accumulates in the skin, the characteristic slate colour is imparted by increased melanin pigmentation and not the iron.

The pathogenesis of the tissue injury is very poorly understood. Haemochromatosis has proved to be very difficult to reproduce experimentally. This may be partly because it takes much longer than can easily be achieved in laboratory animals and partly because iron when given parenterally, tends to be located in the reticuloendothelial system. Nevertheless, iron must be regarded as the main aetiological agent for the following reasons[5]:

(1) Similar changes are seen regardless of the cause of the iron overload.

(2) The degree of fibrosis is directly proportional to the tissue iron concentration.

(3) There may be significant regression following phlebotomy.

(4) Chelation therapy in congenital anaemias prevents or reduces iron overload and fibrosis.

Signs of necrosis or inflammation are virtually never seen. Collagen deposition in portal tracts appears to occur without obvious cell injury as though excess iron is directly stimulating collagen formation, possibly through the release of enzymes by unduly fragile lysosomes in iron-damaged hepatocytes[13]. Recent evidence with cultured fibroblasts showed a direct link between lipid peroxidation and fibrogenesis.[14] Iron loading above the cells' capacity for detoxification leads to the release of free radicals and lipid peroxidation which cause fibrosis directly without prior hepatocyte damage[15]. The organelle changes noted above may themselves be secondary to this process. In most cases nodular regeneration is a relatively late phenomenon, as in biliary cirrhosis.

The liver is usually enlarged, micronodular and quite distinctly brown in colour (Figure 14.3). The high iron concentration can easily be confirmed by the Prussian blue reaction on tissue slices. Microscopically there may be an established micronodular cirrhosis, but frequently there is merely an advanced portal fibrosis with an overall pattern resembling that seen in biliary obstruction. Portal tracts are expanded due to fibrosis (Figures 14.4, 14.5 and 14.6), which often sends short spurs into the parenchyma giving them an overall holly-leaf shape[16]. These tend to link with one another and surround individual lobules and groups of lobules. Iron accumulation is usually marked and predominantly parenchymal (Figure 14.5), although in portal tracts it may also be found in the biliary epithelium (Figure 14.7), phagocytes and deposited on collagen fibres. Because of its tendency to aggregate around bile canaliculi, the latter may be clearly outlined in iron-stained material. The expanded portal tracts may show striking ductular proliferation, but inflammation is conspicuously slight or absent altogether. There is no

piecemeal necrosis and there is no evidence of liver cell necrosis or intralobular inflammation. There may be minor fatty change. Liver cells often have a marked increase in non-iron pigment which is lipofuscin and this may also be seen in portal tract structures. There are often large haemosiderin-filled Kupffer cells scattered randomly through the parenchyma. In the absence of nodular regeneration, iron depletion therapy can be followed by disappearance not only of the iron but also of the excess fibrous tissue (Figures 14.6 and 14.8). The lipofuscin pigment may then be much more conspicuous.

Presymptomatic disease

Because treatment of precirrhotic disease is so successful[12], it is important that all relatives of patients over 10 years should be screened. Although as already stated normal values of serum iron, IBC and ferritin will exclude disease, if any are abnormal, liver biopsy is essential and the examination should include a chemical estimation of tissue iron. Fibrosis does not occur when the hepatic iron concentration is below 14 000 μg/g (about 252 μmol/g) dry weight[17]. The hepatic iron index[17] (defined as the hepatic iron concentration in μmol/g divided by the age in years) has proved to be an effective way of discriminating presymptomatic homozygotes from heterozygotes or alcoholics with iron overload. Even when negative, screening should be repeated every few years. Microscopically, there may be any quantity of iron, which is mainly parenchymal and commences in the periportal cells and then gradually comes to involve the majority of liver cells (Figure 14.9). The earliest signs of damage are seen as increasing portal fibrosis which gradually progresses to the fully developed changes outlined above. It is important to stress that in idiopathic hereditary haemochromatosis iron overload precedes fibrosis and thus significant architectural damage is unlikely unless there is grade IV siderosis. There is no evidence that heterozygotes are at increased risk of hepatic fibrosis[17].

Malignancy

Haemochromatosis carries a definite risk of hepatocellular carcinoma (HCC) which is generally considered in excess of 15%, a relative risk of 200 compared to the general population[18]. Some patients may even present for the first time with carcinoma; in others it may be responsible for sudden deterioration of their condition (Figure 14.10). The tumour itself is indistinguishable from any other hepatocellular carcinoma and is usually iron-free. The frequency of HCC in IHC exceeds that in other forms of cirrhosis, suggesting that iron itself may be directly carcinogenic. Support for this proposal comes from *in vitro* studies[19], and from occasional cases where HCC arises in precirrhotic individuals[20].

SECONDARY IRON OVERLOAD

Iron accumulation in congenital and refractory anaemias, such as thalassaemia and sideroblastic anaemia (erythropoietic haemochromatosis, EHC), occurs through two mechanisms. The accelerated or ineffective erythropoiesis causes an increased absorption of iron and the regular blood transfusions that are required add still further to the iron accumulation. Absorbed iron is deposited in parenchymal cells whilst red-cell-derived iron is taken up by the Kupffer cells. Thus the iron overload tends to affect parenchymal cells and reticuloendothelial cells in roughly equal proportions. The development of fibrosis and cirrhosis is very similar to that in IHC[21], although there is some evidence that true cirrhosis may develop more rapidly in the congenital anaemias[22]. However, this type

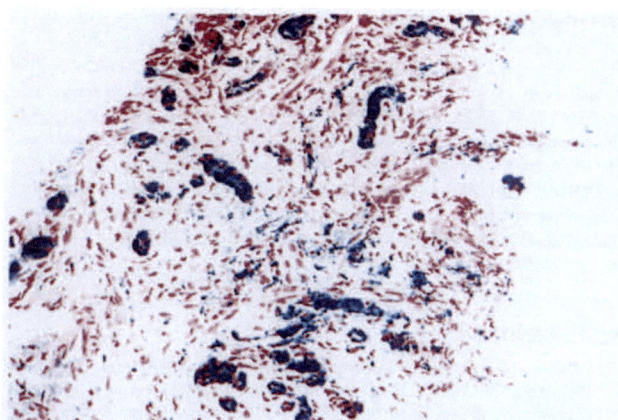

Figure 14.7   Primary haemochromatosis. Another case showing striking deposition of iron in biliary epithelium in this expanded and fibrotic portal tract. Perl's Prussian blue.

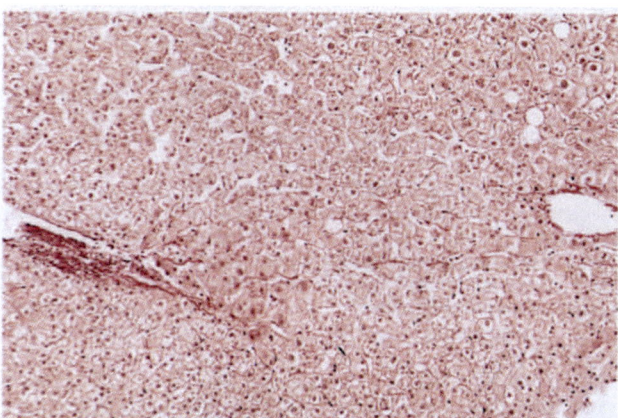

Figure 14.8   Primary haemochromatosis. Same patient as Figure 14.6. After diagnosis, the patient was treated by regular venesection. His liver was rebiopsied 13 years later and this shows that not only has the excess iron completely disappeared but there has also been almost total resolution of the portal fibrosis. Elastic van Gieson.

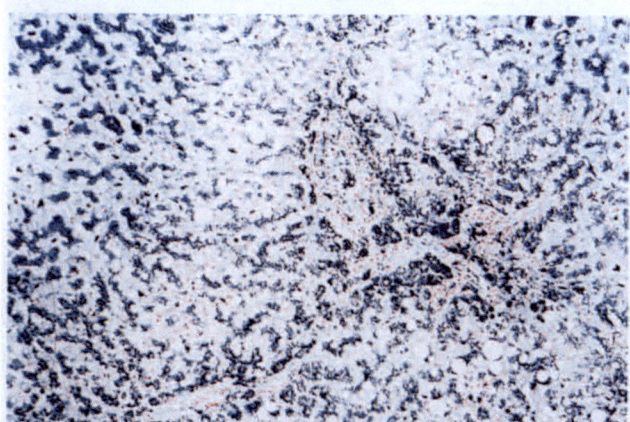

Figure 14.9   Primary haemochromatosis, presymptomatic. A 45-year-old man whose liver was biopsied following the discovery that the serum transferrin was fully saturated. It shows heavy parenchymal deposition of iron, but not yet any evidence of portal fibrosis. Subsequent regular venesection completely removed the iron. Perl's Prussian blue.

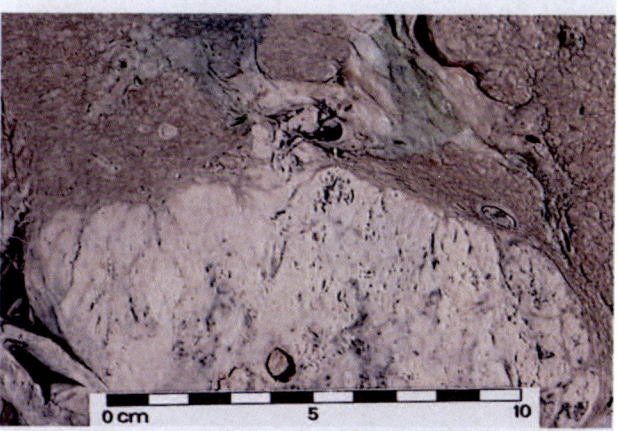

Figure 14.10   Primary haemochromatosis, hepatocellular carcinoma. This patient, who was known to have IHC, suddenly deteriorated and died. Post-mortem examination revealed this tumour mass, confined to the liver, and histologically a typical hepatocellular carcinoma. Note the brown micronodular cirrhosis in the adjacent liver.

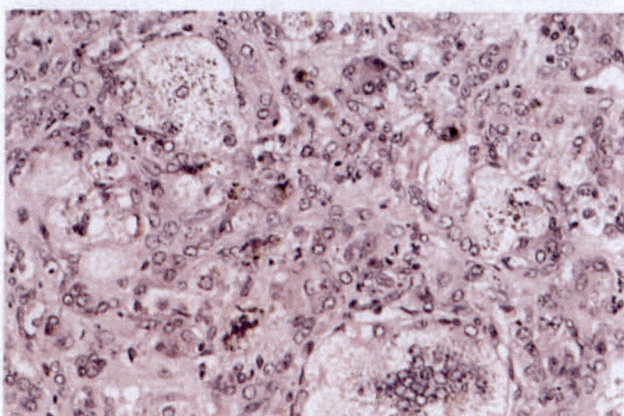

Figure 14.11   Neonatal haemochromatosis. A male baby showed some growth retardation combined with oligohydramnios during pregnancy. Full-term delivery followed by the rapid onset of liver failure with severe coagulation defect. Liver removed at time of transplantation, aged six weeks, was small and showed widespread multilobular necrosis (not shown) with giant-cell hepatitis and prominent brown pigmentation.

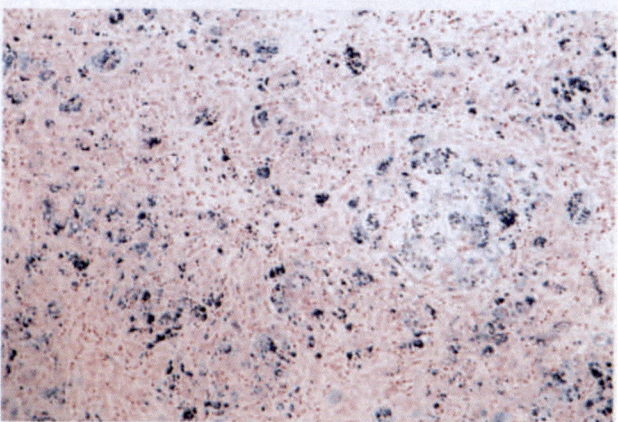

Figure 14.12   Neonatal haemochromatosis. Same case as Figure 14.11, confirming grade III/IV siderosis. Perl's Prussian blue.

of disease can be, and now is, largely avoided by the regular use of chelating agents such as desferrioxamine.

Iron accumulation secondary to established liver disease is relatively common[7,12], although usually only slight, and is probably seen most often in alcoholic cirrhosis. Portacaval shunt causes increased hepatic iron deposition in experimental animals and thus may well be the mechanism in cirrhosis as a result of both intra- and extrahepatic shunting of blood. Perhaps the bypass of liver cells causes relative hypoxia, leading to increased uptake of iron from the blood by hepatocytes, which itself will lead to increased absorption from the gut. Gastrointestinal haemorrhage and deficiencies of factors such as folate and vitamin B12 by causing increased erythropoietic activity, may also be contributory factors. In these cases, although liver iron is increased, there is no evidence that total body iron stores are elevated. Significant iron accumulation only occurs after cirrhosis is fully established; in contrast to the situation in IHC and EHC where the iron deposition precedes fibrosis and architectural disturbance, and thus probably plays little part in tissue damage. The connective tissue septa are often relatively iron-free. Evidence of other aetiological factors, for example alcoholic hepatitis and centrilobular fibrosis, should always be sought, but if there is no previous history or biopsy it may not always be possible to exclude IHC on morphological grounds alone. It is important to stress that there is a documented increased prevalence of alcoholism in patients with IHC[12]. Family studies should be undertaken in all such cases.

Finally, iron accumulation in the liver is commonly seen amongst the Bantu in southern Africa[23,24] and is generally attributed to dietary excess derived from alcoholic drinks brewed in iron cooking utensils. Sporadic cases, usually caused by excessive ingestion of therapeutic iron preparations, are seen in other populations[25]. When large quantities of iron are absorbed, the capacity of transferrin may be exceeded and so there will be both parenchymal and reticuloendothelial deposition of iron. Fibrosis resembles that in IHC and the development of cirrhosis is uncommon.

DIFFERENTIAL DIAGNOSIS

If iron is found only in Kupffer cells, previous haemolysis, blood transfusion or hepatitis should be suspected. If iron is found only in parenchymal cells, especially if significant in amount and in the absence of fibrosis, it is almost certainly IHC in an early phase. Iron in smaller quantities, maximal in zone 1 hepatocytes, may or may not be significant in this context. If it is maximal in centrilobular cells, previous congestive heart failure should be considered. If fibrosis is marked, especially if other than portal, and siderosis is relatively minor, this argues in favour of secondary iron accumulation. If both cirrhosis and siderosis are marked, secondary accumulation is statistically the more likely, especially if accompanied by significant inflammation.

Reticuloendothelial and parenchymal iron in roughly equivalent amounts suggests EHC, and the presence of fully developed cirrhosis, congenital anaemia. However, some reticuloendothelial iron may also be seen in otherwise typical IHC, but it is usually focal and not evenly spaced as in EHC.

NEONATAL HAEMOCHROMATOSIS

Iron may accumulate in the neonatal liver secondary to a number of haematological disorders, and is usually neither severe nor significant[9]. Quite distinct from this group is a rare sporadic condition associated with massive deposition of iron not only in the liver but also in a variety of other parenchymal tissues[26,27]. The condition has been called neonatal or perinatal haemochromatosis and is associated with a typical neonatal hepatitis (Figure 14.11) combined with heavy, usually grade IV, iron deposition in the liver (Figure 14.12). There is frequently extensive fibrosis and even cirrhosis. Infants are usually born prematurely and the prognosis is very poor. It remains uncertain whether the condition is a specific entity, or whether it is merely a response to severe intrauterine liver injury with subsequent derangement of iron metabolism[26].

REFERENCES

1. Walker, R. J., Miller, J. P. G., Dymock, I. W., Shilkin, K. B. and Williams, R. (1971). Relationship of hepatic iron concentration to histochemical grading and to total chelatable body iron in conditions associated with iron overload. Gut, 12, 1011–1014
2. Brissot, P., Bourel, M., D, H., Verger, J.-P., Messner, M., Beaumont, C., Regnouard, F., Ferrand, B. and Simon, M. (1981). Assessment of liver iron content in 271 patients: a reevaluation of direct and indirect methods. Gastroenterology, 80, 557–565
3. Cavill, I., Wormwood, M. and Jacobs, A. (1975). Internal regulation of iron absorption. Nature, 265, 328–329
4. Halliday, J. W., Russo, A. M., Cowlishaw, J. L. and Powell, L. W. (1977). Serum ferritin in diagnosis of haemochromatosis: study of 43 families. Lancet, 2, 621–624
5. Powell, L. W., Bassett, M, L. and Halliday, J. W. (1980). Haemochromatosis: 1980 update. Gastroenterology, 78, 374–381
6. Kier, R. (1990). Quantification of hepatic iron with CT and MRI: practical considerations. Hepatology, 12, 1441–1442
7. Kent, G. and Popper, H. (1968). Liver biopsy in diagnosis of haemochromatosis. Am. J. Med., 44, 837–841
8. Bonkovsky, H. L., Slaker, D. P., Bills, E. B. and Wolf, D. C. (1990). Usefulness and limitations of laboratory and hepatic imaging studies in iron-storage disease. Gastroenterology, 99, 1079–1091
9. Burt, A. D. and MacSween, R. N. M. (1993). Fat, alcohol, iron. In Wight, D. G. D. (ed). Liver, Biliary Tract and Exocrine Pancreas. 11. Systemic Pathology. Symmers, W. S. C., series ed. 3rd edn. Edinburgh: Churchill Livingstone
10. Sciot, R., van Eyken, P., Facchetti, F. et al. (1989). Hepatocellular transferrin receptor expression in secondary siderosis. Liver, 9, 52–61
11. Olynyk, J., Hall, P., Sallie, R., Reed, W., Shilkin, K. and Mackinnon, M. (1990). Computerized measurement of iron in liver biopsies: a comparison with biochemical iron measurement. Hepatology, 12, 26–30
12. Powell, L. W. (1992). Haemochromatosis and related iron storage diseases. In Millward-Sadler, G. H., Wright, R. and Arthur, M. J. P. (eds). Wright's Liver and Biliary Disease. edn. 976–994. London: WB Saunders
13. Peters, T. J. and Seymour, C. A. (1976). Acid hydrolase activities and lysosomal integrity in liver biopsies from patients with iron overload. Clin. Sci. Mol. Med., 50, 75–78
14. Chojkier, M., Houghin, K., Solis-Herruso, J. and Brenner, D. A. (1989). Stimulation of collagen gene expression by ascorbic acid in cultured human fibroblasts. J. Biol. Chem., 264, 16597–16962
15. Bacon, B. R. and Britton, R. S. (1990). The pathology of hepatic iron overload: a free radical-mediated process? Hepatology, 11, 127–137
16. Scheuer, P. J. (1988). Disturbances of copper and iron metabolism. In (eds). Liver Biopsy Interpretation. 4th edn. pp. 207–217. London: Baillière Tindall
17. Sallie, R. W., Reed, W. D. and Shilkin, K. B. (1991). Confirmation of the efficacy of hepatic tissue iron index in differentiating genetic haemochromatosis from alcoholic liver disease complicated by alcoholic haemosiderosis. Gut, 32, 207–210
18. Bradbear, R. A., Bain, C., Siskind, V. et al. (1985). Cohort study of internal malignancy in genetic hemochromatosis and other nonalcoholic liver diseases. J. Natl. Cancer Inst., 75, 81–84
19. Loeb, L. A., James, E. A., Waltersdorph, A. M. and Klebanoff, S. J. (1988). Mutagenesis by the autoxidation of iron with isolated DNA. Proc. Natl. Acad. Sci. USA., 85, 3918–3922
20. Fellows, I. W., Stewart, M., Jeffcoate, W. J., Smith, P. G. and Toghill, P. J. (1988). Hepatocellular carcinoma in primary haemochromatosis in the absence of cirrhosis. Gut, 29, 1603–1609
21. Schafer, A. I., Cheron, R. C., Dluhy, R., Cooper, B., Gleason, R. E., Soeldner, J. S. and Bunn, H. F. (1981). Clinical consequences of

acquired transfusional iron overload in adults. N. Engl. J. Med, 304, 319–324

22. Iancu, T. C., Landing, B. H. and Neustein, H. B. (1977). Pathogenetic mechanisms in hepatic cirrhosis of thalassemia major: light and EM studies. In Sommers, S. C. and Rosen, P. P. (eds). Pathology Annual. pp. 171–200. New York: Appleton Century Crofts

23. Buchanan, W. M. (1969). Bantu siderosis/a review. Centr. Afr. J. Med., 15, 105–120

24. Bothwell, T. H. and Charlton, R. W. (1982). Hemochromatosis. In Schiff, L. and Schiff, E. R. (eds). Diseases of the Liver. 5th edn. pp. 1003–1042. Philadelphia: Lippincott

25. Hennigar, G. R. (1979). Haemochromatosis caused by excessive vitamin iron intake. Am. J. Pathol., 96, 611

26. Witzelben, C. L. (1989). Perinatal haemochromatosis: entity or end result. Hum. Pathol., 20, 335–340

27. Moerman, P., Pauwels, P., Vandenberghe, K., Devlieger, H., Fryns, J. P., Verresen, H., Jaekaen, J., Lauweryns, J. and Eggermont, E. (1990). Neonatal haemochromatosis. Histopathology, 17, 345–351

Wilson's Disease

15

Wilson's disease, or hepatolenticular degeneration, is a lethal condition due to an inborn error of metabolism with recessive inheritance resulting in the abnormal accumulation of copper within the body. The gene, recently localized to the long arm of chromosome 13[1], is worldwide with a carrier frequency of roughly 1:90 and a disease incidence of approximately 1:30 000[2]. Most patients present between the ages of 6 and 25, the younger ones usually with liver disease; the older ones with neurological or neuropsychiatric disturbance.

Copper is essential for life, but the supply of dietary copper relative to biological needs is superabundant and the liver plays a central homeostatic role. Normally about 60–90% of the average daily intake of 2–5 mg of copper is absorbed from the gut by a specific transport mechanism[3]. It is then transported, loosely bound to albumin, to the liver where it is rapidly cleared and most becomes associated with specific copper-binding proteins in the liver cell cytosol: superoxide dismutase (hepatocuprein), metallothionein and cuprophilin. These proteins incorporate about 80% of the absorbed copper; 0.5–1.0 mg of copper per day is re-exported from the liver attached to newly synthesized caeruloplasmin. Copper balance, however, depends upon the excretion of some 1.5 mg per day in the bile, apparently following sequestration in hepatocyte lysosomes. In Wilson's disease both these mechanisms are impaired[2,4] and copper accumulates in the liver at the rate of 10–20 mg per year. Although caeruloplasmin is reduced or absent in 95% of affected individuals, this is almost certainly secondary to the liver disease and not a primary defect[5].

Initially the liver can bind the excess copper, up to 50 times as much as normal, without overt disease. Eventually, usually around puberty, this capacity is exceeded and copper is released into the circulation. Since it is only loosely associated with plasma proteins, some is excreted in the urine, but copper also diffuses from the vascular compartment into other tissues such as brain, cornea, kidneys and joints. It is the rate of the copper release from the liver which seems to determine the nature of the clinical presentation. When the capacity of the liver to sequester the excess copper is overcome suddenly, perhaps the result of fulminant liver cell necrosis or acute hepatitis, the free non-caeruloplasmin bound copper rises to as much as ten times normal and may causes acute haemolysis. Even when presentation is very acute, cirrhosis is already fully established[6]. More usually, the patient presents with insidious onset of cirrhosis and associated disorders such as portal hypertension and hypersplenism. Less commonly presentation may be with a chronic active hepatitis syndrome[7]. However, in many patients there are no symptoms referable to the liver at all, and presentation is then at a slightly older age, most often in the late teens, with the insidious onset of neurological disease due to copper deposition in the basal ganglia of the brain. In the cornea copper deposition is seen as Kayser-Fleischer rings. All untreated patients with Wilson's disease develop cirrhosis, albeit at different rates[5], and the hepatic changes are frequently more advanced than suspected from the length of the clinical history[5].

Pathogenesis

The mechanism of action and primary cellular site of copper toxicity remain to be determined. Virtually all components of the cell are susceptible to damage and may show ultrastructural abnormalities. Mitochondrial damage[8] may lead to diminished lipid oxidation and consequent accumulation of triglyceride in hepatocytes, one of the earliest visible signs of damage. Evidently the lipid or the copper or both induce a discrete mobilization of mesenchymal cells and fibrogenesis in the absence of significant hepatocellular necrosis or inflammation[5], although detailed mechanisms remain to be defined.

Diagnosis

The main diagnostic features are demonstration of Kayser-Fleischer (K-F) rings, low serum caeruloplasmin (< 200 mg/l or 1.5 μmol/l) and high liver copper concentration (> 250 μg/g dry weight)[2]. Each of the biochemical results may be abnormal in other conditions. For example, asymptomatic heterozygotes or any liver disease associated with hepatocyte necrosis may occasionally have low levels of caeruloplasmin. Similarly, diseases associated with the failure of bile flow, for example prolonged biliary obstruction or primary biliary cirrhosis, may show considerable accumulation of copper in the liver, and even have K-F rings[9]. However, only in Wilson's disease are both abnormalities present. In equivocal cases, dynamic studies with radio-copper can provide diagnostic results[10].

Histopathology

Morphological studies in Wilson's disease are rarely diagnostically decisive, but, since liver biopsy for copper estimation is mandatory, material is usually available for histological study. As Walshe has stated[11,12], the diagnosis is often missed because it is not even considered until a second sibling develops symptoms. The first child may have been considered to be suffering from, for example, hepatitis, juvenile or cryptogenic cirrhosis, or idiopathic neurological disease. It is thus vital for Wilson's disease to be actively considered in all cases of unexplained liver disease, especially in late childhood and adolescence. All patients with established neurological disease have fully developed cirrhosis, which is often clinically silent. Even when patients have clinical evidence of liver disease, the liver changes are frequently more advanced than would be predicted from the history.

There is a number of histological features which are suggestive, if not pathognomonic, of Wilson's disease.

Presymptomatic Wilson's disease

When siblings of affected individuals are screened, changes may be seen in the liver long before the appearance of symptoms. Foci of fatty change of variable intensity are commonly found (Figure 15.1). Although occasionally this may just take the form of a few large fat droplets randomly scattered through the liver, sometimes the fat is finely divided and distributed around the periphery of the cell without displacement of the nucleus (Figure 15.6). Glycogen vacuolation of periportal liver cell nuclei is almost invariable (Figure 15.1), but this is not an unusual finding in any adolescent liver (Figure 15.3). Yet despite the high tissue concentration, copper stains are

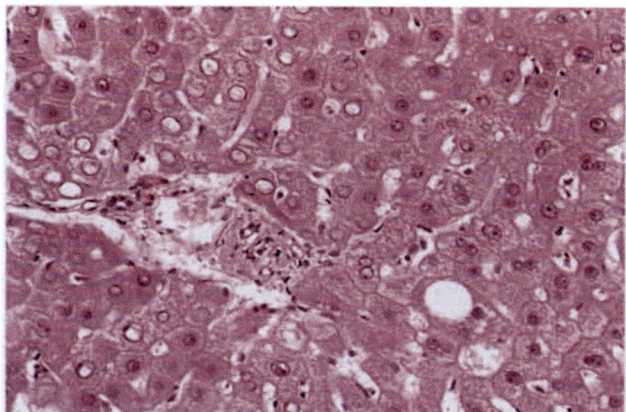

Figure 15.1 Presymptomatic Wilson's disease. A 15-year-old-female, with affected sibling, shown to have a very high hepatic copper. Biopsy shows a normal liver architecture with occasional lipid droplets and striking glycogen vacuolation of periportal hepatocyte nuclei. Although characteristic this appearance is not pathognomonic of Wilson's disease (Figure 15.3). Despite the high tissue copper (shown chemically), stains for copper were negative, a common experience in presymptomatic disease.

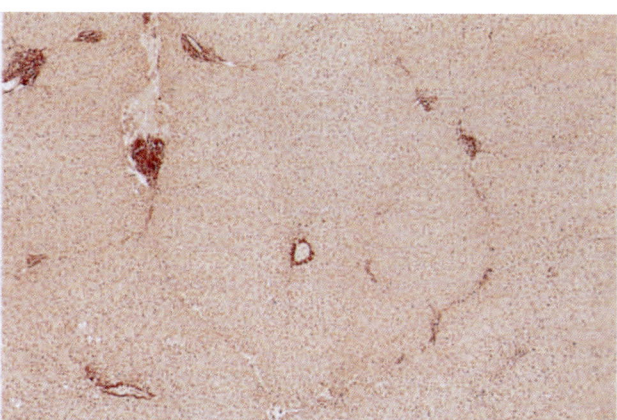

Figure 15.2 Presymptomatic Wilson's disease. Another patient, a 12-year-old boy, with an affected sibling, also has presymptomatic disease shown biochemically. This biopsy shows very early portal fibrosis which tends to accentuate the lobular outlines. Elastic van Gieson.

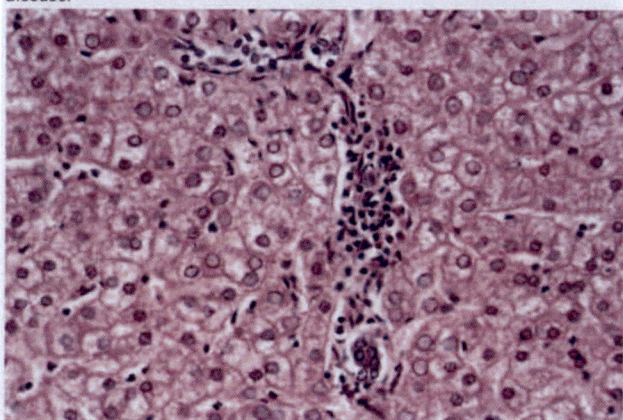

Figure 15.3 Normal control. A 15-year-old male, killed in a road traffic accident. This section shows mild non-specific portal chronic inflammation and striking periportal glycogen vacuolation of hepatocyte nuclei. Tissue copper levels were normal. This section emphasizes that this appearance is common in livers of this age group and is not specific for Wilson's disease.

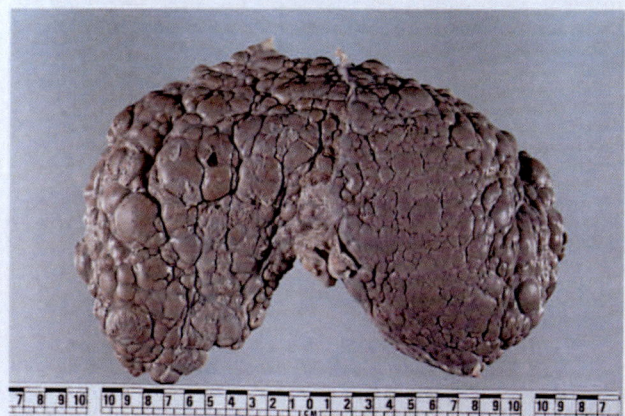

Figure 15.4 Wilson's disease. Fully developed macronodular cirrhosis in this 22-year-old patient with untreated Wilson's disease who died following massive haemorrhage from oesophageal varices.

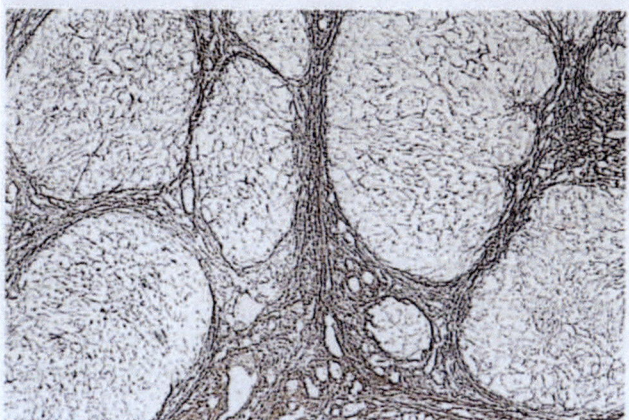

Figure 15.5 Wilson's disease. Another patient with fully developed cirrhosis died of gastrointestinal haemorrhage after only a few months of chelation therapy. This section of post-mortem liver shows rather smaller nodules than in Figure 15.4, each surrounded by fibrous tissue septa. In contrast to iron overload states the cirrhosis appears nodular from the start in Wilson's disease. Reticulin.

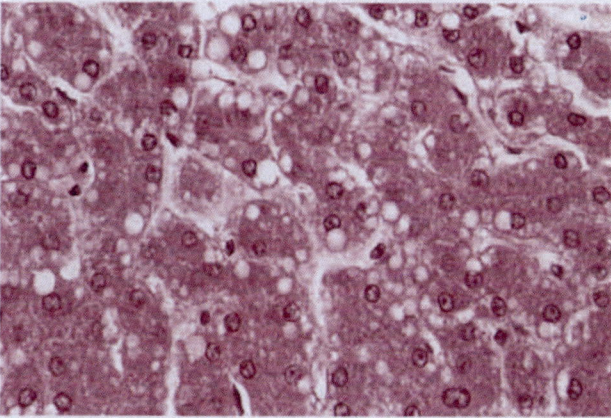

Figure 15.6 Wilson's disease. Another fatal case of Wilson's disease in an 11-year-old boy. Post-mortem liver shows the distinctive pericellular fat droplets often seen.

usually negative because the copper is diffusely distributed throughout the cytosol. Ultrastructural studies reveal striking changes in the mitochondria which show marked heterogeneity of size and shape, increased matrix density, separation of inner and outer mitochondrial membranes and enlarged intercristal spaces. They may also contain vacuolated, crystalline or dense inclusions[13]. These changes are characteristic but probably not entirely pathognomonic and are probably related to the fat infiltration. Large irregular granules of lipofuscin may sometimes be seen in periportal liver cells[14]. There is occasionally prominence of Kupffer cells laden with iron pigment, possibly secondary to an episode of haemolysis. Later, thin fibrous septa accentuating rather than destroying lobules may be seen (Figure 15.2). Portal inflammation is usually not conspicuous. Most untreated patients thereafter seem to progress insidiously to the development of cirrhosis, and indeed up to 50% of children in the presymptomatic stage are already cirrhotic[15].

Cirrhosis

The cirrhosis seen in Wilson's disease is typically macronodular (Figures 15.4 and 15.5) with often quite variable nodular size. Septa are usually thin. but they may be broad with areas of collapse and bile ductular proliferation. Histologically, unless the diagnosis is actively considered, there may be no particular pointers towards Wilson's disease. Commonly, however, liver cells show similar fatty change (Figure 15.6) and glycogen vacuolation to that in the pre-cirrhotic liver, as described above. Mallory's hyalin may be abundant in the peripheral liver cells in late disease (Figure 15.7)[14]. Although the total liver copper may be lower than in the presymptomatic phase, it is at this stage that stains for copper are more reliably positive since most of the liver copper is now sequestered in lysosomes. However, even now only about 50% of cases will be positive with the rhodamine or rubeanic acid stains[16,17]. The copper is seen as granular deposits staining reddish or greenish black (Figure 15.9) respectively, maximal in the peripheral liver cells, but also distributed throughout the hepatocytes in some nodules (Figure 15.10), a pattern almost never seen in cholestatic diseases (where the copper protein is exclusively peripheral). Even at this advanced stage, some nodules contain no stainable copper and thus its absence does not exclude the diagnosis. The orcein stain for copper-associated protein is positive in even fewer cases (Figure 15.8). Ultrastructurally, the mitochondria may have returned to normal. Unlike in many other types of cirrhosis the risk of hepatocellular carcinoma appears to be very low in Wilson's disease[3].

Acute disease

If the capacity of the liver to bind copper is suddenly exceeded, the disease may be much more acute. Occasionally an acute haemolytic anaemia coincident with acute hepatic failure may be the first manifestation of disease and may lead to death within a few days. Other patients may present with the clinical and biochemical features of chronic active hepatitis[7]. Morphologically most of these patients already have an established cirrhosis with nodule formation[6]. Superimposed upon this, there may be varying degrees of activity ranging from severe liver cell damage with piecemeal necrosis at the limiting plates (Figure 15.11) and ballooning of liver cells throughout the parenchyma to a more moderate periportal and septal chronic hepatitis. Inflammation is patchy and disproportionately light compared to the amount of liver damage. There is usually at least one additional feature such as fatty change, glycogen vacuolation of nuclei or

positive copper stains to give at least a pointer towards Wilson's disease.

Treatment

Wilson's disease is thus a condition which may present in many different ways. Although rare, it must be considered in all cases of otherwise unexplained liver disease in patients under 40 years of age. It is never too late to start treatment with copper chelating agents and even in the presence of already established cirrhosis there may be considerable clinical improvement with return of the serum biochemistry to normal[18]. Even portal hypertension appears capable of regression and the cirrhosis becomes compensated. When treatment is initiated prior to the development of cirrhosis, life expectancy is normal. If medical treatment fails or is started too late, liver transplantation is curative[19].

INDIAN CHILDHOOD CIRRHOSIS (ICC)

ICC is an unexplained form of chronic liver disease which affects young children in most parts of the Indian subcontinent but is almost unknown in other parts of the world[20]. Typically it presents between the ages of 9 months and 5 years with progressive abdominal distension[21]. Jaundice is often the symptom which finally brings the child to hospital and death usually follows within weeks or months from infection, haemorrhage or liver failure.

Histologically the appearances in advanced cases are characteristic (Figure 15.12). Virtually every liver cell is abnormal, showing ballooning, vacuolation or necrosis. Many also contain clumped Mallory's hyalin. There is little regenerative activity and this, together with the aggressive pericellular fibrosis, gives rise to a micro-micronodular cirrhosis in many cases. Cholestasis and bile ductular proliferation may be prominent, but inflammatory cells are usually not numerous. One of the most interesting recent discoveries is the finding of a very high liver copper in ICC, and that almost every cell contains multiple coarse dark brown orcein positive granules. This is in contrast to copper accumulation in Wilson's disease and chronic cholestasis where it tends to be much more focal[22,23].

This has led to the suggestion that copper is directly responsible for the tissue damage in ICC, apparently confirmed by the observation that copper chelation causes significant histological improvement[24]. The mechanism of copper accumulation, however, remains unknown. Although up to 30% of cases have a family history, there is no clear pattern of inheritance[25] and thus it could as easily be explained by an increased environmental copper. Other possibilities include increased availability of copper in food, perhaps through interaction with other substances, or even defective hepatic excretion of copper. However it accumulates, the copper itself may cause further interference with excretion, especially in an immature liver[18]. There is no evidence that hepatitis A or B, malnutrition or α_1-antitrypsin deficiency play any part in the pathogenesis.

REFERENCES

1. Bowcock, A. M., Farrer, L. A., Hebert, J. M. et al. (1988). Eight closely linked loci place the Wilson's disease within 13q14-q21. Am. J. Hum. Gen., 43, 667–674
2. Scheinberg, I. H. and Sterlieb, I. (1984). Wilson's Disease. Major Problems in Internal Medicine. Philadelphia: W B Saunders
3. Sterlieb, I. and Scheinberg, I. H. (1992). Wilson's Disease. In Millward-Sadler, G. H., Wright, R. and Arthur, M. J. P. (eds). Wright's Liver and Biliary Disease. 3rd edn. pp. 965–975. London: W B Saunders

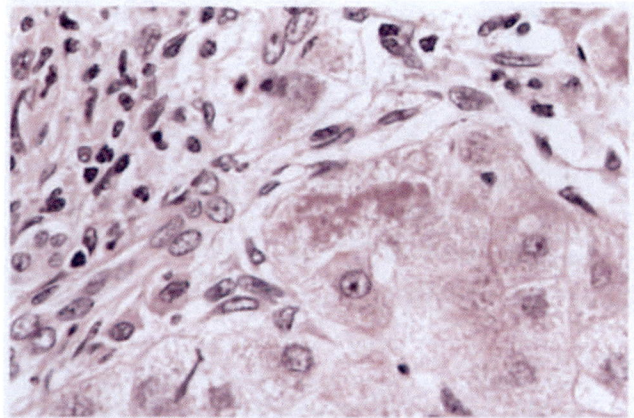

Figure 15.7 Wilson's disease. This section, from a liver removed at transplantation, shows well–developed Mallory's hyaline as strongly eosinophilic irregular aggregates in the cytoplasm of a few hepatocytes at the periphery of a nodule.

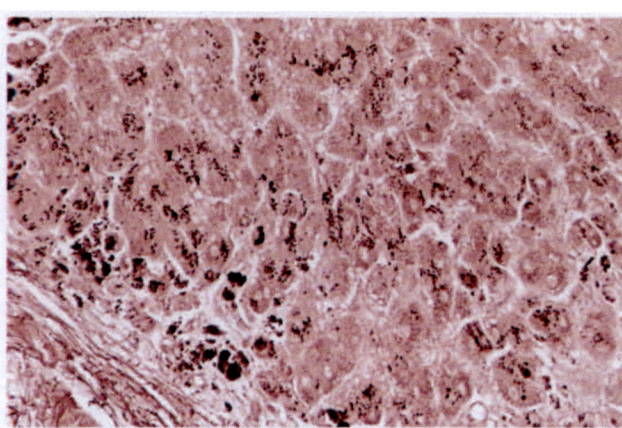

Figure 15.8 Wilson's disease. Same case as Figure 15.6 . Accumulation of dark brown granules of copper-associated protein at the periphery of a nodule. Orcein.

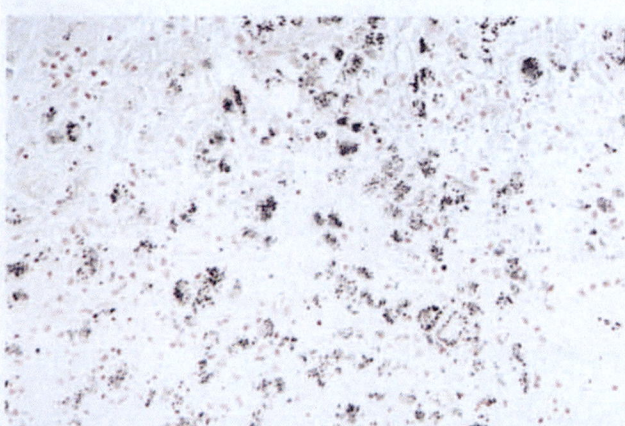

Figure 15.9 Wilson's disease. Another case with fully established cirrhosis. Rubeanic acid reveals abundant greenish–black granular deposits of copper within hepatocytes. Rubeanic acid.

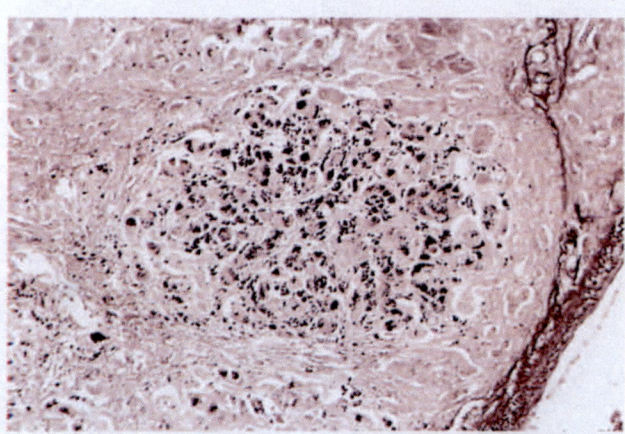

Figure 15.10 Wilson's disease. Another late case treated by liver transplantation. Note the uniform distribution of orcein-positive copper-associated protein throughout this small nodule, a pattern almost never seen in cholestatic liver disease.

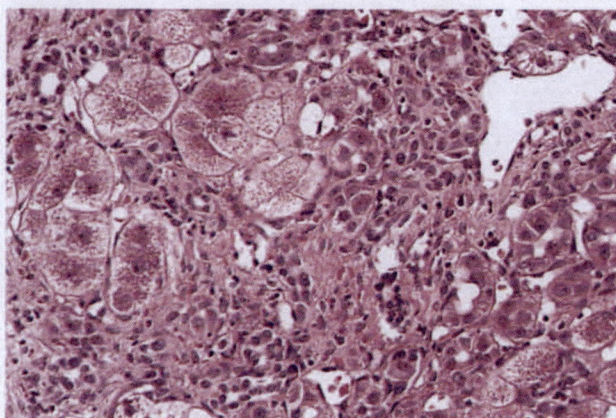

Figure 15.11 Wilson's disease. A 10-year-old female who presented with a lupoid hepatitis syndrome, subsequently proved to be due to Wilson's disease. Biopsy shows an aggressive chronic hepatitis indistinguishable histologically from CAH, although inflammatory cells are perhaps not as prominent as in true CAH. Note the portal tract expansion with piecemeal necrosis leading to isolation of small groups of ballooned hepatocytes.

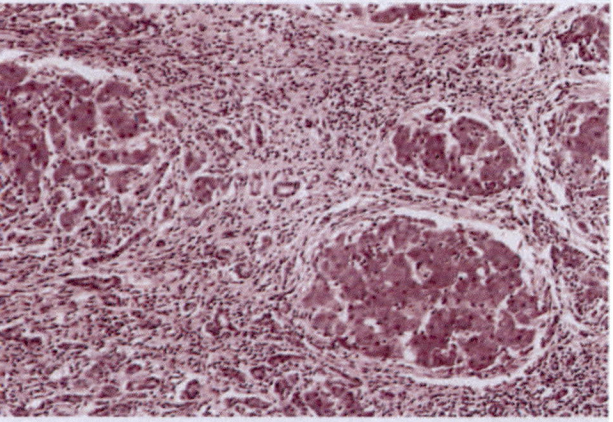

Figure 15.12 Indian childhood cirrhosis. Liver of a three-year old child showing a fully developed micronodular cirrhosis in which there was a very high copper content.

4. Frommer, D. J. (1974). Defective biliary excretion of copper in Wilson's disease. Gut, 15, 125–129

5. Sternlieb, I. (1990). Perspectives on Wilson's disease. Hepatology, 12, 1234–1239

6. Davies, S. E., Williams, R. and Portmann, B. (1989). Hepatic morphology and histochemistry of Wilson's disease presenting as fulminant hepatic failure: a study of 11 cases. Histopathology, 15, 385–394

7. Scott, J., Gollan, J. L., Samourian, S. and Sherlock, S. (1978). Wilson's disease presenting as chronic active hepatitis. Gastroenterology., 74, 645–651

8. Seymour, C. A. (1987). Copper toxicity in man. In Howell, J. M. and Gawthorne, J. M. (eds). Copper in animals and man. pp. 79–106. Boca Raton: CRC Press

9. Fleming, C. R., Dickson, E. R., Wahner, H. W. et al. (1977). Pigmented corneal rings in non-Wilsonian liver disease. Ann. Intern. Med., 86, 285–288

10. Sternlieb, I. and Scheinberg, I. H. (1979). The role of radiocopper in the diagnosis of Wilson's disease. Gastroenterology., 77, 138–142

11. Walshe, J. M. (1975). Missed Wilson's disease. Lancet, 2, 405

12. Walshe, J. M. (1989). Wilson's disease presenting with symptoms of hepatic dysfunction: a clinical analysis of eighty-seven patients. Quart. J. Med., 70, 253–263

13. Sternlieb, I. and Feldman, G. (1976). Effect of anticopper therapy or hepatocellular mitochondria in patients with Wilson s disease. Gastroenterology, 71, 457–461

14. Stromeyer, F. W. and Ishak, K. G. (1980). Histology of the liver in Wilson's disease. Am. J. Clin. Pathol., 73, 12–24

15. Levi, A. J., Sherlock, S., Scheuer, P. J. and Cumings, J. N. (1967). Presymptomatic Wilson's disease. Lancet., 2, 575–579

16. Irons, R. D., Schenk, E. A. and Lee, J. C. K. (1977). Cytochemical methods for copper. Arch. Pathol. Lab. Med., 101, 298–301

17. Jain, S., Scheuer, P. J., Archer, B., Newman, S. P. and Sherlock, S. (1978). Histological demonstration of copper and copper-associated protein in chronic liver diseases. J. Clin. Pathol., 31, 784–790

18. Danks, D. M. (1991). Copper and liver disease. Eur. J. Pediatr., 150, 142–148

19. Peleman, R. R., Gavaler, J. S., Van Thiel, D. H., Esquivel, C., Gordon, R., Iwatsuki, S. and Starzl, T. E. (1987). Orthotopic liver transplantation for acute and subacute hepatic failure in adults. Hepatology, 7, 484–489

20. Adamson, M., Reiner, B., Olson, J. L., Goodman, Z., Plotnick, L., Bernardini, I. and Gahl, W. A. (1992). Indian childhood cirrhosis in an American child. Gastroenterology, 102, 1771–1777

21. Tanner, M. S. and Portmann, B. (1981). Indian childhood cirrhosis. Arch. Dis. Child., 56, 4–6

22. Tanner, M. S., Portmann, B., Mowat, A. P., Williams, R., Pundit, A. N., Mills, C. F. and Bremner, I. (1979). Increased hepatic copper concentration in Indian childhood cirrhosis. Lancet, 1, 1203–1205

23. Popper, H., Goldfischer, S., Sternlieb, I., Nayak, N. C. and Madhavan, T. V. (1979). Cytoplasmic copper and its toxic effects. Studies in Indian childhood cirrhosis. Lancet, 1, 1205–1208

24. Bhusnurmath, S. R., Walia, B. N., Singh, S., Parkash, D., Radotra, B. D. and Nath, R. (1991). Sequential histopathologic alterations in Indian childhood cirrhosis treated with d-penicillamine [see comments]. Hum. Pathol., 22, 653–8

25. Nayak, N. C., Marwaha, N., Kalra, V., Roy, S. and Ghai, O. P. (1981). The liver in siblings of patients with ICC: a light and EM study. Gut, 22, 295–300

Cholestasis denotes a disturbance in the normal bile secretory mechanism, although clinicians and pathologists each view the problem from a different standpoint. The clinician thinks in terms of jaundice with a diminished or absent flow of bile. The pathologist expects to see morphological evidence of bile retention in the form of inspissated plugs of bile in canaliculi as well as accumulation of bile pigment in Kupffer cells and hepatocytes.

In addition to water and electrolytes, bile also includes bile salts, bilirubin, phospholipid, cholesterol and a number of enzymes. Various exogenous compounds including many drugs influence the secretory process and/or are excreted by this pathway. There is evidence that the organic anions such as bilirubin and dyes like bromsulphthalein have a transport system separate from that of bile acids and it is the accumulation of the latter in the skin which gives rise to pruritus, one of the most significant clinical features of cholestasis.

Cholestasis may be functional or mechanical, involving obstruction of the extrahepatic or intrahepatic bile ducts, or both (Table 16.1). It may be caused by malfunction at any point between the uptake of bile salts by the basolateral membrane of the liver cell to delivery of bile to the

Table 16.1 Classification of functional cholestasis*

PURE CHOLESTASIS

Hyperbilirubinaemias
Unconjugated
Physiological
Crigler-Najjar Type I
Crigler-Najjar Type II
Gilbert's syndrome

Conjugated
Dubin Johnson syndrome
Rotor syndrome

Children	Byler's syndrome
	THCA syndrome
	Zellweger's syndrome
	Norwegian cholestasis
Adults	Benign recurrent intrahepatic cholestasis
	Pregnancy

CHOLESTASIS SECONDARY TO OTHER CONDITIONS

Congenital	Alagille's syndrome
	α_1-Antitrypsin deficiency
	Galactosaemia
	Hereditary fructose intolerance
	Tyrosinaemia
	Erythropoietic protoporphyria
Acquired	Drugs and Toxins (including alcohol) (Chapters 10, 13)
	Viral hepatitis (Chapter 2)
	Postoperative cholestasis
	Congestion and shock (Chapter 18)
	Sepsis
	Parenteral nutrition
	Haemolysis
	Malignant lymphoma (Chapter 25)

duodenum. Detailed pathogenic mechanisms of functional cholestasis have been reviewed in a number of

Table 16.2 Causes of intrahepatic bile duct damage*

	With duct loss	*Little or no duct loss*
Developmental	Biliary atresia Alagille's syndrome	Cystic/dysplastic disease
Familial/genetic	Adult ductopenia	Cystic fibrosis α_1-Antitrypsin deficiency
Immunological	PBC PSC Graft-versus-host Chronic rejection Sarcoidosis?	
Vascular	Arterial occlusion	Non-cirrhotic portal hypertension
Infective	Chronic rejection 5-FUDR for metastases Bacterial cholangitis	Viral hepatitis (Hepatitis C) CMV Parasites
Drugs and chemicals	Scolicides	Drugs Toxins

* Based on Wight, D. G. D. (1993). Cholestasis and extrahepatic bile ducts. In Wight, D. G. (ed.). *Liver, Biliary Tract and Exocrine Pancreas.* Vol. II: Systemic Pathology. Symmers, W. S. C., series ed. 3rd edn. Edinburgh: Churchill Livingstone

recent publications[1-6]. The causes of intrahepatic bile duct damage are shown in Table 16.2. With individual causes, it may be very difficult to establish whether the observed changes are primarily due to that agent or merely themselves secondary to the cholestasis. Also many aetiological agents may have an effect at more than one point in the process.

Although the risk of biliary peritonitis following needle biopsy of the liver in obstructive jaundice is a small one, the modern approach to the differential diagnosis of cholestasis includes a search for dilated intrahepatic bile ducts by non-invasive imaging techniques, principally ultrasound examination. Only if these fail to demonstrate dilatation is needle biopsy performed (although the technique of transjugular liver biopsy has been recommended for this group of patients, the quality of the specimen cannot always be assured). However, even when these investigations are negative, a proportion of biopsied patients will subsequently be shown to have large duct obstruction.

THE MORPHOLOGY OF CHOLESTASIS

Bile deposition, at least initially, occurs principally in zone 3 of the acinus. Involvement may not always be concentric around central venules but rather paracentral (Figure 16.1), possibly because of variable involvement of different acini. Additionally, tissue processing and embedding may leach out much of the accumulated bile pigment and so make the observed changes less marked than expected. Ultrastructurally the first and most constant change appears to be dilatation of the bile canaliculus with a decrease in the number of microvilli. The typical light microscopic appearance is of dilated bile capillaries filled with inspissated refractile bile which stains yellow-brown in H&E-stained sections and greenish with Fouchet reagent (Figure 16.2). The bile plugs often have one or two branches within the plane of section. Their composition varies but the bilirubin is mainly conjugated and in some cases, possibly the older ones, may stain positively with PAS after diastase digestion, suggesting participation of membrane and/or glycocalyx fragments.

Secondary phenomena

These depend upon the degree and the duration of the jaundice. *Liver cells* may have an eosinophilic ground glass appearance of the cytoplasm, due to an 'induced' increase of smooth endoplasmic reticulum (Figure 16.3) (Chapter 10). There may also be evidence of hypertrophy and hyperplasia reflected by an increased number of binucleate or even multinucleate liver cells (Figure 16.4). Bile retention may be seen as finely granular pigment associated with rarefaction of the cytoplasm. As this progresses, the liver cell cytoplasm comes to appear almost empty apart from brown stained residual strands– an appearance known as feathery degeneration (Figures 16.5 and 16.6). This affects single or small groups of cells in the centrilobular region and may be a consequence of the detergent action of bile, since its intensity parallels the tissue content of dehydroxy bile salts. Typical acidophil bodies may also be seen[7]. Possibly following necrosis of such cells there is a focal *reactive inflammation* which consists of macrophages or Kupffer cells laden with granular pigment composed principally of bilirubin and lipofuscin and staining positively with PAS (Figure 16.1). This is missing in early or mild cholestasis and must be distinguished from an accompanying hepatitis. In cholestasis the inflammatory changes are confined to the cholestatic zones, whereas in hepatitis, even if more marked in zone 3, they are also found elsewhere. In hepatitis, the pigment within Kupffer cells is usually finer and browner, being composed mainly of lipofuscin and ceroid. With prolongation of cholestasis, bile thrombi may also be found in periportal parenchyma (Figure 16.7), possibly due to mechanical obstruction by portal fibrosis, and here there is usually symmetrical involvement around individual portal tracts. Occasionally, in addition to the typical thrombi between two liver cells, much larger thrombi in the lumen of tubules or acini of liver cells, so-called secondary canaliculi, may be found at this stage (Figure 16.8).

Bile ductular proliferation and fibrosis in the portal tracts may be found in any type of cholestasis. Accompanying inflammatory cells, including neutrophil polymorphs, probably follow leakage of bile into the portal tract connective tissue and do not necessarily indicate the presence of bacterial infection. The portal tract changes sometimes persist after subsidence of cholestasis of any aetiology.

None of the changes so far described are in any way helpful in assessing the cause of the cholestasis.

Cholestasis without jaundice implies focal disease such as a tumour deposit. It is sometimes also seen in cirrhosis of any cause and less commonly in conditions such as congenital hepatic fibrosis and sclerosing cholangitis. Ductal cholestasis, where portal bile ducts and ductules contain concretions of bile, may also be encountered in the same conditions in the absence of jaundice.

FUNCTIONAL CHOLESTASIS

A great variety of different conditions may be associated with intrahepatic cholestasis. These may be classified into those with pure cholestasis and those secondary to other conditions (Table 16.1).

Pure cholestasis

Hyperbilirubinaemias

The conditions characterized by impairment only of bilirubin excretion but with normal handling of bile acids are not associated with morphological cholestasis, but will be briefly considered here.

In the first few days of life, the *physiological* mechanisms for the metabolism of bile pigments are not fully developed, and thus there may be a mild unconjugated hyperbilirubinaemia, which reaches a peak 2 to 5 days after birth. *Crigler-Najjar syndrome* is a genetic disorder due to reduced or absent levels of bilirubin-UDP glucuronyl transferase, which usually leads to death in infancy or soon after. Histologically, the only abnormality is an occasional bile plug in an otherwise normal liver. *Gilbert's syndrome* is the commonest of the familial hyperbilirubinaemias, and is characterized by unconjugated bilirubinaemia of modest degree, often aggravated by stress or intercurrent infection. The liver is usually histologically normal.

In *Dubin-Johnson syndrome* there is an intermittent rise in the serum levels of conjugated bilirubin due to a familial defect in its canalicular excretion. Bile salts, however, are handled normally and thus there is no morphological cholestasis. The hallmark of the condition is the presence of a complex dark brown pigment within hepatocytes, which can usually be recognized macroscopically by the greenish-black colour it imparts to a biopsy. The pigment has many features in common with lipofuscin, both in its pericanalicular position in the hepatocyte and in its staining reactions (usually PAS-positive) (Figure 16.9). Ultrastructurally it is rather different and thus electron microscopy can be used in cases of doubt. Interestingly, viral hepatitis can cause mobilization and excretion of the pigment, which then takes time to reaccumulate. *Rotor syndrome* is a very similar condition, except that there is no pigment accumulation and thus liver biopsy is normal.

Other pure cholestasis

There are several rare autosomal recessive cholestatic syndromes, which generally present in the neonatal period (Table 16.1)[6]. In all cases, the histological picture is of canalicular cholestasis without special features, diagnosis being dependent on clinical and family studies. Benign familial recurrent cholestasis[8], and benign recurrent intrahepatic cholestasis of pregnancy[9], are similarly not distinctive histologically. The latter patients are also liable to develop jaundice when taking oral contraceptives.

Secondary cholestasis.

Various inherited metabolic liver diseases may present as cholestatic syndromes in childhood (Table 16.1). These are separately discussed in Chapters 8 and 9.

The many causes of acquired functional cholestasis are listed in Table 16.1, and discussed further in the appropriate chapters. *Postoperative cholestasis* is not a single entity and probably many different mechanisms are operative, including bilirubin overload, shock, bacterial infection, and the effects of drugs such as halothane[10]. *Sepsis*–pure cholestasis complicating lobar pneumonia– was once common, but is also seen as a complication of any serous bacterial infection[11], and of the toxic shock syndrome[12]. Microscopically, ductular cholestasis is a particularly distinctive feature of systemic infection[13]. Here proliferated ductules at the margins of portal tracts are filled with inspissated, PAS-positive bile-stained material mixed with neutrophil polymorphs (Figure 16.10). *Total parenteral nutrition* (TPN), especially when prolonged, may be complicated by cholestasis which may

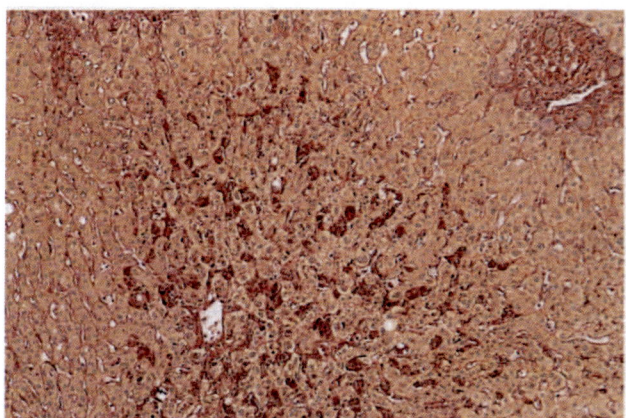

Figure 16.1 Cholestasis, Kupffer cell reaction. Kupffer cells are hypertrophied and filled with PAS-positive bile and ceroid pigment, in this case of centrilobular cholestasis. Note the very uniform Kupffer cell involvement, confined to the cholestatic zone, as compared to that in hepatitis which tends to be focal (see Chapter 2). Note also that the cholestatic zone is paracentral and not precisely central. (From a case of biliary obstruction due to pancreatic carcinoma). PAS diastase.

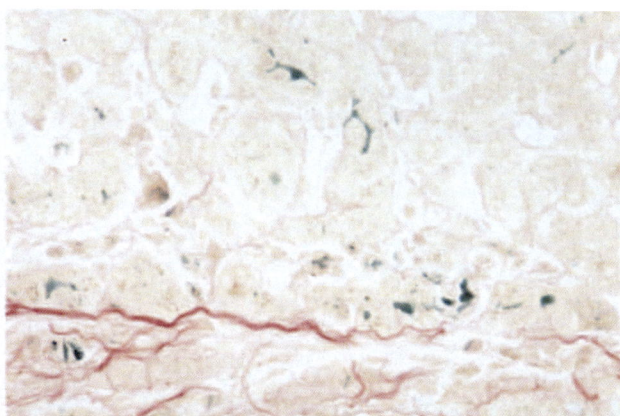

Figure 16.2 Cholestasis. Cholestasis showing dilated bile canaliculi filled with inspissated bile. Note that several of the greenish bile plugs are branched. (From a case of sclerosing cholangitis). Fouchet van Gieson.

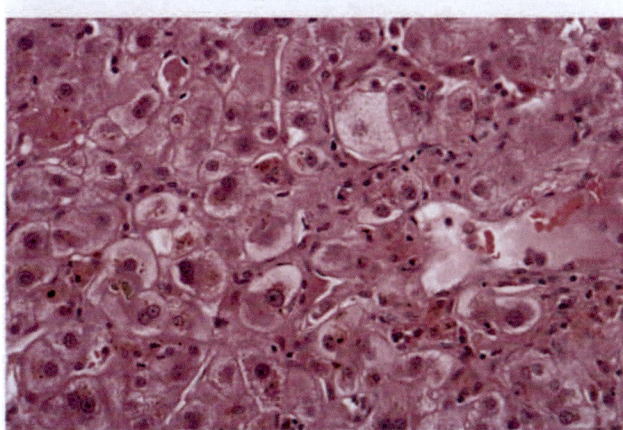

Figure 16.3 Cholestasis, 'induced' hepatocytes. Several of the hepatocytes have, in addition to distended bile canaliculi, a pale, homogeneous eosinophilic 'ground glass' or 'induced' appearance (see also Chapter 10). Note also that many Kupffer cells contain brown pigment. (From a case of biliary obstruction by a bile duct carcinoma).

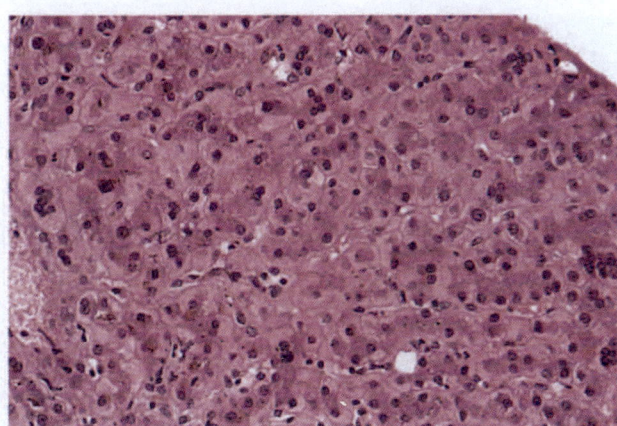

Figure 16.4 Cholestasis, multinucleate cells. Several hepatocytes contain multiple nuclei, in addition to bile thrombi. (From a case of drug-induced cholestasis, same case as Figure 8.2).

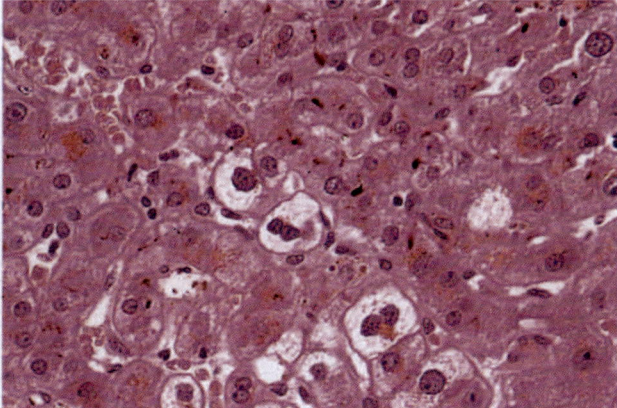

Figure 16.5 Cholestasis, feathery degeneration. There is pronounced rarefaction of the cytoplasm of several hepatocytes, some of which also contain granular bile pigment (same case as Figure 16.3).

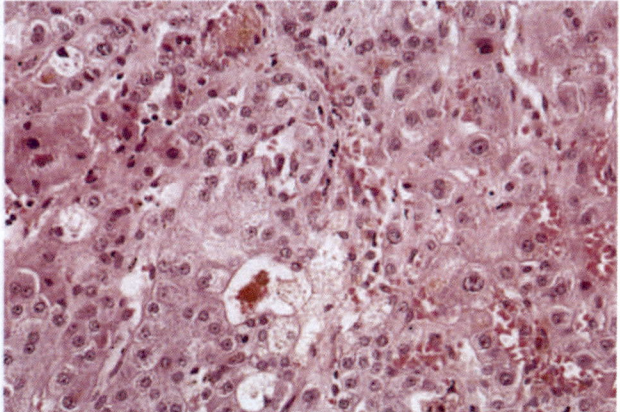

Figure 16.6 Cholestasis, feathery degeneration. Here there is even more extreme bile damage to hepatocytes, in one of which the cytoplasm has completely disappeared; in others it is reduced to a few wispy strands. (Same case as Figures 16.3 and 16.5).

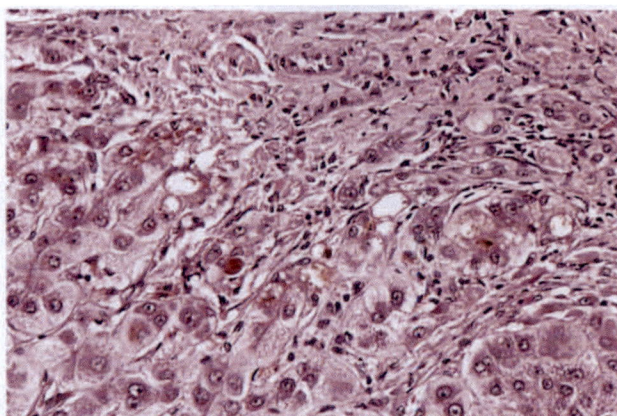

Figure 16.7 Cholestasis, peripheral. Bile plugs are seen at the periphery of the lobule, in this case of prolonged cholestasis due to primary biliary cirrhosis.

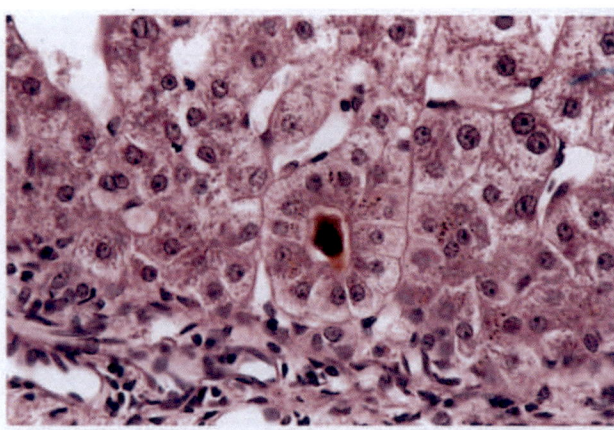

Figure 16.8 Cholestasis, secondary canaliculi. Here a group of liver cells are arranged as an acinus or rosette around a greatly distended bile canaliculus containing a bile thrombus. (From a case of cirrhosis following chronic active hepatitis).

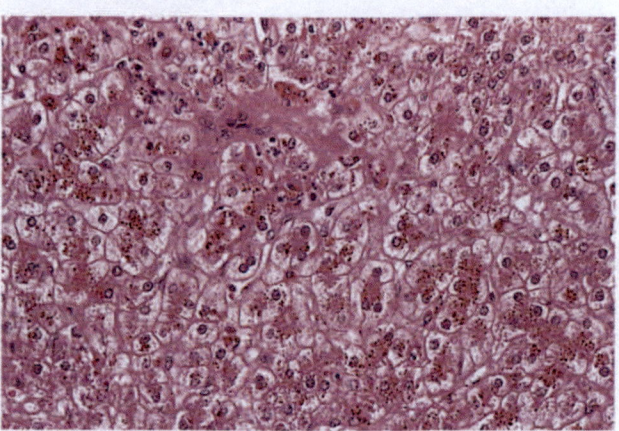

Figure 16.9 Dubin-Johnson syndrome. A 30-year-old female with intermittent conjugated hyperbilirubinaemia. The biopsy was strikingly dark in colour macroscopically, and it shows the typical pericanalicular granules of brown pigment, a little larger than lipofuscin, maximal in the centre of the lobule.

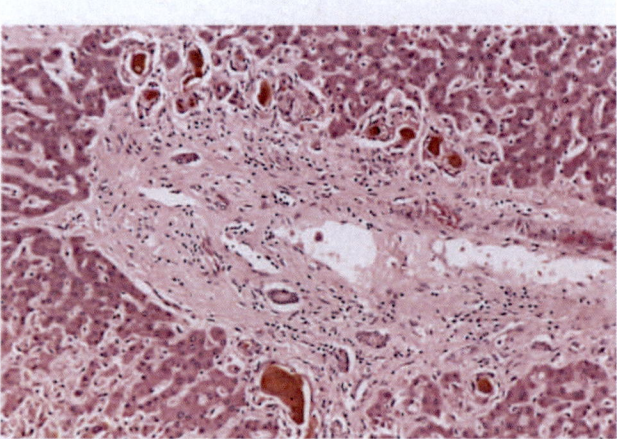

Figure 16.10 Ductular cholestasis secondary to systemic sepsis. There was no evidence of bile duct obstruction.

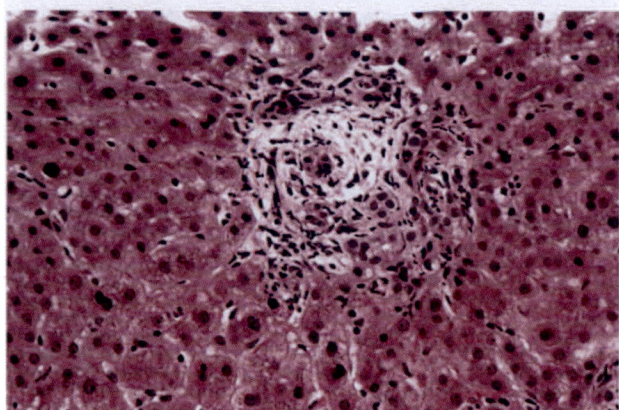

Figure 16.11 Extrahepatic biliary obstruction. Biliary obstruction of about 3 weeks duration, subsequently shown to be due to gallstones. Biopsy shows rounding of this portal tract and striking oedema, particularly around the central bile duct. There is also some marginal ductular proliferation associated with neutrophilic infiltration.

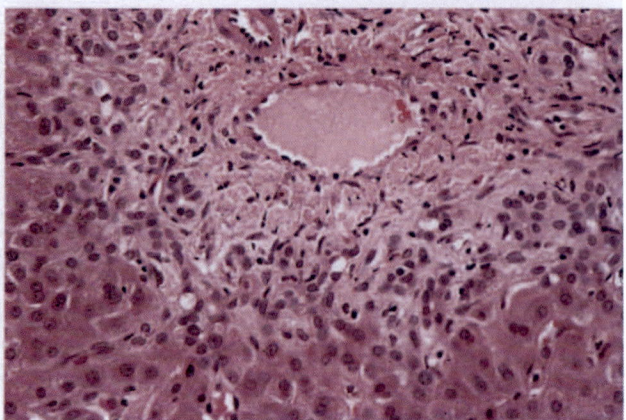

Figure 16.12 Extrahepatic biliary obstruction. Same case as Figure 16.3, 16.5 and 16.6. This moderate-sized portal tract shows very typical marginal bile ductular proliferation. Each has a small but definite lumen, in contrast to those seen in primary biliary cirrhosis.

go on to progressive portal fibrosis and cirrhosis[14]. The pathogenesis of the cholestasis in sepsis and TPN is not well understood.

MECHANICAL CHOLESTASIS

This may be caused by damage to or obstruction of bile ducts in any part of the biliary tree, both outside and within the liver.

Extrahepatic biliary obstruction

Mechanical obstruction of large bile ducts may be due to calculi, inflammatory strictures and tumours of any part of the biliary tree. Macroscopically the liver is enlarged, swollen and green in colour. In complete obstruction, the bile will eventually become clear, due to suppression of its secretion.

Initially centrilobular cholestasis may be the only change seen. This will be followed by the secondary phenomena described above. Only after a week or two of uninterrupted obstruction will more nearly pathognomonic changes be seen in portal tracts and periportal regions.

Portal tracts become expanded and often rounded due to oedema, cellular infiltration and bile ductular proliferation in varying degrees (Figure 16.11). The rounding and the oedema, said to be due to the toxic effect of bile constituents, occur relatively early, especially in small portal tracts. Initially there may be some dilatation of interlobular or septal ducts with flattening of their epithelium, although this is not always easy to assess. The most consistent change is bile ductular proliferation (Figure 16.12) which was found in all biopsies from one series of surgically verified large duct obstruction[7]. Characteristically the bile ductules seen around the periphery of the portal tract are lined by cuboidal epithelium and usually have a definite but fine lumen. They often run parallel to the limiting plate before bending towards it. Although bile ductular proliferation is seen in most portal tracts of all sizes in a biopsy, it is most marked in the large tracts and here its marginal location is most obvious. Connective tissue or elastic stains such as orcein are often very helpful in both delineating the former unexpanded portal tract (Figure 16.13) and demonstrating the proliferated bile ductules as rather characteristic empty spaces (Figure 16.14). Light infiltration with chronic inflammatory cells, mainly lymphocytes and histiocytes, is also seen in nearly all portal tracts in most biopsies. Neutrophils are rather less common but their presence is helpful, especially when found adjacent to the basement membranes of proliferating ductules (Figure 16.15), although, as already stated, they may be seen in any cholestasis. Oedema too may only be found in a proportion of portal tracts and, in common with neutrophil infiltration, probably increases in incidence and severity with the degree and duration of jaundice. As obstruction persists, fibroblasts lay down new collagen fibres which often have a striking concentric arrangement around septal and interlobular ducts (Figure 16.16), a finding which may cause confusion with Primary Sclerosing Cholangitis (Chapter 20)[15]. With the passage of time, the rather delicate collagen laid down initially is replaced by refractile hard collagen. It is the fibrosis which probably causes extension of the cholestasis to the lobular periphery by mechanical interference with bile flow at the entry of canaliculi into the portal tract, cholestasis is thus a relatively late phenomenon. Peripheral (zone 1) cholestasis is also associated with increased numbers of secondary canaliculi, which may or may not contain recognizable bile in their lumens.

The portal tract findings are generally the most helpful in confirming the diagnosis of biliary obstruction. Much less commonly other changes may be found. Although many can be quite helpful diagnostically (since they are near pathognomonic), they tend to be late and sporadic and thus are seldom seen in biopsy material. *Bile infarcts* are usually in periportal zones near to portal tracts (Figure 16.17). They represent groups of adjacent cells undergoing feathery degeneration and those involving more than two or three cells are diagnostic of extrahepatic obstruction. As the lesions evolve, the cells round off, reticulin staining disappears, the bile gradually fades and liver cells are replaced by macrophages with foamy cytoplasm and often containing clumped bile pigment. *Bile lakes* are another unusual finding which, although often said to be diagnostic, may also be seen in the late stages of primary biliary cirrhosis. These are the consequence of rupture of ducts with bile leakage and thus are found in or near portal tracts. They are rounded pools of bile, often quite dark in colour, surrounded by a vigorous macrophage response which often includes foreign body type giant cells (Figure 16.18). Prolonged obstruction may be associated with heaping up and even micropapilla formation of the bile duct epithelium. Occasional macrophages containing PAS positive material within their cytoplasm tend to accumulate in portal tracts as a late phenomenon. These are found following liver cell necrosis of any cause and may persist long after resolution of the initiating condition.

Infection is a common but not inevitable accompaniment of extrahepatic obstruction. Neutrophils are often regarded as an indication of infection, but this is clearly not always the case. However, in infection, neutrophils may be more prominent and seen also between epithelial cells and in the lumen of ducts (Figures 16.16 and 16.19). Oedema may also be more marked. In severe cases there is abscess formation (Figure 16.20) with destruction of ducts and even whole portal tracts. Occasionally there may be relative dissociation of ascending infection from cholestatic morphological changes, indicating perhaps an increased susceptibility to infection in recurrent or incomplete obstruction. Suppurative inflammation may be followed by fibrous scars ('secondary sclerosing cholangitis') indistinguishable from those of primary sclerosing cholangitis (Chapter 20).

Mallory's hyalin (Chapter 13), in the form of irregular clumps of refractile eosinophilic material within the cytoplasm of liver cells and quite indistinguishable from that found in alcoholic liver disease, is an occasional finding in periportal liver cells[16]. Orcein-positive granules in the cytoplasm of periportal liver cells are frequently seen. The orcein-positive material is a copper-metallothionein complex which accumulates when copper cannot be excreted in the bile. It is much more frequently seen in primary biliary cirrhosis (Chapter 17) but in both conditions correlates best with long-standing cholestasis complicated by portal fibrosis.

Differential diagnosis of biliary obstruction

The diagnosis is seldom based on morphological evidence alone, but the most helpful features in the presence of cholestasis are the following:

oedema and rounding of portal tracts;
cholangitis with neutrophil infiltration;
marginal bile duct proliferation;
ductular cholestasis (Figure 16.21);
concentric periductal fibrosis;
bile infarcts;
bile lakes.

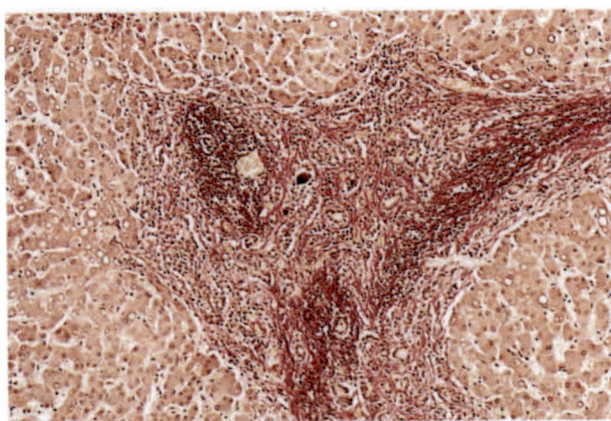

Figure 16.13 Extrahepatic biliary obstruction. Another case of prolonged obstruction due to pancreatic tumour. The pre-existing unexpanded portal tract can be seen in this connective tissue stain as the denser and darker red areas at the centre of the field. These are surrounded by a band of peripheral ductular proliferation where collagen fibres are less numerous and elastic absent. Elastic van Gieson.

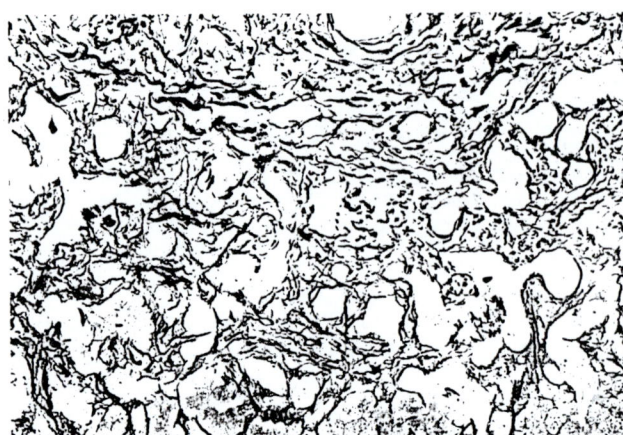

Figure 16.14 Extrahepatic biliary obstruction. Proliferating bile ductules in this portal tract have a characteristic profile. Reticulin, neutral red.

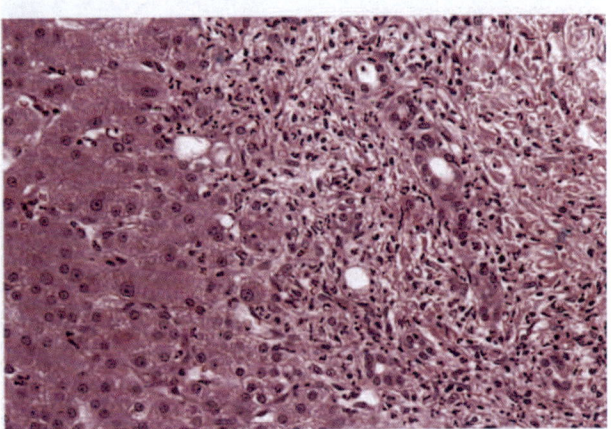

Figure 16.15 Extrahepatic biliary obstruction. Same case as Figures 16.3, 16.5, 16.6 and 16.12. The proliferating marginal bile ductules in this portal tract are surrounded by neutrophil polymorphs, many of which are intimately related to the ductular basement membranes.

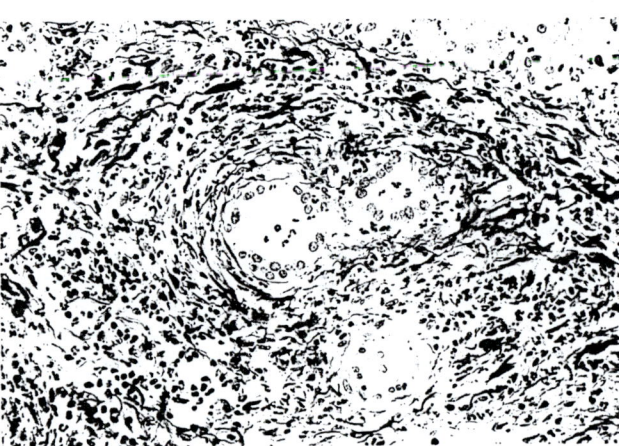

Figures 16.16 Extrahepatic biliary obstruction. Same case as Figures 16.3, 16.5, 16.6, 16.12 and 16.15. This central interlobular bile duct is surrounded by concentrically arranged collagen fibres, separated from one another by oedema and inflammatory cells. Note also the neutrophils around, within the epithelium and within the lumen of the bile duct, all highly suggestive of ascending infection. Elastic van Gieson.

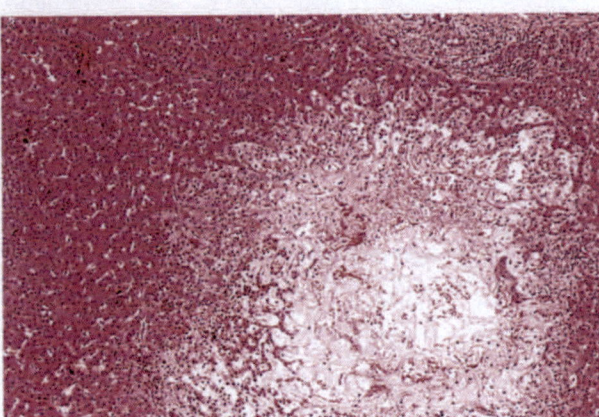

Figure 16.17 Extrahepatic biliary obstruction, bile infarct. Same case as Figure 16.14. This section shows a large bile infarct with a central clear space surrounded by faintly bile-stained necrotic debris. A lesion of this size is pathognomonic of biliary obstruction.

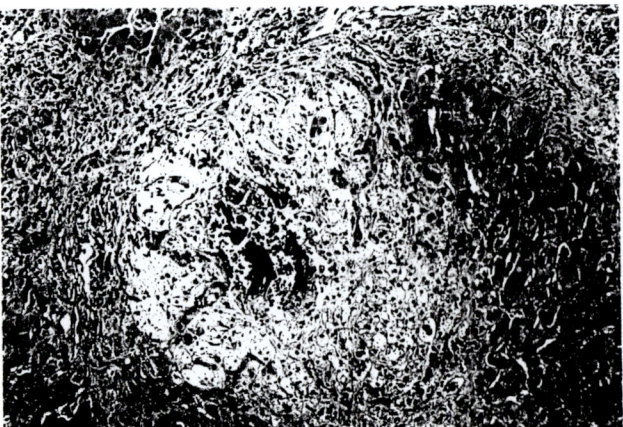

Figure 16.18 Extrahepatic biliary obstruction, bile lake. Same case as Figures 16.3, 16.5, 16.6, 16.12, 16.15 and 16.16. There is a central pool of bile surrounded by foamy macrophages. These are occasionally seen in PBC as well as in biliary obstruction (see Chapter 17).

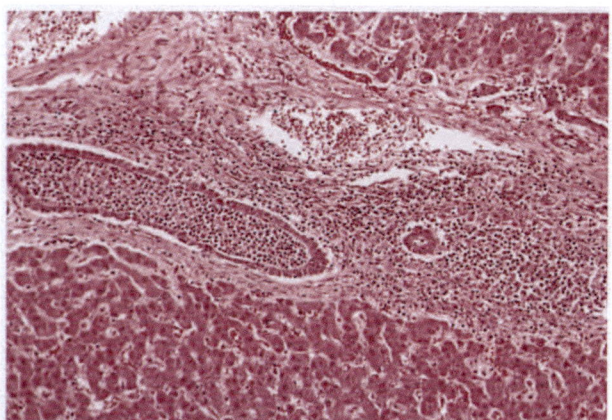

Figure 16.19 Extrahepatic biliary obstruction, cholangitis. This inter lobular bile duct is distended and filled with neutrophil polymorph which are also present in the portal connective tissue.

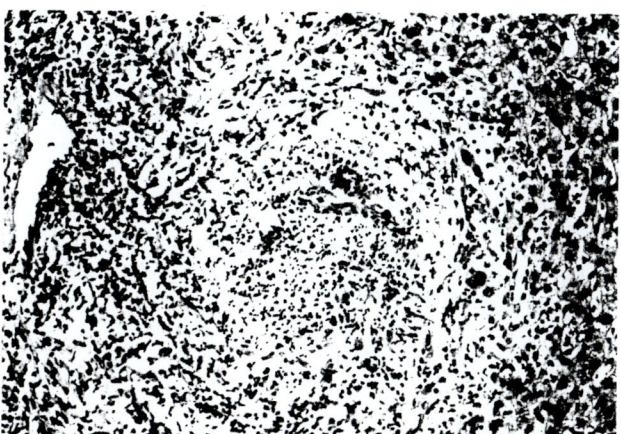

Figure 16.20 Extrahepatic biliary obstruction, cholangitis. Recurrent biliary obstruction due to gallstones. The patient presented on this occasion with fever. Biopsy shows an abscess at the centre of an expanded portal tract.

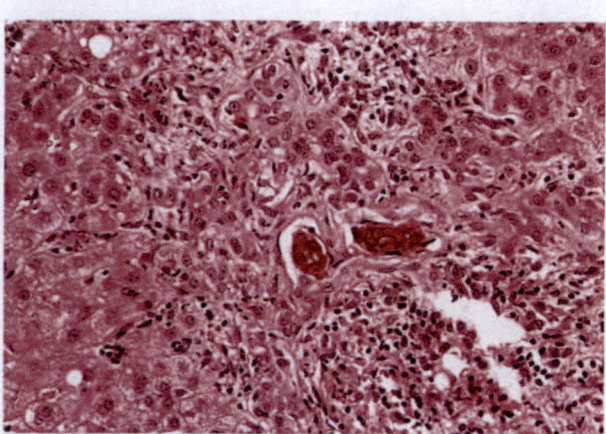

Figure 16.21 Extrahepatic biliary obstruction. Another case due t bile duct carcinoma. This biopsy shows bile calculi within the lumen an interlobular bile duct. The expanded portal tract also shows margin: bile duct proliferation and inflammatory cell infiltration.

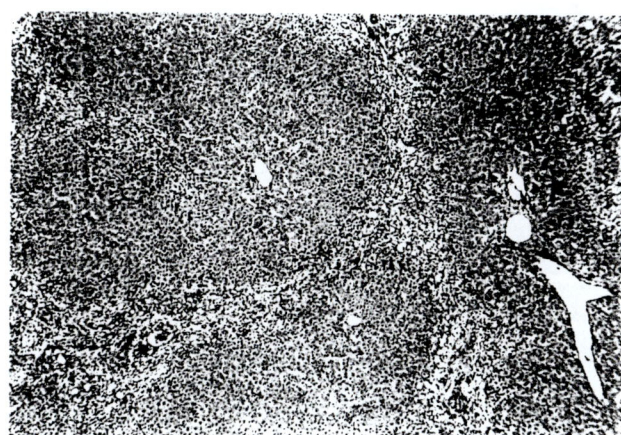

Figure 16.22 Secondary biliary cirrhosis. A 28-year-old female with cholangiocarcinoma which led to biliary cirrhosis. The section shows intercommunication of expanded portal tracts forming septa which surround relatively normal lobules. There is no nodule formation and this would thus be more properly called biliary fibrosis (compare congenital hepatic fibrosis, Chapter 8).

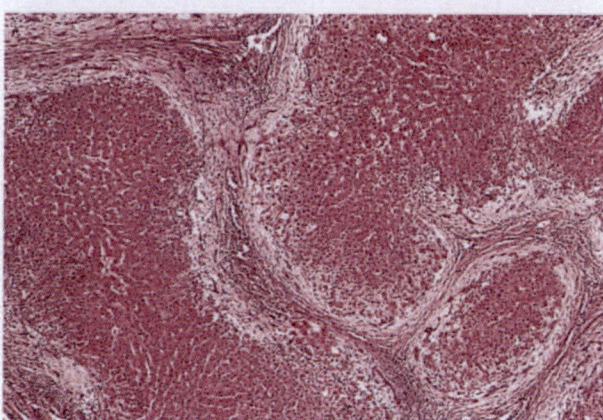

Figure 16.23 Secondary biliary cirrhosis. More advanced than Figur 16.22, the septa are now lined by a layer of oedematous connectiv tissue whose fibres run parallel to the limiting plate. There is still littl nodular regeneration even at this late stage.

Figure 16.24 Secondary biliary cirrhosis. Same case as Figure 16.23. A 43-year-old female with recurrent biliary stricture which eventually led to the development of cirrhosis. Note the intensely bile-stained dark green micronodular cirrhosis.

Secondary biliary cirrhosis

The development of true cirrhosis is generally considered a late and relatively uncommon occurrence in prolonged biliary obstruction, although in one series it was found as early as 6 months after onset. The common aetiological associations are duct stricture and stones, occasionally tumours. It is also an inevitable complication of congenital biliary atresia, when its onset may be more rapid than in adult patients.

As obstruction persists, portal tracts continue to expand with replacement of peripheral liver cells by bile ductules, possibly by a process of tubular transformation. closely paralleled by an increase in fibrous tissue. Eventually portal-to-portal fibrous septa cause a perilobular biliary fibrosis (Figure 16.22). True nodular regeneration is a late phenomenon and the final result is a liver composed of single or multiple nodules with an outline said to resemble the pieces of a jigsaw. There is often a highly characteristic thin layer of oedematous connective tissue separating the parenchyma from the septa with the collagen fibres running parallel to that junction (Figure 16.23). The other changes of biliary obstruction may or may not be present, but the disease is now in a progressive phase even if the obstruction is relieved[17]. As in cirrhosis of any cause the septa may contain dilated lymphatics and a sprinkling of chronic inflammatory cells (but rarely lymphoid aggregates). Quite consistently septal and inter-lobular bile ducts are reduced in number and thus a relative absence of ducts should not be regarded as evidence of primary biliary cirrhosis. Macroscopically the liver is dark green in colour and has a nodular cut surface (Figure 16.24). Dilatation of the main ducts may be marked, but the bile may or may not be green.

Intrahepatic bile duct damage

The causes are shown in Table 16.2 and most are discussed in the relevant chapters.

REFERENCES

1. Phillips, M. J., Poucell, S. and Oda, M. (1986). Biology of disease: mechanisms of cholestasis. Lab Invest, 54, 593–608
2. Desmet, V. J. (1987). Cholestasis: extrahepatic obstruction and secondary biliary cirrhosis. In MacSween, R. N. M., Anthony, P. P. and Scheuer, P. J. (eds). Pathology of the Liver. 2nd edn. pp. 364–423. Edinburgh: Churchill Livingstone
3. Reichen, J. and Simon, F. R. (1988). Cholestasis. In Arias, I. M., Jakoby, W. B., Popper, H., Schacter, D. and Shafritz, D. A. (eds). The liver: biology and pathobiology. 2nd edn. pp. 1105–1124. New York: Raven Press Limited
4. Sellinger, M. and Boyer, J. L. (1990). Physiology of bile secretion and cholestasis. Progr Liver Dis, 9, 237–259
5. Schaffner, F. (1992). Cholestasis. In Millward-Sadler, G. H., Wright, R. and Arthur, M. J. P. (eds). Wright's Liver and Biliary Disease. edn. pp. 371–396. London: W B Saunders
6. Wight, D. G. D. (1993). Cholestasis and extrahepatic bile ducts. In Wight, D. G. D. (eds). Liver, Biliary Tract and Exocrine Pancreas. 11. Systemic Pathology. Symmers, W. S. C. Series ed. 3rd edn. pp. Edinburgh: Churchill Livingstone
7. Christoffersen, P. and Poulsen, H. (1970). Histological changes in human liver biopsies following extrahepatic biliary obstruction. Acta Pathol Microbiol Scand., 212, 150–157
8. Lovisetto, P., Raviolo, P., Rizzetto, M., Marchi, L., Actis, G. C. and Verme, G. (1990). Benign recurrent intrahepatic cholestasis. A clinico-pathologic study. Ric. Clin. Lab., 20, 19–27
9. Reyes, H. (1982). The enigma of intrahepatic cholestasis of pregnancy: lessons from Chile. Hepatology, 2, 87–96
10. Koff, R. S. (1975). Postoperative jaundice. Med. Clin. NA., 59, 823–829
11. Miller, D. J., Keeton, G. R., Webber, B. L. and Saunders, S. J. (1976). Jaundice in severe bacterial infections. Gastroenterology, 71, 94–97
12. Gourlay, G. R., Chesney, P. J., Davis, J. P. and Odell, G. B. (1981). Acute cholestasis in patients with toxic-shock syndrome. Gastroenterology, 81, 928–931
13. Lefkowitch, J. H. (1982). Bile ductular cholestasis: an ominous histopathological sign related to sepsis and 'cholangitis lenta'. Hum. Pathol., 13, 13–24
14. Balistreri, W. F. and Bove, K. E. (1990). Hepatobiliary consequences of parenteral alimentation. Progr. Liver Dis., 9, 567–601
15. Scheuer, P. J. (1988). Biliary Disease. In (eds). Liver Biopsy Interpretation. 4th edn. pp. 207–217. London: Baillière Tindall
16. Gerber, M. A., Orr, W., Denk, H., Schaffner, F. and Popper, H. (1973). Hepatocellular hyalin in cholestasis and cirrhosis: its diagnostic significance. Gastroenterology., 64., 89–98
17. Scobie, B. A. and Summerskill, W. H. J. (1965). Hepatic cirrhosis secondary to obstruction of biliary system. Am. J. Dig. Dis., 10., 135–146

Primary Biliary Cirrhosis **17**

Primary biliary cirrhosis (PBC) is a form of chronic obstructive non-suppurative granulomatous cholangitis. Females are afflicted eight times as often as males and the typical patient is in her fifth or sixth decade.

Most patients present clinically with cholestasis, frequently preceded by intense itching. Patients may, however, present with established cirrhosis, for example, with portal hypertension or, increasingly, the disease may be presymptomatic at the time of discovery.

Approximately 98% of patients have in their serum an antibody to the inner membrane of mitochondria, the M2 fraction. This is a highly useful method for distinguishing primary biliary cirrhosis from other forms of cholestasis, although a small proportion of patients with other liver diseases, particularly chronic active hepatitis and cryptogenic cirrhosis, may also be positive. Relatives of patients with PBC may also have the antibody. There is no correlation between immunological status and either the clinical state or histological stage of the disease[1]. Although the disease is slightly commoner amongst first-degree relatives, there is no link with histocompatibility antigens nor with blood groups. Presymptomatic disease may remain histologically static for many years (Figure 17.1), but once symptoms appear, the course is identical to that of patients diagnosed after the onset of symptoms, and ranges from 4 to 7 years. It is not possible to predict when presymptomatic patients will become symptomatic and whether the course will be short or long[2]. Histologically the diagnostic lesions of stage 1 (see below) are found in about 75% of presymptomatic cases.

The pathogenesis as yet remains unresolved[3], but a great range of possible mechanisms has been proposed. A number of studies has shown geographical clustering of cases, in one instance apparently related to a common water supply[4]. All attempts to induce the disease by stimulating the appearance of mitochondrial antigens have failed[5]. It has been suggested that antibodies to mitochondria may be primarily directed against enterobacterial antigens, resulting from intestinal infection, with which they cross-react[6]. Whether or not it is initiated by an environmental or infective agent, many features of the disease suggest immunological involvement. As well as the morphological features, described below, and the serum antibodies, there is a number of associated conditions, many of which have an autoimmune basis; namely, rheumatoid arthritis, Sjögren's syndrome, systemic sclerosis, Addisonian pernicious anaemia, thyroid disease and coeliac disease. There is some evidence that biliary epithelium in PBC shows altered expression of both class I and class II HLA determinants[7]. The similarities between the bile duct lesion of PBC and graft-versus-host disease on the one hand and chronic rejection of liver transplants on the other provide additional circumstantial support for the concept that the bile duct lesion is immunologically mediated. PBC might perhaps represent a breakdown of the self-recognition between the lymphocyte and bile duct[8]. Of particular interest is the fact that injection of lymphocytes from patients with PBC into mice with severe combined immunodeficiency leads to development of PBC-like morphological lesions[9]. This suggests that the defect might be in the lymphocytes rather than the bile ducts.

HISTOPATHOLOGY

The liver is usually deep green in colour and often enlarged. The surface may be finely nodular or smooth, for primary biliary cirrhosis is a misnomer with only the advanced disease showing true cirrhosis. A number of histological grading schemes has been devised[10-13], all of which have certain limitations. The most durable classification is the first[10,11], which divides the disease into four stages; only the earlier ones are histologically distinctive.

Stage 1. Florid duct lesion. There is focal damage to septal and large interlobular bile ducts, of a size which are not necessarily seen in every biopsy. The earliest lesions affect medium-sized bile ducts, 45–75μ in diameter. Chronic inflammatory cells can be seen infiltrating into the collar of connective tissue which normally surrounds the bile duct. They may then apparently disrupt the basement membrane and invade the epithelium where they are often surrounded by vacuoles (Figure 17.1). This process has been called 'piecemeal necrosis of biliary epithelium'[14]. Although it may become very irregular, the epithelium usually remains single-layered. Further sections may reveal the distinctive duct ruptures which are virtually diagnostic (Figure 17.2). Affected ducts may be surrounded by a cellular infiltrate which includes lymphocytes, plasma cells and occasional eosinophils, and, especially at points of rupture, the inflammation may be granulomatous (Figures 17.1–17.4). This may range from ill-defined faintly epithelioid macrophages through to well-defined non-caseating epithelioid and giant cell granulomas which are usually quite small. Granulomas are very occasionally found in the parenchyma. Other portal tracts may or may not show a similar infiltrate or may contain lymphoid aggregates, occasionally with germinal centres (Figure 17.2). It is the smaller portal tracts which are the most likely to be normal, but they may also show changes similar to those described.

In stage 1 the limiting plates are usually intact. Occasional lymphocytes may be found in sinusoids in other parts of the parenchyma. Morphological cholestasis, as opposed to biochemical cholestasis, is, surprisingly, generally absent. Occasional twin celled liver cell plates may be seen as an expression of liver cell proliferation.

Stage 2. The characteristic lesions of stage 1 regress and diminish in number. The portal tracts are now expanded with chronic inflammatory cells and there may be destruction of limiting plates, typically with biliary piecemeal necrosis, but occasionally of classic type. Ductular proliferation is usual but is commonly very focal in distribution, and thus there may be none in a needle biopsy. The ductules are often described as atypical (Figure 17.5) in the sense that they tend to be smaller and more angular than in other diseases and have only a very small or no lumen. The cellular infiltrate may be similar to that found in stage 1, but often also includes macrophages, which sometimes ingest large quantities of lipid to become foam cells. These may form small aggregates under the capsule or within lobules as well as in portal tracts (Figure 17.6). Neutrophils are also common at this stage. Cholestasis may or may not be present; when it is, it usually takes the form of small granules of bile pigment within periph-

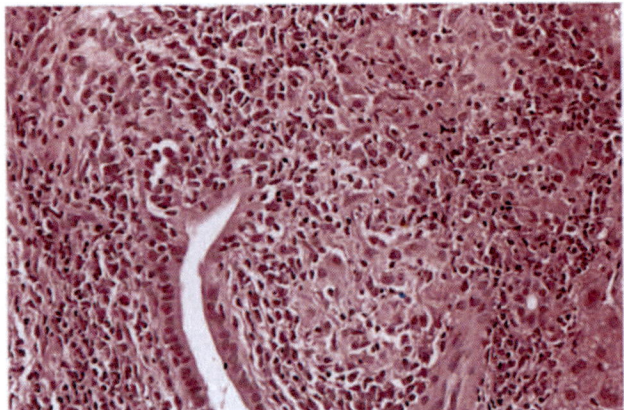

Figure 17.1   Primary biliary cirrhosis. Asymptomatic 51-year-old female. Liver biopsy shows this portal lesion which is almostidentical to that in Figure 17.3. The interlobular bile duct shows focal rupture of its epithelium with an ill-defined epithelioid granuloma related to it at this point. There is also an intense inflammatory cell infiltrate in which lymphocytes and plasma cells predominate. This is a pathognomonic picture and antimitochondrial antibodies were subsequently shown to be present.

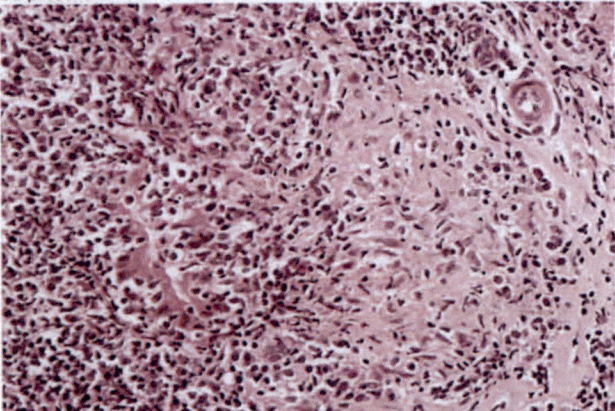

Figure 17.3   Primary biliary cirrhosis. A 45-year-old female with clinically typical symptomatic primary biliary cirrhosis. Liver biopsy shows that the epithelium of the interlobular bile duct on the left of the field has been almost totally destroyed. It is surrounded by inflammatory cells which are predominantly lymphocytes and plasma cells. To the right of the duct is a large ill-defined epithelioid granuloma.

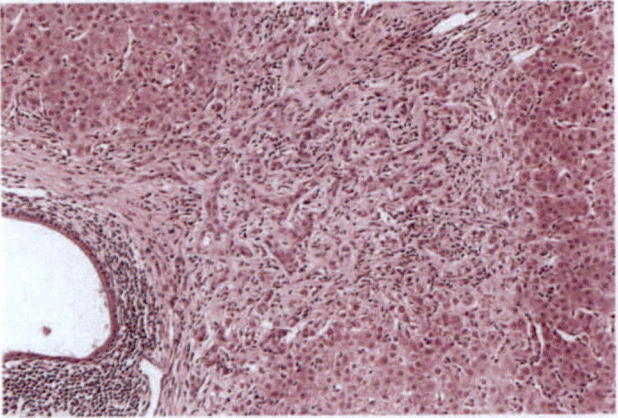

Figure 17.5   Primary biliary cirrhosis. Another typical case with severe portal hypertension and treated by liver transplantation. This section shows the very characteristic ductular proliferation. Note that the ductules are small, angular and intercommunicate with one another. Most have no lumen. To the left is an intact septal bile duct surrounded by lymphocytes.

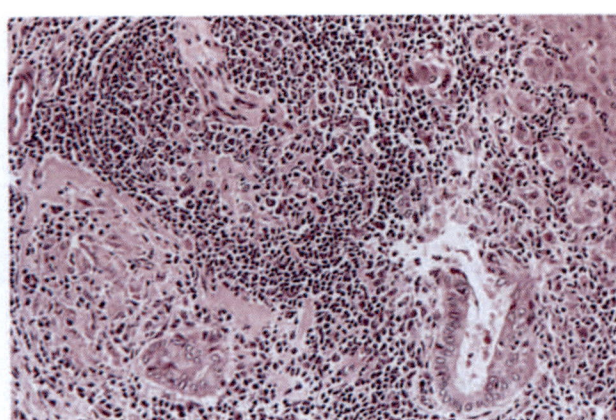

Figure 17.2   Primary biliary cirrhosis. An expanded portal tract contains a ruptured bile duct (below right), ill-defined epithelioid granuloma (below left) and a lymphoid aggregate (above).

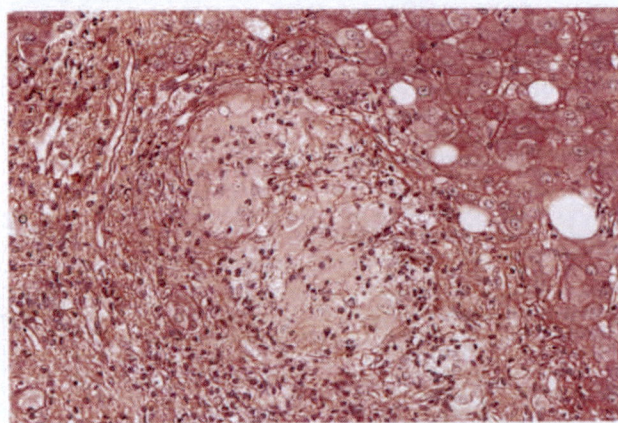

Figure 17.4   Primary biliary cirrhosis. Another typical case. This portal tract contains a well-formed epithelioid granuloma not apparently related to a bile duct. The appearances here are thus not diagnostic. Note that PAS stain demonstrates granulomas very well. PAS diastase.

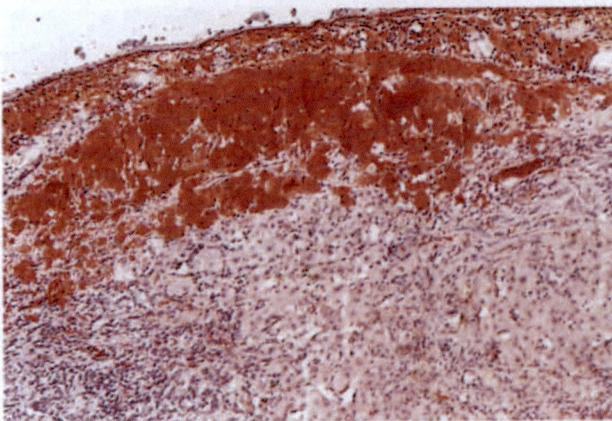

Figure 17.6   Primary biliary cirrhosis. Same case as Figure 17.5. There were several bright yellow patches beneath the capsule of the liver. These proved to be aggregates of foam cells which this frozen section shows to be filled with neutral lipid. Sudan III and IV.

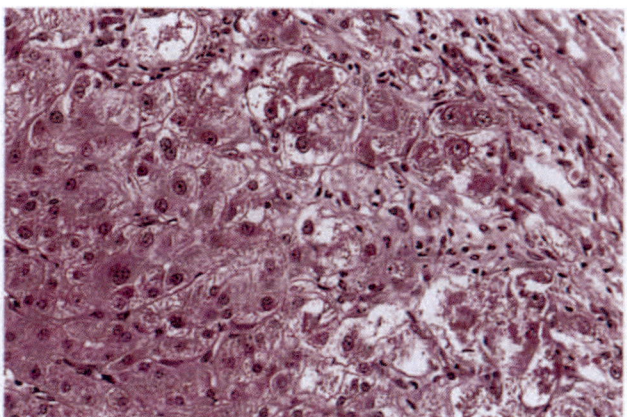

Figure 17.7   Primary biliary cirrhosis. Another typical case in stage 3/4. At the periphery of the nodules many hepatocytes contain clumped eosinophilic masses of Mallory's hyalin.

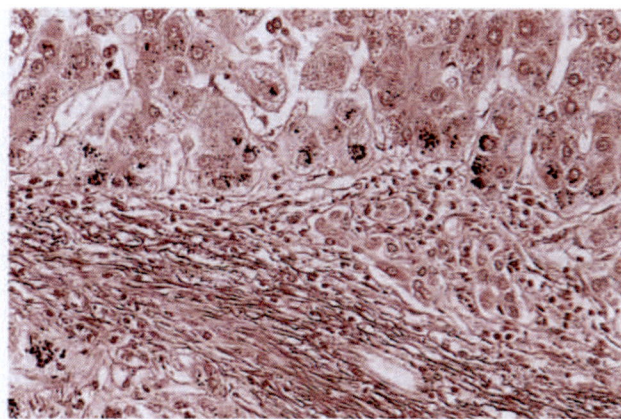

Figure 17.8   Primary biliary cirrhosis. Another typical case, stage 3. The periportal liver cells contain granular aggregates of black copper-associated protein. Orcein.

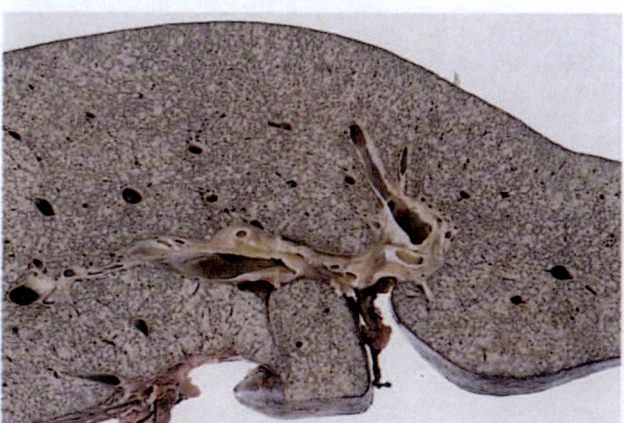

Figure 17.9   Primary biliary cirrhosis. A 51-year-old female who came to transplantation 3 years after diagnosis. The liver was enlarged and shows a typical green micronodular cut surface.

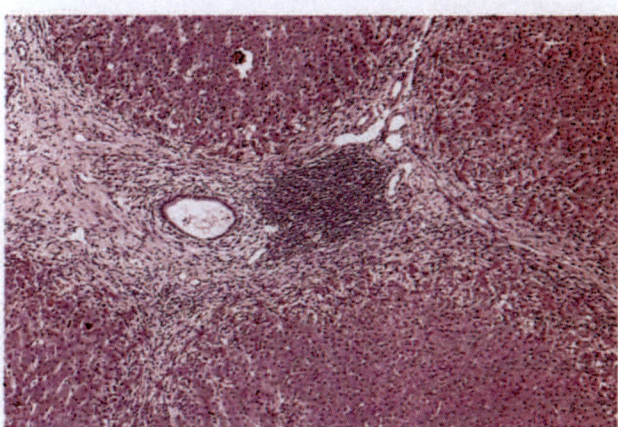

Figure 17.10   Primary biliary cirrhosis. Another typical case treated by liver transplantation. The section shows stage 4 disease with the nodules surrounded by fibrous septa. Aggregates of lymphocytes as seen here are characteristic but not diagnostic. Note preservation of the larger septal bile duct.

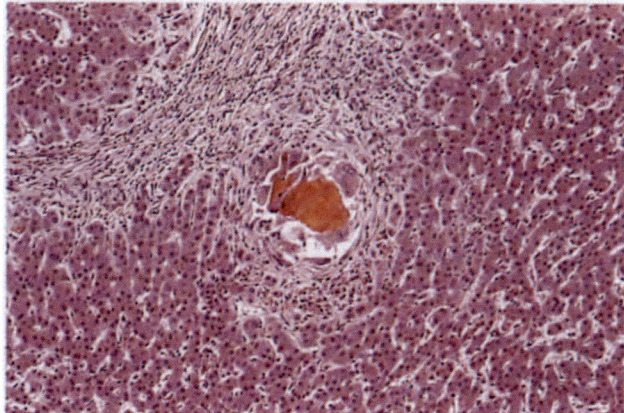

Figure 17.11   Primary biliary cirrhosis. Another typical case. This section shows a small periportal bile lake surrounded by foreign body giant cells. The large bile ducts were fully patent.

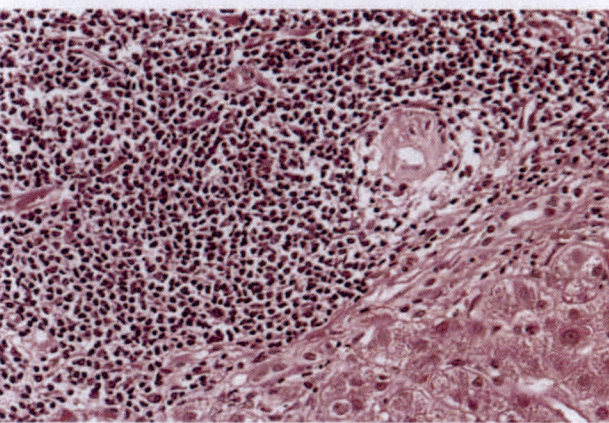

Figure 17.12   Primary biliary cirrhosis/chronic active hepatitis overlap syndrome. The patient had anti-smooth muscle antibodies and hyper-gammaglobulinaemia as well as antimitochondrial antibodies. The epithelium of the interlobular bile duct is again degenerate, but there is no related granuloma. Note the very intense portal chronic inflammation, but the limiting plate is intact in this field.

eral liver cells which may also show feathery degeneration. The same periportal cells may contain clumped eosino-philic masses of Mallory's hyalin (Figure 17.7). There is also irregular portal fibrosis with some distortion of architecture and linkage of adjacent portal tracts but preservation of lobules.

Stage 3. Fibrosis increases in concert with periportal cholestasis. At this stage there may be accumulation of granular brownish-black orcein-positive material in periportal liver cells (Figure 17.8). This has been shown to be a copper-metallothionein complex[15] which accumulates because of a failure of copper excretion through its normal biliary route. Similar accumulation is seen in other types of prolonged cholestasis (see Chapter 16). Bile duct lesions are relatively uncommon at this stage. Instead, the site of former bile ducts may be marked by fibrosis or a lymphoid aggregate.

Stage 4. True cirrhosis supervenes with regeneration nodules.

There is considerable overlap between different stages and, indeed, more than one stage may be seen in different parts of the same liver. For example, granulomas may be seen in stage 4, and, even quite late in the disease, when many portal tracts have reached the scar stage, other portal tracts may still be normal.

DIFFERENTIAL DIAGNOSIS

The main conditions which should be considered[3] include chronic active hepatitis, primary sclerosing cholangitis (PSC), large duct obstruction and granulomatous disease. Although bile duct rupture is characteristic of PBC it is not always seen. When bile duct lesions are not found, proliferating atypical ductules in association with absent medium-sized bile ducts, especially when accompanied by scattered lymphoid aggregates, are strong pointers to the diagnosis. Periportal cholestasis, especially with hyalin and orcein-positive granules, are usually present in late disease but are not diagnostic since they are found in most forms of cirrhosis late in the natural history. Distinction from *chronic active hepatitis* is not always easy[14] and indeed the two diseases may be related (Figure 17.12). There can be considerable clinical and histological overlap between the two conditions in as many as 20 % of cases of PBC[16]. In chronic active hepatitis, destruction of the limiting plate and piecemeal necrosis are usually more marked and inflammatory changes more likely to have a lobular as well as periportal distribution. Most patients with the overlap syndrome, or who have PBC in association with other connective tissue disorders, have antibodies to the M4 component of the mitochondrial antigen[16]. Bile duct damage may be seen in acute and chronic hepatitis C, where there may also be periductal lymphoid aggregates[17], and thus may cause some diagnostic difficulties (Chapter 2). However, the pattern is usually rather different in that the epithelium of affected ducts is more likely to show nuclear stratification and vacuolation. Prolonged *extrahepatic biliary obstruction* (secondary biliary cirrhosis) may cause confusion (see below). Here periductal fibrosis is more marked than duct destruction, and proliferating ductules tend to be larger and located more uniformly at the peripheries of the portal tracts. Piecemeal necrosis and periportal or lobular inflammation are usually insignificant, whereas cholest-asis with or without hyalin may be more striking. Bile infarcts and large bile lakes (see below) are diagnostic, but small bile lakes are occasionally seen in PBC. *Primary sclerosing cholangitis*, with or without ulcerative colitis, may affect larger as well as smaller ducts the remnants of

which usually leave a recognizable scar[18]. *Drug-induced cholestasis* may only be recognized in the clinical context. A chronic cholangitis may be found in *liver fluke* infes-tation, although usually with many eosinophils. Portal infiltrates in *malignant lymphomas*, particularly Hodgkin's disease, may also cause confusion from time to time. Other forms of *granulomatous disease* can often be excluded by the presence of any of the other features of PBC. In cases of doubt, clinical and biochemical correl-ation are essential. The presence of antimitochondrial antibody, especially if the subtype M2 is present, is a strong pointer to the diagnosis.

TREATMENT AND PROGNOSIS

Symptomatic disease is relentlessly progressive. A recent large international prospective trial showed that the most unfavourable sign was the rapid onset of severe cholest-asis[19]. This was always associated with rapid progression of disease, whatever the histological stage. Other factors which seemed to have prognostic value were age, histo-logical stage and the serum bilirubin level. In contrast, the patient's sex, the duration of symptoms and the mode of presentation seemed to have no prognostic importance.

PBC is the second most frequent indication for hepatic transplantation in adults. A recent large series of 161 patients treated by transplantation[20] showed a one year survival of 75% and 5 year survival of 70%. This was considerably better than that predicted using the Mayo Clinic survival model.[21] This uses clinical and biochemical parameters rather than histological, with age, serum biliru-bin, serum albumin, prothrombin time, and the severity of oedema as the main criteria. A study from Glasgow, using histological criteria, found that hepatic fibrosis, bilirubinostasis and Mallory's hyalin were all independent risk factors.[22] Other prognostic models are similarly effec-tive,[23,24] and thus choosing the right moment for trans-plantation is rapidly becoming the treatment of choice in otherwise suitable patients. It remains an open question whether PBC recurs after transplantation (Chapter 26), but if it does, it clearly does so only very rarely.

Of the more conventional treatments, azathioprine does not appear to be beneficial, despite the apparently immu-nological nature of PBC[25]. Tissue copper levels in PBC frequently reach the sort of level found in Wilson's disease, but there is no evidence that it is directly hepatotoxic[26]. Recent controlled trials have show very promising results both with cyclosporin[27], and with ursodeoxycholic acid, the major bile acid in the brown bear[28].

REFERENCES

1. Hadziyannis, S., Scheuer, P. J., Feizi, T., Naccarato, R., Doniach, D. and Sherlock, S. (1970). Immunological and histological studies in primary biliary cirrhosis. J. Clin. Pathol., 23, 95–98
2. Beswick, D. R., Klatskin, G. and Boyer, J. L. (1985). Asymptomatic primary biliary cirrhosis–long term follow-up and natural history. Gastroenterology, 89, 267–271
3. Wight, D. G. D. (1993). Cholestasis and extrahepatic bile ducts. In Wight, D. G. D. (ed.). Liver, Biliary Tract and Exocrine Pancreas. Vol. 11. Systemic Pathology. Symmers, W. S. C., series ed. 3rd edn. Edinburgh: Churchill Livingstone
4. Triger, D. R. (1980). Primary biliary cirrhosis: an epidemiological study. Br. Med. J., 281, 772–775
5. Krams, S. M., Surh, C. D., Coppel, R. L., Ansari, A., Ruebner, B. and Gershwin, M. E. (1989). Immunization of experimental animals with dihydrolipoamide acetyltransferase as a possible purified recombi-nant polypeptide generates mitochondrial antibodies but not primary biliary cirrhosis. Hepatology, 9, 411–416
6. Hopf, U., Moller, B., Stemerowicz, R., Lobeck, H., Rodloff, A., Freudenberg, M., Galanos, C. and Huhn, D. (1989). Relation between Escherichia coli rough-forms in gut, lipid A in liver and primary biliary cirrhosis. Lancet, 2, 1419–1421
7. Nakanuma, Y. and Kono, N. (1991). Expression of HLA-DR antigens

on interlobular bile ducts in primary biliary cirrhosis and other hepatobiliary diseases: an immunohistochemical study. Hum. Pathol., 22, 431–436

8. Epstein, O., Thomas, H. C. and Sherlock, S. (1980). Primary biliary cirrhosis is a dry gland syndrome with features of chronic graft-vs-host disease. Lancet, 1, 1166–1168

9. Krams, S. M., Dorshkind, K. and Gershwin, M. E. (1989). Generation of biliary lesions after transfer of human lymphocytes into severe combined immuno-deficient (SCID) mice. J. Exp. Med., 170, 1919–1930

10. Rubin, E., Schaffner, F. and Popper, H. (1965). Primary biliary cirrhosis. Chronic non-suppurative destructive cholangitis. Am. J. Pathol., 46, 387–407

11. Scheuer, P. J. (1967). Primary biliary cirrhosis. Proc. Roy. Soc. Med., 60, 1257–1260

12. Ludwig, J., Dickson, E. R. and McDonald, G. S. A. (1978). Staging of chronic non-suppurative destructive cholangitis (syndrome of primary biliary cirrhosis). Virch. Arch. A. Path. Anat. Histol., 379, 103–112

13. Portmann, B., Popper, H., Neuberger, J. and Williams, R. (1985). Sequential and diagnostic features in primary biliary cirrhosis. Gastroenterology, 88, 1777–1790

14. MacSween, R. N. M. and Portmann, B. C. (1987). Diseases of the intrahepatic bile ducts. In MacSween, R. N. M., Anthony, P. P. and Scheuer, P. J. (eds). Pathology of the liver. 2nd edn. pp. 424–453. Edinburgh: Churchill Livingstone

15. Janssens, A. R., Bosman, F. T., Ruiter, D. J. and Van den Hamer, C. J. (1984). Immunohistochemical demonstration of the cytoplasmic copper-associated protein in the liver in primary biliary cirrhosis: its identification as metallothionein. Liver, 4, 139–147

16. Berg, P. A., Weber, P., Oehring, J., Lindenborn-Fotinos, J. and Stechemesser, E. (1985). Significance of different types of mitochondrial antibodies in primary biliary cirrhosis. In Brunner, H. and Thaler, H. (eds). Hepatology: a Festschrift for Hans Popper. pp. 231–242. New York: Raven Press

17. Scheuer, P. J., Ashrafzadeh, P., Sherlock, S., Brown, D. and Dusheiko, G. (1992). The pathology of hepatitis C. Hepatology, 15, 567–571

18. Harrison, R. F. and Hübscher, S. G. (1991). The spectrum of bile duct lesions in end-stage primary sclerosing cholangitis. Histopathology, 19, 321–327

19. Christensen, E., Crowe, J., Doniach, D., Popper, H., Ranek, L., Rodes, J., Tygstrup, N. and Williams, R. (1980). Clinical pattern and course of disease in PBC based on an analysis of 236 patients. Gastroenterology, 78, 286–246

20. Markus, B. H., Dickson, E. R., Grambsch, P. M., Fleming, T. R., Mazzaferro, V., Klintmalm, G. B. C., Wiesner, R. H., Van Thiel, D. H. and Starzl, T. E. (1989). Efficacy of liver transplantation in patients with primary biliary cirrhosis. N. Engl. J. Med., 320, 1709–1713

21. Dickson, E. R., Grambsch, P. M., Flemming, T. R., Fisher, L. D. and Langworthy, A. (1989). Prognosis in primary biliary cirrhosis: model for decision making. Hepatology, 10, 1–7

22. Goudie, B. M., Burt, A. D., Macfarlane, G. J., Boyle, P., Gillis, C. R., MacSween, R. N. M. and Watkinson, G. (1989). Risk factors and prognosis in primary biliary cirrhosis. Am J Gastroenterol., 84, 713–716

23. Neuberger, J. M. (1989). Predicting prognosis in primary biliary cirrhosis. Gut, 30, 1519–1522

24. Bonsel, G. J., Klompmaker, I. J., Van'T Veer, F., Habbema, J. D. F. and Slooff, M. J. H. (1990). Use of prognostic models for assessment of value of liver transplantation in primary biliary cirrhosis. Lancet, 335, 493–497

25. Crowe, J., Christensen, E., Smith, M., Cochrane, M., Ranek, L., Watkinson, G., Doniach, D., Popper, H., Tygstrup, N. and Williams, R. (1980). Azathioprine in PBC: a preliminary report of an international trial. Gastroenterology, 78, 1005–1010

26. Vierling, J. M. (1990). Primary biliary cirrhosis. In Zakim, D. and Boyer, T. D. (eds). Hepatology. A textbook of liver disease. 2nd edn. pp. 1158–1205. Philadelphia: Saunders

27. Wiesner, R. H., Ludwig, J., Lindor, K. D., Jorgensen, R. A., Baldus, W. P., Homburger, H. A. and Dickson, E. R. (1990). A controlled trial of cyclosporin in the treatment of primary biliary cirrhosis. N. Engl. J. Med., 322, 1419–1424

28. Poupon, R. E., Balkau, B., Eschwege, E. and Poupon, R. (1991). A multicenter, controlled trial of ursodiol for the treatment of primary biliary cirrhosis. UDCA-PBC Study Group. N. Engl. J. Med., 324, 1548–1554

The liver receives between one-fifth and one-quarter of the cardiac output at rest. Of this the portal vein contributes between 65 and 80% of the blood, although less than 50% of the oxygen. In some animals the liver plays an important role in regulating blood flow in general by acting as a reservoir. There is some evidence that a similar system may operate in humans so that the liver may discharge blood to maintain cardiac output or retain it in congestive heart failure, when it greatly increases in volume. Interruption or reduction of flow through any of the major vessels may be followed by a variety of distinctive responses by the liver.

INFARCTS OF ZAHN OR PSEUDOINFARCTS

These are foci of liver cell atrophy usually attributable to obstruction of branches of the portal vein, although additional factors such as hypovolaemia may also be necessary[1]. They are not true infarcts, since there is no necrosis, but represent atrophy of hepatocytes due to deprivation of growth factors, mainly insulin, normally present in the portal blood. The commonest cause of portal vein occlusion is thrombosis as a complication of tumour deposits, either by direct invasion or by compression of the vessel. Alternatively, embolism may occur, especially following ligation of the splenic vein at splenectomy. Pseudoinfarcts give rise to no symptoms or signs during life and thus are usually an incidental post-mortem finding. Their fate is uncertain but may well be reversible. Pseudoinfarcts do not appear to occur in cirrhotic livers, probably because of the great alteration in vascular architecture which occurs in cirrhosis.

Macroscopically the affected part of the liver may be shrunken and tends to retract away from the cut surface. The colour is usually a darker red-brown than the normal liver (Figure 18.1) and a lobular pattern is often discernible, although the lobules are smaller than normal. Microscopically liver cells are smaller than normal with abundant lipofuscin. Sinusoids are usually dilated and filled with blood (Figure 18.2), possibly due to cross-over between the territories of the portal vein and hepatic veins[2]. The occluded portal vein may be visible in the same section, although occasionally no vascular lesion can be found.

INFARCTION

True infarcts of the liver are not common, but when they do occur they resemble anaemic infarcts in other organs. They are mostly attributable to hepatic artery occlusion. Polyarteritis nodosa was the commonest cause in the older literature, but more recently hepatic artery ligation and atherosclerosis of the aorta and/or hepatic artery have become the predominant causes. They are also seen as a result of hepatic artery thrombosis, an occasional complication in liver transplantation[3]. Most series include several cases in which the portal vein contains the only demonstrable thrombus, although the significance of this has been questioned[4], since the thrombosis may have followed the infarction. Other cases have no vascular lesion at all, but most of these have associated cardiovascular or biliary disease or some other reason for hepatic hypoperfusion[5,6]. Clinically infarcts may give rise to local

pain and even fever and jaundice[6].

Macroscopically, they are similar to anaemic infarcts in other organs, with a yellowish opaque cut surface, surrounded by a rim of hyperaemia (Figure 18.3). Microscopically they vary greatly in size and show coagulative necrosis of all parts of the acinus (Figure 18.4). Sinusoidal cells, central veins and portal tracts, although spared initially[4], are included in the necrosis by about 48 hours, at least in the central part of the lesion. Around the periphery there may be prolonged sparing of portal tracts and periportal liver cells. From two days onwards an acute inflammatory response becomes more apparent, with vasodilatation and neutrophil infiltration at the border of the necrotic zone (Figure 18.4). There is collapse of the lobular stroma at about one week and eventually replacement by granulation tissue and ultimately a fibrous scar.

Hepatic artery occlusion, particularly involving peripheral branches, may be a cause of biliary cysts and von Meyenburg complexes (Chapter 22)[7].

THE LIVER IN CIRCULATORY FAILURE
Congestive cardiac failure

There is a marked contrast between biopsy and necropsy specimens. At post-mortem the typical nutmeg liver is a common occurrence, although usually patients have no symptoms or signs referable to the liver other than a variable degree of hepatic enlargement. Microscopically hepatic venous radicals and adjacent sinusoids are engorged and liver cells shrink, dissociate and often disappear completely[8]. The liver cells adjacent to these congested centrilobular zones frequently show loss of glycogen and fatty change (Figure 18.5), hence even greater contrast with the dark areas of congestion when seen with the naked eye.

In biopsies the changes are much less conspicuous and minor atrophy of centrilobular parenchymal cells may be all that is seen. However, in more severe cases sinusoidal dilatation and congestion are present, although fatty change is rare, suggesting that it may be a terminal event when found at post-mortem[9].

The liver in hypoperfusion and shock

Anything which causes hypoperfusion of the liver may lead to centrilobular necrosis associated with a clinical syndrome of mild to moderate jaundice with elevation of serum transaminases and alkaline phosphatase. The syndrome may follow recognizable shock, for example after myocardial infarction, pulmonary embolism, prolonged surgery and anaesthesia, sepsis or severe trauma[10,11], but it may also follow left heart failure, either alone[12] or in conjunction with congestive failure. In a few patients the hepatic necrosis may be so acute as to mimic acute virus hepatitis[13,14] and may even obscure the primary condition[12]. A minority of patients present with a predominantly cholestatic biochemical picture[15].

Microscopically the extent of the changes can be related to the duration of the shock state. Shock of less than 10 hours duration is unlikely to be associated with necrosis, whilst if it is prolonged beyond 24 hours, necrosis is almost constant. There is congestion of the terminal

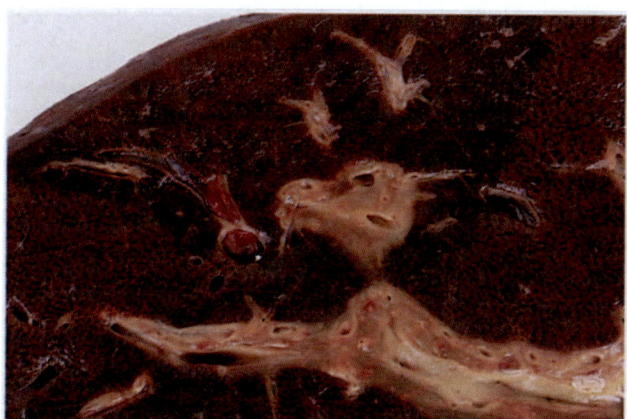

Figure 18.1 Infarct of Zahn. This shows a wedge-shaped area of darker parenchyma. An hepatic vein thrombus is also clearly visible in this photograph and was thought to be secondary to the portal vein thrombus (not visible).

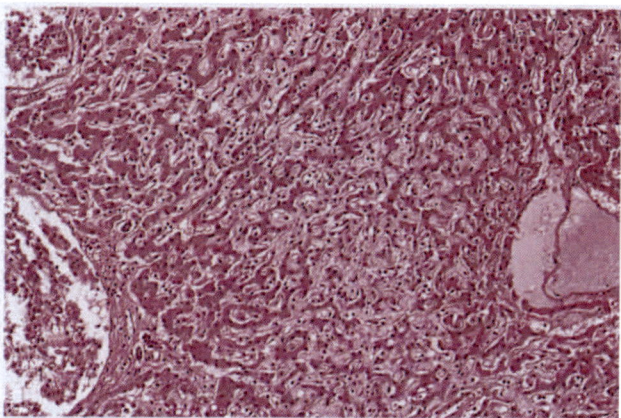

Figure 18.2 Infarct of Zahn. This 57-year-old man died with a renal carcinoma which had metastasized to the liver. At autopsy a wedge-shaped subcapsular area of congestion was seen. Section of this shows thinning of liver cell plates and congestion of sinusoids which transcends lobular boundaries. Renal carcinoma can be seen permeating the portal vein (to the left).

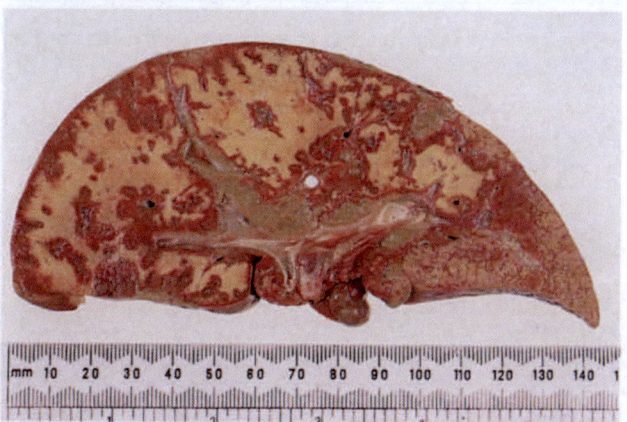

Figure 18.3 Infarct. Recent hepatic transplantation complicated by hepatic artery thrombosis. The photograph shows extensive yellow infarction, bordered by a zone of vasodilatation.

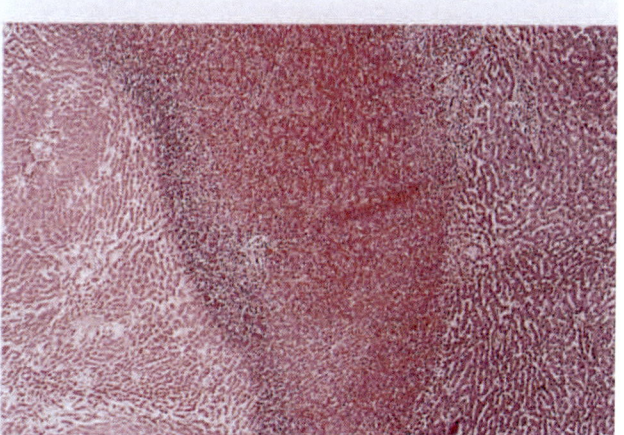

Figure 18.4 Infarct. The section shows a classic infarct with coagulative necrosis (left) and a zone of haemorrhage and neutrophil infiltration at its junction with viable liver.

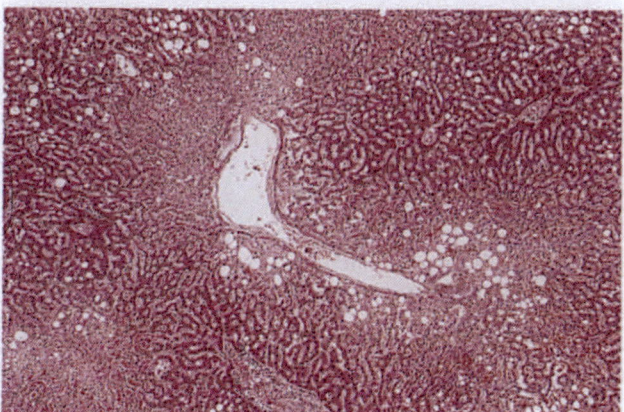

Figure 18.5 Congestive heart failure, nutmeg liver. Classic nutmeg liver in an elderly patient at post–mortem showing centrilobular congestion and liver cell atrophy, with focal fatty change at the interface with the normal parenchyma.

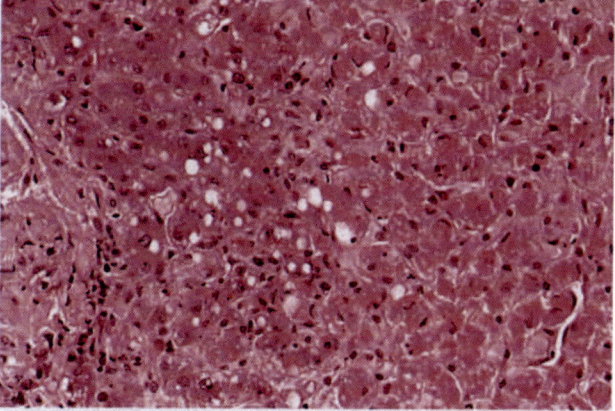

Figure 18.6 Shock liver. Recent hepatic transplantation complicated by profound haemorrhage. Liver biopsy shows a sharply demarcated zone of coagulative necrosis of hepatocytes in the centrilobular region (right). Peri-portal liver cells are normal. Note that the sinusoidal cell nuclei remain viable.

hepatic venule with local haemorrhage from it and patchy liver cell necrosis, which is usually centrilobular but occasionally apparently mid-zonal[16], affects a variable proportion of the acinus, sometimes even causing bridging necrosis[17]. The necrotic zone is often quite sharply defined with affected cells showing eosinophilic necrosis with pyknosis, karyorrhexis or karyolysis of nuclei (Figure 18.6). Frequently the cells lining sinusoids remain intact (Figure 18.6)[4]. The reticulin framework usually stays intact and complete recovery is possible (Figure 18.7). A neutrophil response develops after a few days but is often patchy and inconspicuous. Occasionally swollen Kupffer cells filled with ceroid pigment are prominent in the areas of necrosis. Rarely centrilobular sinusoids appear dilated but empty, whilst the adjacent liver cell plates are replaced by red blood cells[18], due to entry of red blood cells into the space of Disse, something which can also be seen in severe cardiac failure and in Budd-Chiari syndrome (Figure 18.11). At the periphery of the lesion the blood-filled liver cell plates merge with atrophic liver cells, often containing an abundance of lipochrome pigment. Morphological cholestasis in the form of bile plugs is sometimes seen and correlates with the biochemical cholestasis referred to above[15].

There is some controversy over the relative importance of congestion as compared to hypoperfusion in the development of changes in the liver in congestive heart failure[17]. In all probability it is merely a matter of degree, and it is impossible to confidently distinguish between the changes attributable to congestive heart failure on the one hand and those due to left heart failure and shock on the other. Typical congestive failure is rarely seen in biopsy material, since there are few indications for biopsy.

Differential diagnosis

Despite the clinical difficulties sometimes encountered[12], heart failure is usually easily distinguished from viral hepatitis on biopsy. It may be less easy to recognize injury due to necrotizing hepatotoxins such as paracetamol (Chapter 10), but in heart failure there are usually no transitional stages of injury. Heat stroke may lead to changes identical to those in heart failure[19].

Shock states in the presence of cirrhosis, for example following bleeding from varices, may give rise to a pseudolobular necrosis involving liver cells in the central parts of nodules (Figure 18.8) which is otherwise identical to that described above.

BUDD-CHIARI SYNDROME

The most severe acute venous congestion occurs in the Budd-Chiari syndrome. This is a condition in which the major hepatic veins are occluded by tumour or more commonly thrombus. The latter occurs most often in young women, in whom it has been linked with the contraceptive pill, in association with various coagulation disorders (such as polycythaemia[20], sickle cell disease) or after trauma. It is becoming increasingly clear that a much higher proportion of patients than hitherto appreciated have evidence of an underlying myeloproliferative disorder at the time of presentation[20,21]. In Budd-Chiari syndrome most of zones 2 and 3 of the acinus become replaced by blood (Figures 18.9 and 18.10) with only a narrow rim of surviving zone 1 periportal liver cells leading to so-called reversed lobulation (Figure 18.10). Much more commonly than in heart failure or shock, there may be replacement of liver cell plates by blood, the intervening sinusoids appearing empty (Figure 18.11), a change seen particularly in the midzones[22]. The latter authors suggest that this unexpected picture may represent extra-sinusoidal flow of blood through Disse's space to a plexus of small vessels running coaxially in the adventitia of the central veins. These are often quite conspicuous in outflow block and would enable the block to be bypassed if it were localized. There are variable numbers of pigment-containing phagocytes and occasionally free iron may be demonstrated. Bile thrombi are sometimes seen and surviving liver cells may show regenerative activity in the form of twinning of liver cell plates or even the formation of an occasional nodule.

Budd-Chiari syndrome is rapidly fatal in about one-third of cases[20], but if the patient survives the changes vary considerably from one part of the liver to another. There are often large blood-filled cysts and areas of infarction, as well as the changes described above. In addition, there may be relative sparing of the caudate and quadrate lobes, because of their independent venous drainage directly into the inferior vena cava, leading to localized hypertrophy of the posterior part of the liver and a cottage-loaf profile (Figure 18.12). A few patients go on to develop a true cirrhosis (see below).

VENO-OCCLUSIVE DISEASE

Veno-occlusive disease affects principally the small veins and only occasionally medium-sized vessels. This is a disease which affects mainly children between 18 months and 5 years of age and is attributable to ingestion of pyrrolizidine alkaloids usually in the form of bush tea. Irradiation of the whole liver[23] and treatment with certain chemotherapeutic agents, especially alkylating agents such as azathioprine[24] cause similar changes. It may also be part of the graft-versus-host disease following bone marrow transplantation (Figure 18.13)[25].

The onset is usually abrupt with rapid development of ascites and histologically there is severe centrilobular congestion and necrosis similar to that seen in the Budd-Chiari syndrome, but in addition, central veins are abnormal. They are often very inconspicuous, but connective tissue stains show the outline of the wall with the lumen reduced or obliterated by sub-endothelial oedematous connective tissue which later becomes dense[26] (Figures 18.14 and 8.15). The initiating event appears to be obliteration of the outlets of sinusoids into efferent veins by deposition of fibrin and platelets.

Some patients make a prompt and unexpected recovery; others progress to chronic liver disease and cirrhosis. In an endemic area such as Jamaica, it is thought to account for up to 30% of all cases of cirrhosis.

CARDIAC FIBROSIS AND CIRRHOSIS

If venous congestion is prolonged, whatever the cause, centrilobular sinusoidal collagenization is liable to occur. The fibrosis is most severe in chronic venoocclusive disease and chronic Budd-Chiari syndrome (Figure 18.16), but may also follow heart failure, especially when there are recurrent acute episodes. Proliferation of small bile ductules in these scarred central zones may be so conspicuous that they may simulate portal tracts and thus the true nature of the condition may not be appreciated. Although initially centrilobular, in a proportion of cases fibrous bands eventually link adjacent terminal venules (Figure 18.17) and terminal venules to portal tracts and a true nodular cirrhosis may develop, although this is rare.

SINUSOIDAL DILATATION

Although sinusoidal dilatation in liver biopsies is most often seen in zone 3 and attributable to disturbances of the circulation, it may also be seen in a number of other unrelated conditions. Periportal sinusoidal dilatation has been clearly linked to oral contraceptive usage[27] (Chapter

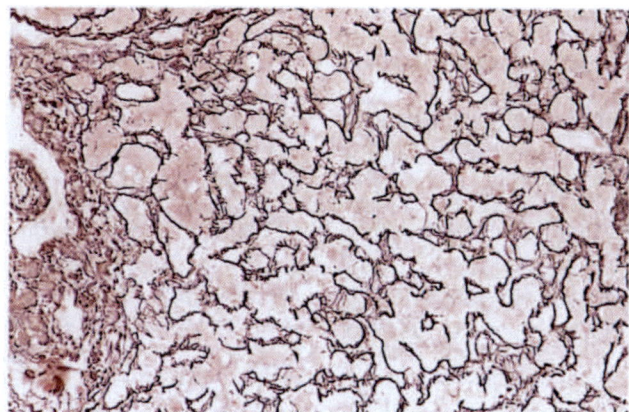

Figure 18.7 Shock liver. Same field as Figure 18.6. This section shows that the reticulin framework of the necrotic zone is completely preserved. Reticulin.

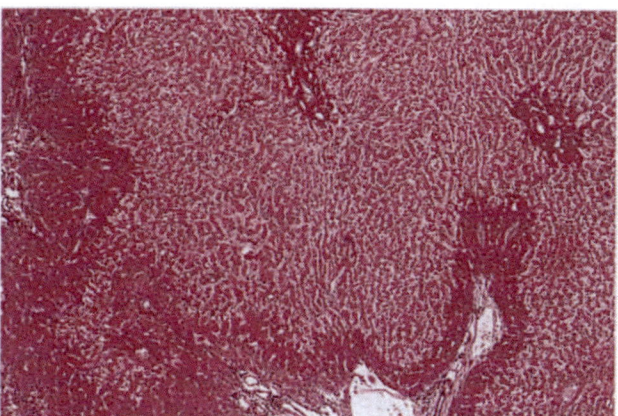

Figure 18.8 Cirrhosis, pseudolobular necrosis. An 18-year-old male who presented with massive gastrointestinal haemorrhage from bleeding varices which were due to HBsAg-positive cirrhosis. Biopsy shows irregular areas of coagulative necrosis involving much of the central parts of the nodules but sparing a peripheral rim of liver cells.

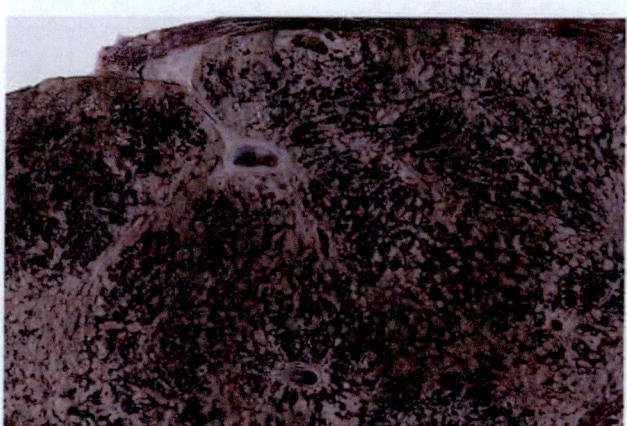

Figure 18.9 Acute Budd-Chiari syndrome. A 42-year-old man with idiopathic hepatic vein thrombosis received a liver transplant. The excised liver showed changes of varying ages, but this field shows the classic acute congestion resembling an exaggerated nutmeg pattern. Note the occluded hepatic vein tributary (above centre).

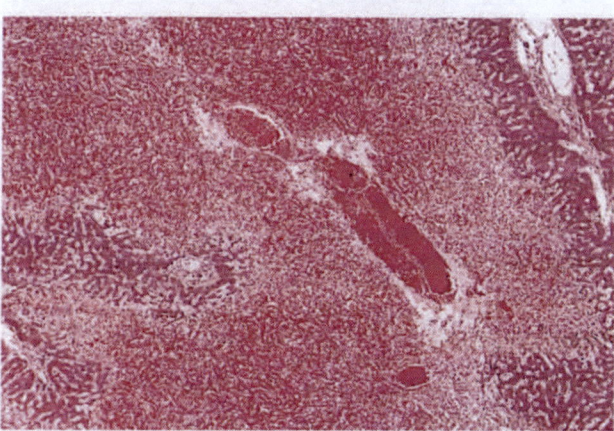

Figure 18.10 Acute Budd-Chiari syndrome. A 53-year-old female who presented with ascites and was shown radiologically to have occlusion of the inferior vena cava at the level of the hepatic veins. At autopsy there was also extensive hepatic vein thrombosis, but no cause was discovered. The liver section shows massive congestion of central venules and the majority of the parenchyma leading to 'reversed lobulation'.

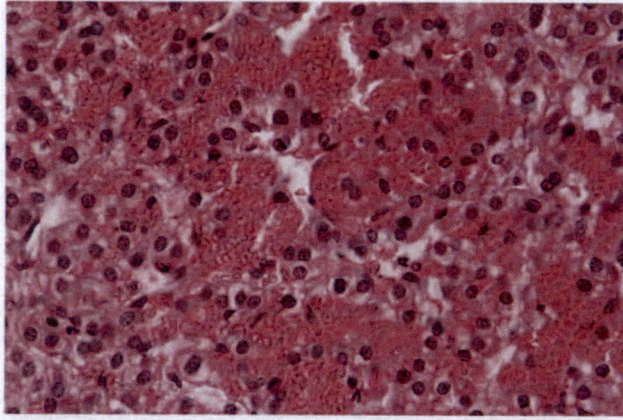

Figure 18.11 Acute Budd-Chiari syndrome. A 10-year-old male presented with ascites, again due to idiopathic hepatic vein thrombosis. Biopsy shows, in this case, extensive replacement of liver cell plates by red cells, the sinusoids remaining empty. Although most often seen in venous outflow obstruction, this appearance is also found in cardiac failure and shock states.

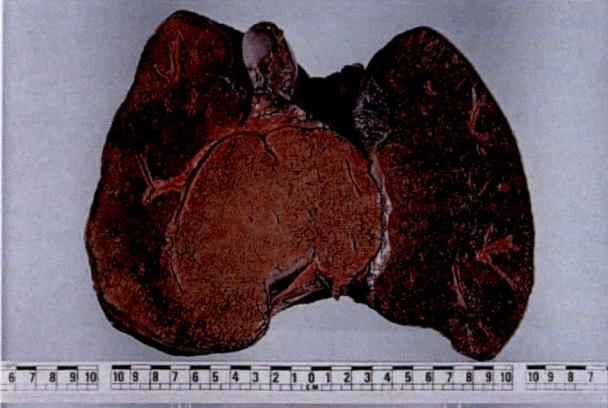

Figure 18.12 Acute Budd-Chiari syndrome. The liver has been sliced transversely and the light brown hypertrophied caudate/quadrate lobe can be clearly seen centrally. This is relatively spared from the acute congestion seen peripherally.

22). Dilatation accompanies cellular infiltrations in leukaemia, malaria, extramedullary haemopoiesis and sickle cell disease.

In a series of 906 biopsies[28], sinusoidal dilatation unrelated to any of the above factors was found in 3%. In half the sinusoidal dilation was of random distribution, but in the remainder it was mid-zonal with sparing of the centrilobular sinusoids (Figure 18.18). The majority of cases were associated with malignant disease (metastatic carcinoma, Hodgkin's disease and primary cancer) or granulomatous disease (tuberculosis, brucellosis, Crohn's disease), but these diseases were actually visualized in the biopsy in only half of the cases. The pathogenesis of the sinusoidal dilatation is unknown. In at least some cases it may represent the first stage of peliosis hepatis. The discovery of sinusoidal dilatation as an isolated finding should prompt a search for malignant or granulomatous disease by other parameters.

PELIOSIS HEPATIS

This is a pathological entity that is usually an incidental finding at autopsy or laparotomy and takes the form of blood cysts up to 3-4 mm in diameter (Figure 18.19). Until recently the majority of cases were associated with wasting diseases such as tuberculosis or terminal malignancy, but it is now regularly associated with the use of the contraceptive pill or anabolic steroids[29].

The pathogenesis of peliosis remains a matter of dispute. Some authors believe that it commences as focal liver cell necrosis, causing damage to the reticulin and allowing inflow of blood to form a cyst[30], whilst others believe that damage may be primarily to the sinusoidal lining[29]. Paradinas and his colleagues[31] noted that prolapse of hepatocytes into the central veins (Figure 10.21) was a constant finding in their series of cases due to anabolic steroids and proposed that this might interfere with drainage of blood from the sinusoids.

Microscopically peliosis is characterized by multiple blood-filled cysts of variable size, usually not lined by endothelium (Figure 18.19) and communicating either with sinusoids or central veins. Occasionally they are filled with thrombus. Sinusoidal dilatation is also quite commonly seen elsewhere in an affected liver.

VASCULAR DISEASE

Primary blood vessel disease may occasionally be encountered in liver biopsies.

Hyalinization of the small branches of the hepatic artery is seen in the liver, as in vessels of comparable size in other organs, in *systemic hypertension* (Figure 18.20). *Amyloidosis* when confined to these vessels may produce a picture which is indistinguishable without the use of special stains (Chapter 21).

Polyarteritis nodosa affects medium-sized arteries and according to the older literature[32] affects the liver in up to two-thirds of cases. Liver biopsy occasionally is helpful in detecting an unexpected arteritis in obscure inflammatory conditions (Figure 18.21). Thrombosis of these vessels may lead to infarction (see above). Aneurysms may give rise to haemobilia. Liver involvement is described in *giant cell arteritis*[33] but is essentially non-specific.

Hereditary haemorrhagic telangiectasia (Osler-Rendu-Weber disease). Hepatomegaly is frequent and the liver contains randomly distributed fibrovascular foci (Figure 18.22). These may take the form of a peliosis-like meshwork of dilated sinusoids accompanied by a variable amount of collagenous stroma or more typically tortuous venous channels embedded in fibrous tissue and often accompanied by wide calibre arteries coursing through the liver. Communications between these, and between

enlarged portal tracts, may surround liver lobules, giving a false impression of cirrhosis[34], although a link with true cirrhosis cannot be excluded[35].

SICKLE CELL DISEASE

Liver abnormalities are common in patients with sickle cell disease[36], the majority of whom have a clinically enlarged liver. Microscopically, Kupffer cells are enlarged and contain haemosiderin, ceroid and often phagocytosed red cells (Figure 18.23). Sickling can usually quite easily be recognized in sinusoids and this may very occasionally be of diagnostic value when unsuspected clinically. In sickle cell crisis vessels and sinuses are packed with red cells, especially in centrilobular regions, and this leads to sinusoidal dilatation throughout the acinus. Focal parenchymal necrosis is also quite common.

Parenchymal iron accumulation and/or portal fibrosis are seen in up to half of all patients[36], but in only a small proportion is there progression to cirrhosis.

PORTAL HYPERTENSION

Traditionally, the causes of portal hypertension are divided into pre-hepatic, hepatic and post-hepatic according to the site of greatest resistance to flow. This classification (see Table 18.1) has some merit in terms of management, since patients with pre-hepatic portal hypertension tend to suffer less from ascites and post-shunt encephalopathy than the other groups. Most of the listed conditions are discussed elsewhere.

Table 18.1   Causes of portal hypertension

A. Presinusoidal	
Congenital	Congenital hepatic fibrosis
Infections	Schistosomiasis, Kala azar
Portal vein thrombosis	
Splenomegaly	Myeloproliferative disorders
	Gaucher's disease
	Felty's syndrome
	Tropical splenomegaly syndrome
Drugs and toxins	Arsenic, Copper, Vinyl Chloride
Miscellaneous	Partial nodular transformation
	Nodular regenerative hyperplasia
	Idiopathic portal hypertension
	Sarcoidosis

B. Sinusoidal	
Cirrhosis	
Non-cirrhotic	Acute alcoholic hepatitis
	Cytotoxic drugs
	Vitamin A intoxication

C. Postsinusoidal
Central hyaline necrosis (alcohol)
Venous outflow obstruction
Cardiac disease

Idiopathic portal hypertension

A proportion of patients have no detectable cause for portal hypertension and are sometimes labelled primary (synonyms include: hepatoportal cirrhosis, non-cirrhotic portal fibrosis and Banti's syndrome. There may also be overlap with nodular regenerative hyperplasia (see Chapter 22).). Morphologically the portal veins may be normal or may show sclerosis of the intrahepatic branches[37] (Figure 18.24), coupled with distortion of the lobular architecture. The long-term outlook in some of these patients is surprisingly good[38]. A similar disorder is widespread in India where it accounts for about one-third of all portal hypertension[37]. These Indian authors have described thickening of the walls of large-and

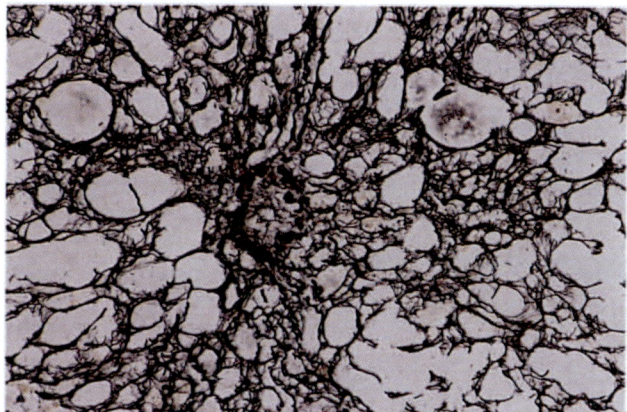

Figure 18.13 Acute veno-occlusive disease. A seventeen-year-old boy was treated with chemotherapeutic agents for acute myeloid leukaemia and subsequently by bone marrow transplantation. Although technically successful this was followed by the development of acute VOD. Note the complete obliteration of the small terminal hepatic venules, and condensation of adjacent reticulin. Reticulin stain.

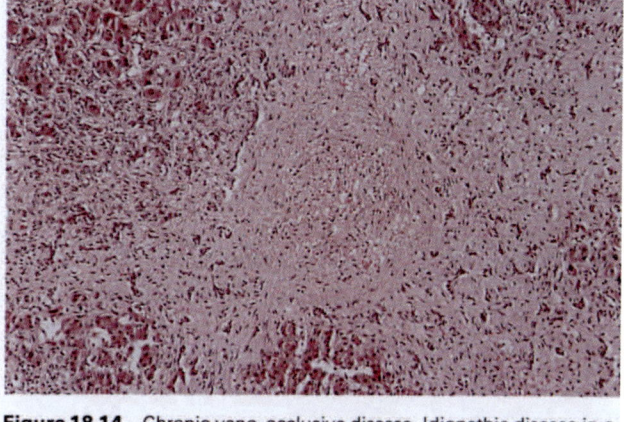

Figure 18.14 Chronic veno-occlusive disease. Idiopathic disease in a 31-year-old British farm labourer who gave a 6-month history of progressive ascites. The post-mortem liver shows complete fibrous obliteration of this efferent vein (centre) so that its outline can barely be seen. Note the numerous proliferating bile ductules which can be confusing when present in the centrilobular region.

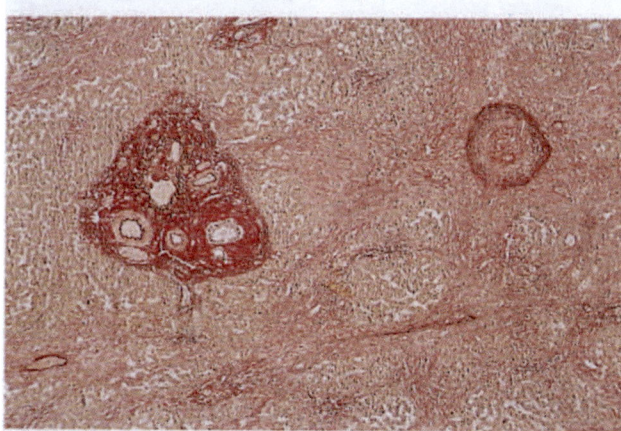

Figure 18.15 Chronic veno-occlusive disease. Same case as Figure 18.14. This adjacent section shows the architectural relationships of the same terminal vein now seen above centre on the right. Its centrilobular position can be seen, and the large portal tract (left) is normal and surrounded by relatively normal periportal parenchyma. Elastic van Gieson.

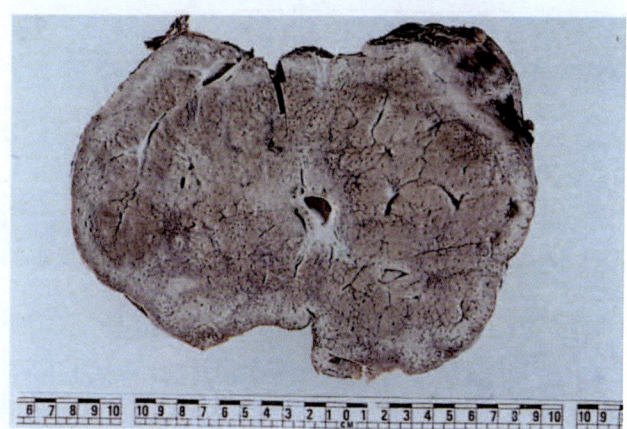

Figure 18.16 Chronic Budd-Chiari syndrome. A 40-year-old female with a 2–year history of hepatic vein occlusion, attributed to the contraceptive pill. The liver was excised at transplantation and shows a nodular cut surface difficult to distinguish from any other cirrhosis. The hepatic vein had almost totally disappeared, leaving only fibrous remnants.

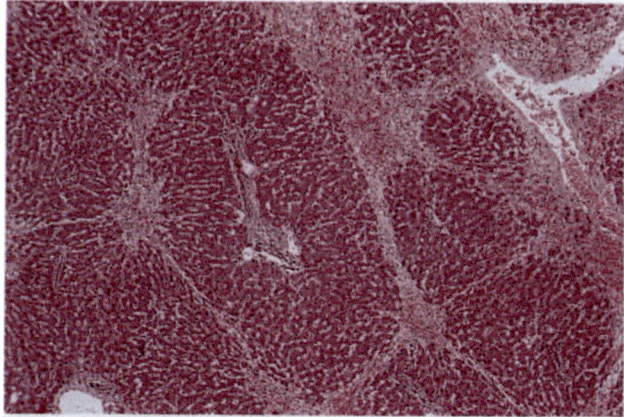

Figure 18.17 Cardiac cirrhosis. A 71-year-old man with 50-year history of chronic lung disease (following poison gas in the First World War) and congestive heart failure. At autopsy the liver was nodular and shows centrilobular fibrosis with thin septa radiating to link with other central veins and surrounding islands of liver with portal tracts at their centre (left of centre). There are no regeneration nodules.

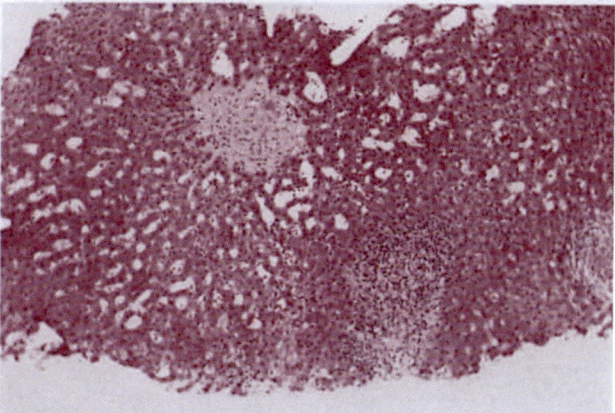

Figure 18.18 Sinusoidal dilatation. Sarcoidosis. Note the striking sinusoidal dilatation which can be seen to be surrounding the granuloma above and to the left of centre.

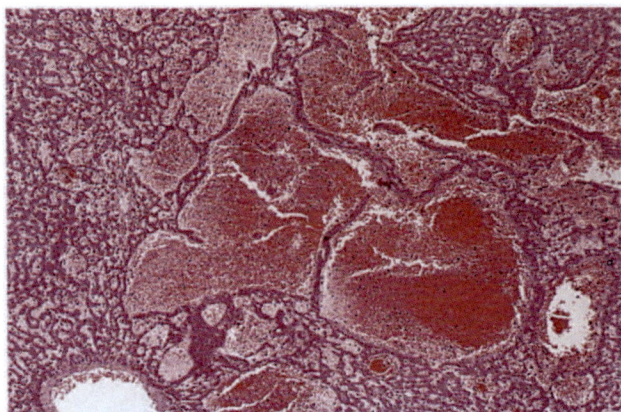

Figure 18.19 Peliosis hepatis. A 25-year-old female died of Hodgkin's disease which had been first diagnosed 10 years previously. At autopsy numerous blood cysts were visible in the liver. Histologically they can be seen to be of varying size and most are completely without a lining.

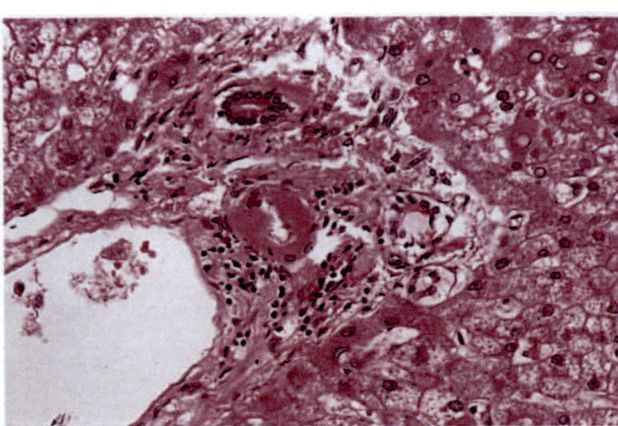

Figure 18.20 Systemic hypertension. A 55-year-old male died of myocardial infarction. He had been a known hypertensive for several years. Arterioles in many organs showed the typical homogeneous hyaline change seen in this hepatic artery branch.

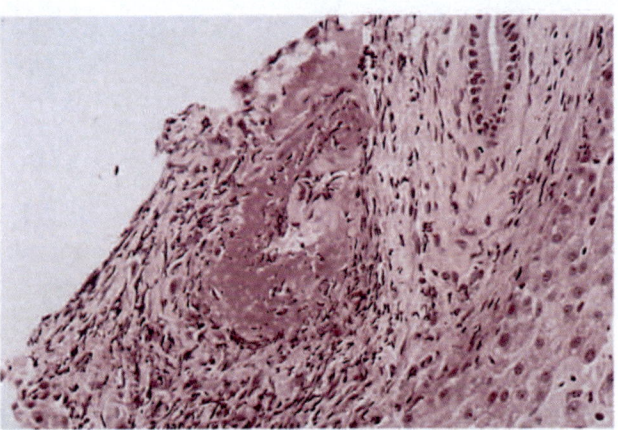

Figure 18.21 Polyarteritis nodosa. A 60-year-old female presented with systemic disease but liver function tests showed a 'hepatitic' picture. Biopsy revealed this acute fibrinoid necrosis of a single hepatic artery branch. Renal biopsy subsequently showed other characteristic lesions of polyarteritis nodosa.

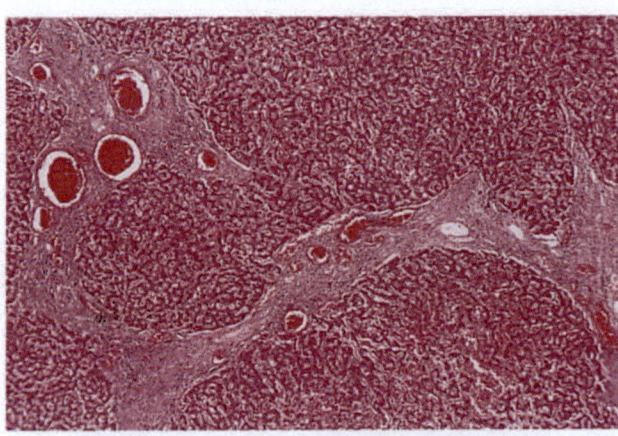

Figure 18.22 Hereditary haemorrhagic telangiectasia. A 71-year-old female known to have this condition for many years suffered repeated gastrointestinal haemorrhages for 35 years. At autopsy the liver was enlarged and coarsely nodular with numerous haemorrhagic foci. The section shows that the parenchyma is divided up by irregularly arranged fibrous septa, many of which contain telangiectatic blood vessels.

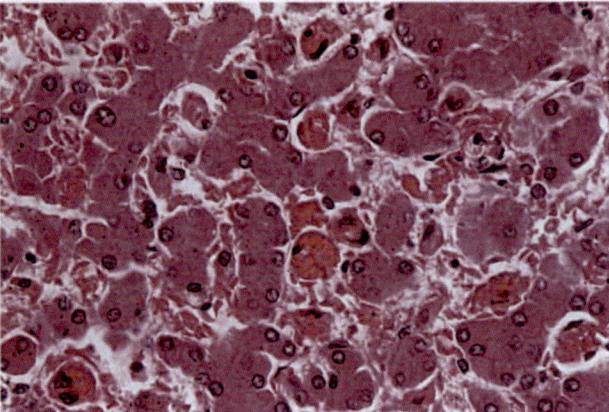

Figure 18.23 Sickle cell disease. Ugandan child with homozygous sickle cell disease. This section of liver at post-mortem shows sickled red cells both in sinusoids and phagocytosed by enlarged Kupffer cells.

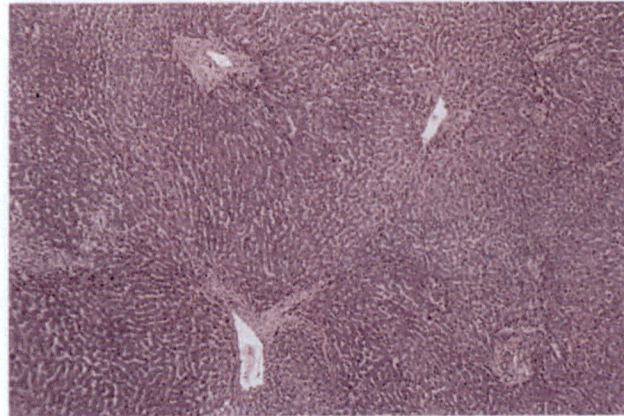

Figure 18.24 Non-cirrhotic portal hypertension. A 33-year-old male with idiopathic portal hypertension which was associated with bleeding oesophageal varices. The liver had a smooth capsule and a normal cut surface. Section shows a normal distribution of portal tracts and central veins, but the former appear a little sclerotic.

medium-sized branches of the portal vein and occasionally recanalized thrombi are also seen. The aetiology is unclear, but toxic metals, infective thrombophlebitis and immunogenic factors have all been implicated[37].

REFERENCES

1. Horrocks, P. and Tapp, E. (1966). Zahn's 'infarcts' of the liver. J. Clin. Pathol., 19, 475–478
2. Weinbren, K. (1978). The liver. In Symmers, W. S. C. (eds). Systemic Pathology. Vol 3. 2nd edn. pp. 1200–1301. Edinburgh: Churchill Livingstone
3. Wight, D. G. D. (1993). The pathology of liver transplantation. In Wight, D. G. D. (eds). Liver, Biliary Tract and Exocrine Pancreas. Vol. 11. Systemic Pathology. Symmers, W. S. C. Series ed. 3rd edn. pp. Edinburgh: Churchill Livingstone
4. Seeley, T., Blumenfeld, C. M., Ikeda, R., Knapp, W. and Ruebner, B. H. (1972). Hepatic infarction. Hum. Pathol., 3, 265–276
5. Woolings, K. R., Baggenstoss, A. M. and Weir, J. F. (1951). Infarcts of the liver. Gastroenterology., 17, 479–493
6. Chen, V., Hamilton, J. and Qizilbash, A. (1976). Hepatic infarction: a clinico-pathological study of seven cases. Arch. Pathol. Lab. Med., 100, 32–36
7. Popovsky, M. A., Costa, J. C. and Doppman, J. L. (1979). Meyenburg complexes of the liver and bile cysts as a consequence of hepatic ischaemia. Hum. Pathol., 10, 425–432
8. Dunn, G. D., Hayes, P., Breen, K. J. and Schenker, S. (1973). The liver in congestive heart failure: a review. Am. J. Med. Sci., 265, 174–189
9. Popper, H. (1948). Significance of agonal changes in the human liver. Arch. Pathol., 46, 132–144
10. Sherlock, S. (1989). Circulatory failure. In (eds). Diseases of the Liver and Biliary System. 8th edn. pp. 221–229. Oxford: Blackwell
11. Birgens, H. S., Hellriksen, J., Matzen, P. and Poulsen, H. (1978). The shock liver. Clinical and biochemical findings in patients with centrilobular liver necrosis following cardiogenic shock. Acta. Med. Scand, 204, 417–421
12. Cohen, J. A. and Kaplan, M. M. (1978). Left-sided heart failure presenting as hepatitis. Gastroenterol, 74, 583–587
13. Bynum, T. E., Boitnott, J. K. and Maddrey, W. C. (1979). Ischemic hepatitis. Dig. Dis. Sci., 24, 129–135
14. Nouel, O., Henrion., J., Bernhuan, J., Degott, C., Rueff, B. and Benhamou, J.-P. (1980). Fulminant hepatic failure due to transient circulatory failure in patients with chronic heart disease. Dig. Dis. Sci., 25, 49–52
15. Nunes, G., Blaisdell, F. W. and Margaretten, W. (1970). Mechanism of hepatic dysfunction following shock and trauma. Arch. Surg., 100, 546–566
16. De la Monte, S. M., Arcidi, J. M., Moore, G. M. and Hutchins, G. M. (1984). Midzonal necrosis as a pattern of hepatocellular injury after shock. Gastroenterol, 86, 627–631
17. Buhac, I., Agrawal, A. B., Park, S. K., Lomotan, A., Lowen, B. and Balin, J. A. (1976). Jaundice and bridging centrilobular necrosis of liver in circulatory failure. N. Y. State J. Med., 76, 678–683
18. Kanel, G. C., Ucci, A. A., Kaplan, M. M. and Wolfe, H. J. (1980). A distinctive perivenular hepatic lesion associated with heart failure. Am. J. Clin. Pathol., 73, 235–239
19. Kew, M., Bersohn, I., Seftel, H. and Kent, G. (1970). Liver damage in heat stroke. Am. J. Med., 49, 192–202
20. Valla, D., Casadevall, N., Lacombe, C. and et al. (1985). Primary myeloproliferative disorder and hepatic vein thrombosis: a prospective study of erythroid colony formation in vitro in 20 patients with Budd-Chiari syndrome. Ann. Int. Med., 103, 329–334
21. Boughton, B. J. (1990). Hepatic and portal vein thrombosis. Br. Med J, 302, 192–193
22. Leopold, J. G., Parry, T. E. and Stoming, F. K. (1970). A change in the sinusoid-trabecular structure of the liver with hepatic venous outflow block. J. Pathol., 100, 87–98
23. Fajardo, L. F. and Colby, T. V. (1980). Pathogenesis of veno occlusive liver disease after radiation. Arch. Pathol. Lab. Med., 104, 584–588
24. Sterneck, M., Wiesner, R. H., Ascher, N., Roberts, J., Ferrel, L., Ludwig, J. and Lake, J. (1991). Azathioprine toxicity after liver transplantation. Hepatology, 14, 806–810
25. Rollins, B. J. (1986). Hepatic veno-occlusive disease. Am. J. Med., 81, 297–306 ·
26. Bras, G. and Hill, K. R. (1956). Veno-occlusive disease of the liver. Essential pathology. Lancet, 2, 161–163
27. Winkler, K. and Poulson, H. (1975). Liver disease with periportal sinusoidal dilatation. A possible complication to contraceptive steroids. Scand J Gastroenterol, 10, 699–704
28. Bruguera, M., Aranginbel, F., Ros, E. and Rodes, J. (1978). Incidence and clinical significance of sinusoidal dilatation in liver biopsies. Gastroenterology, 75, 474–478
29. Nadell, J. and Kosek, J. (1977). Peliosis hepatis. Arch Pathol Lab Med, 101, 405–410
30. Bagheri, S. A. and Boyer, J. L. (1974). Peliosis hepatis associated with androgenic-anacolic steroid therapy. A severe form of hepatic injury. Ann Intern Med, 81, 610–618
31. Paradinas, F. J., Bull, T. B., Westaby, D. and Murray-Lyon, I. M. (1977). Hyperplasia and prolapse of hepatocytes into hepatic veins during long-term methyl testosterone therapy: possible relationships of these changes to the development of peliosis hepatis and liver tumours. Histopathology, 1, 225–246
32. Mowrey, F. H. and Lundbergh, E. A. (1954). The clinical manifestations of essential polyangiitis (periarteritis nodosa) with emphasis on hepatic manifestations. Ann. Intern. Med., 40, 1145–1164
33. McCormack, L. R., Astarita, R. W. and Foroozan, P. (1978). Liver involvement in giant cell arteritis. Am. J. Dig. Dis., 23, 725–745 [Suppl.]
34. Daly, J. J. and Schiller, A. L. (1976). The liver in hereditary haemorrhagic telangiectasia (O.R.W. disease). Am. J. Med., 60, 723–726
35. Feizi, O. (1972). Hereditary haemorrhagic telangiectasia presenting with portal hypertension and cirrhosis of the liver. Gastroenterology, 63, 660–664
36. Bauer, T. W., Moore, G. W. and Hutchins, G. M. (1980). The liver in sickle cell disease – a clinico-pathological study of 70 patients. Am. J. Med., 69, 833–837
37. Sarin, S. K. (1989). Non-cirrhotic portal fibrosis. Gut, 30, 406–415
38. Kingham, J. G. C., Levison, D. A., Stansfeld, A. G. and Dawson, A. M. (1981). Non-cirrhotic intrahepatic portal hypertension: A long-term follow-up study. Quart. J. Med., 50, 259–268

Granulomas are amongst the most easily recognized and common findings in liver pathology, occurring in as many as 10% of all biopsies[1]. The list of potential causes of granulomas is a very long one (Table 19.1), and even taking all clinical and other investigative findings into account, there remains a residuum of cases in which no obvious cause is detected (possibly in as many as 12–15% of cases)[2,3].

Without qualification, the term granuloma usually implies the involvement of at least some epithelioid cells, with or without giant cells (Figure 19.1). However, different pathologists have differing thresholds for the acceptance of epithelioid cells and some may include small focal collections of unmodified macrophages within the meaning of the term (Figure 19.2). This is probably unwise and it should be restricted to lesions containing genuine epithelioid macrophages, often but not invariably with a peripheral cuff of lymphocytes. Lipogranulomas (Chapter 12) are thus not included in this definition. Experimentally, granulomas form in two sets of circumstances. They may be due either to persistence of phagocytosed material for example infectious agents, such as tuberculosis or schistosome ova–or purely hypersensitivity mechanisms, as in the response to a number of drugs.

The liver is the largest parenchymal organ in the body and a prime target for the formation of granulomas because of its large population of fixed macrophages, the Kupffer cells, which clear antigens and immune complexes from the circulation. It is also the place where many drugs and other chemical substances undergo metabolic transformation by the microsomal enzymes of the liver cell into active toxic or allergic metabolites. It is thus not surprising that granulomas in the liver may be either a manifestation of systemic granulomatous disease or a purely local hepatic phenomenon.

Granulomas can occur anywhere in the liver acinus but are most often found in or adjacent to portal tracts. They are sharply defined and usually do not disturb the lobular architecture. The average granuloma measures approximately 50 μm in diameter and thus, if present, should be detected by routine step sections[3]. Serial sections are thus not necessary. Glycogen stains such as PAS may make them more obvious, since they will be surrounded by positively stained liver cells. If there is a significant chance of infective granulomas being present, a portion of the biopsy should be set aside for culture.

Table 19.1 gives lists some of the more common causes of granulomas in the liver. A more exhaustive list can be found in reference[4]. Despite the many conditions that can give rise to granulomas, only a few conditions account for the vast majority of cases in most series; namely sarcoidosis, tuberculosis, intrinsic liver disease (mainly primary biliary cirrhosis) and schistosomiasis[5], but drugs are also playing an increasing role[6], and in recent years the infectious complications of the acquired immunodeficiency syndrome have become much more common (Chapter 3)[7].

DIFFERENTIAL DIAGNOSIS

In a proportion of cases the cause of the granuloma will be visible or at least demonstrable within the section, e.g. tubercle bacilli, fungi or schistosomes. In others the

Table 19.1 Causes of hepatic granulomas

Bacteria
  Mycobacteria
  Leprosy
  Brucellosis
  Tularaemia
  Listeriosis
  Syphilis
Fungi
  Histoplasmosis
  Candidiasis
  Cryptococcosis
  Nocardiosis
  Coccidioidomycosis
  Aspergillosis
Rickettsiae
  Q fever
Viruses
  Cytomegalovirus
Parasites
  Schistosomiasis
  Toxocariasis
  Ascariasis
  Strongyloides
Hypersensitivity
  Berylliosis
  Erythema nodosum
  Drugs
  Vascular diseases
Neoplasia
  Hodgkin's disease
  Metastatic carcinoma
Miscellaneous
  Sarcoidosis
  Primary biliary cirrhosis
  Crohn's Disease
  Haemodialysis

relationships of the granuloma may be sufficiently distinctive, for example, in association with bile duct lesions in primary biliary cirrhosis. Significant numbers of eosinophils associated with the granulomas provide a strong pointer towards drugs[6] or schistosomiasis.

In the majority of cases of granulomas, however, there are no morphological clues to the diagnosis, and then a systematic approach should be adopted. Ideally, cultures should be set up – if not from the liver biopsy, from other suitable specimens from the patient – and a detailed drug history must always be taken. Other investigations, such as skin tests and serology, are performed as appropriate.

SARCOIDOSIS

Sarcoidosis is a disease of unknown cause without any wholly distinctive clinical features and thus is usually diagnosed by its morphological feature of granuloma formation. Granulomas are most often encountered in mediastinal and peripheral lymph nodes, lungs, spleen, skin, eyes, bones and parotid glands, as well as the liver, but almost any other organ or tissue may be involved. It is most often seen for the first time in 20–35-year-old patients of either sex and is ten times as common in blacks as whites in the United States. In London its overall prevalence ranges from 27 per 100 000 amongst the indigenous population to 200 per 100 000 amongst West Indian immigrants.

Liver biopsy is a legitimate method for the diagnosis of suspected sarcoidosis (Figure 19.1) and may be positive in up to 90% of cases[8]. Klatskin has calculated that for a single lesion to be visible in a section of a needle biopsy, the liver would have to contain 15×10^6 granulomas, but since there are on average five per section, the liver must contain 75×10^6 or more. It is surprising, therefore, that there are few clinical or biochemical manifestations of liver involvement in many cases. Indeed, the diagnosis is often unsuspected until granulomas are found in the liver.

Sarcoid granulomas are the prototype of all non-caseating epithelioid granulomas. They vary greatly in size but on the whole tend to be larger in sarcoid (Figure 19.3) than most other conditions and are composed of a sharply circumscribed compact mass of epithelioid cells which are quite haphazardly arranged and intermingled with giant cells (Figure 19.1). There is a cuff of lymphocytes and histiocytes and occasionally there may be a small central core of granular fibrinoid material but never caseation. Schaumann bodies and asteroids, seen quite frequently in sarcoid granulomas elsewhere, appear to be unusual in the liver[5]. Sarcoid granulomas seem especially prone to healing by a process of segmentation, with each of the segments becoming surrounded by its own rim of connective tissue (Figures 19.4 and 19.5)[9], and is ultimately replaced by a fibrous scar. They occur most often in or near to portal tracts. They cause little disturbance to the reticulin framework of the liver, but often possess a rich reticulin network themselves. Special stains for organisms are negative.

None of these features is diagnostic of sarcoidosis. Ultimately the diagnosis depends upon the clinical context and exclusion of other causes of granulomas. The Kveim test can be helpful but is only positive in some 70% of cases[2]. The serum angiotensin-converting enzyme level is another useful marker, but this too is only positive in up to 80% of cases[10]. There is some overlap between sarcoidosis and primary biliary cirrhosis (PBC). Rudzki et al.[11] described a syndrome of intrahepatic cholestasis in sarcoidosis which closely resembled PBC but lacked bile duct lesions and a positive antimitochondrial antibody test. This last is probably the most useful distinguishing feature (see Chapter 17). It should be stressed, however, that most cases of PBC and hepatic sarcoid are quite distinct from each other; the latter, as already stated, being asymptomatic in the majority of cases.

In a small proportion of cases, hepatic sarcoidosis may be progressive and lead to portal hypertension[12] and cirrhosis. These cases usually have multiple granulomas with portal and parenchymal fibrosis. Although partly related to healing of granulomas, not all the fibrosis can be accounted for in this way. Portal hypertension may occur in the absence of cirrhosis, but the mechanism of this is unknown.

TUBERCULOSIS

This is probably the most important diagnosis to make in view of the therapeutic implications. Blind needle biopsy of the liver can be expected to yield granulomas in about 50% of cases of miliary tuberculosis. They are often localized away from portal tracts, near to central veins and in a proportion of cases, but by no means all, show central caseation (Figures 19.6 and 19.7). Organisms are demonstrable in less than 10%[13], except in immunocompromised patients in whom organisms may be very numerous[14]. Non-specific reactive changes may also be seen in the liver in the absence of granulomas.

Mycobacteria have been the most frequent bacteria to infect the liver in patients with AIDS (Chapter 3), and they include atypical organisms such as *Mycobacterium avium-intracellulare* and *M. kansasii* as well as *M. tuberculosis*[15,16]. In the immunodeficient patient, granulomas form poorly or not at all – raising comparisons with lepromatous leprosy – and the bacteria are found in dense clusters within foamy macrophages or even within single sinusoidal Kupffer cells. It is therefore important to use an acid-fast Ziel-Nielsen stain in all biopsies from AIDS patients. *Mycobacterium avium-intracellulare* also stains with silver stains.

Caseating granulomas are also sometimes seen in tularaemia[2] and chronic granulomatous disease of childhood[1]. A recent biopsy site can occasionally produce an appearance reminiscent of tuberculosis in the liver as in any other organ (Figure 19.8). Knowledge of the circumstances should assist in the recognition of this entity. Necrotic tumour deposits may also resemble a hyalinized tuberculous lesion (Figure 19.9).

Atypical mycobacterial infections are commonly encountered in the liver of patients with the acquired immunodeficiency syndrome (AIDS)[7], *Mycobacterium avium intracellulare* being the most common. Here the granulomas are generally poorly formed, have no caseation and contain large numbers of acid/alcohol fast bacteria. In immunocompetent patients *M avium intracellulare* cannot be reliably distinguished from *M. tuberculosis* on histological features alone[14].

OTHER INFECTIONS

Organisms should usually be readily demonstrable in parasitic infestations such as schistosomiasis and larva migrans, in fungal infections and in leprosy. In some cases of Q fever (Chapter 3) the granulomas are characteristic with a central clear space surrounded by neutrophils and a ring of fibrin as well as epithelioid and giant cells[17], although in a recent study identical granulomas were also attributed to other causes such as visceral leishmaniasis, boutonneuse fever and toxoplasmosis[18]. Most cases of infection with *Brucella abortus* are associated with discrete granulomas indistinguishable from those of sarcoidosis. Occasionally, however, numerous microgranulomas composed of spherical collections of histiocytes, up to ten in the plane of section, may be scattered through the parenchyma[19]. In contrast, B. *melitensis* and B *suis* cause areas of necrosis without significant cellular reaction[20].

The liver is frequently affected by opportunist infections during the course of AIDS (Chapter 3) some of which may be granulomatous[14].

DRUG-INDUCED GRANULOMAS

In one recent series of 95 cases of granulomatous hepatitis[6], probable and possible associations with medicinal compounds were detected in 29%. Highly suspect drugs included antihypertensives (especially methyldopa), antirheumatic and analgesics (aspirin), anticonvulsants (phenytoin) and antimicrobial agents (isoniazid, penicillin, sulphonamides and cephalexin).

Drug-induced granulomas exhibited no pathognomonic features, but there were some rather characteristic findings. Although they were seen in all parts of the lobule, some portal tract involvement was consistent. They were discrete or diffuse, with or without giant cells and a peripheral cuff of lymphocytes and plasma cells. Eosinophils, more than five to ten per granuloma and sometimes in large numbers, were the most reliable pointer to drug aetiology, particularly in the early lesions. Also in many instances numerous Kupffer cell granulomas were seen in the parenchyma in association with the portal tract eosinophilic granulomatous reaction. In a few cases, granulomas were intimately associated with interlobular

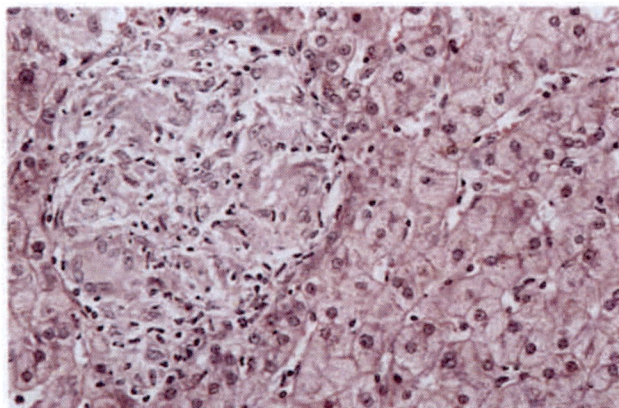

Figure 19.1 Sarcoidosis. A 28-year-old female who presented in a classic way with bilateral hilar lymphadenopathy. Liver biopsy, performed as a diagnostic procedure, contained many epithelioid granulomas. This section shows a classic granuloma, composed of a compact group of epithelioid cells and a single Langhans giant cell with a few lymphocytes around the periphery. This appearance is in no way diagnostic.

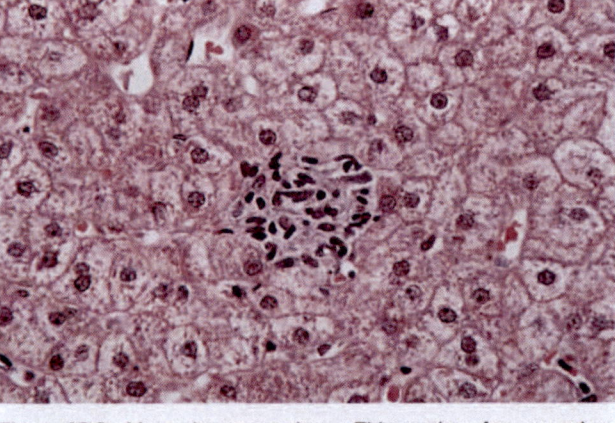

Figure 19.2 Macrophage granuloma. This section, from a patient with non-specific reactive hepatitis, shows a sinusoidal collection of unmodified macrophages together with a few lymphocytes. This is not an epithelioid granuloma and thus if the term granuloma is used, it should always be appropriately qualified.

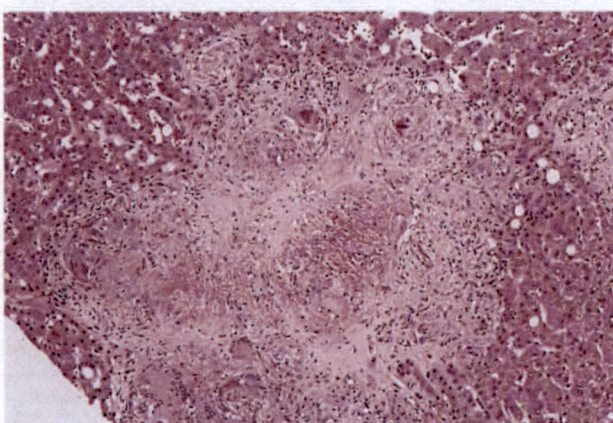

Figure 19.3 Sarcoidosis. A 27-year-old female patient with classic sarcoidosis, subsequently shown to be Kveim-positive. This section shows a portal tract almost completely replaced by a group of confluent granulomas with a focus of fibrinoid change at the centre. This should not be confused with caseation necrosis, which is negative with fibrin stains.

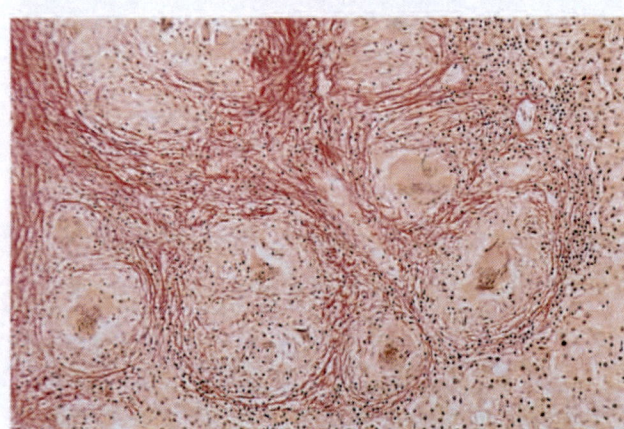

Figure 19.4 Sarcoidosis. The diagnosis in this 59-year-old asymptomatic female was made as an incidental finding at autopsy. The section shows a group of granulomas undergoing healing. Each granuloma is surrounded by a concentric rim of collagen fibres. Elastic van Gieson.

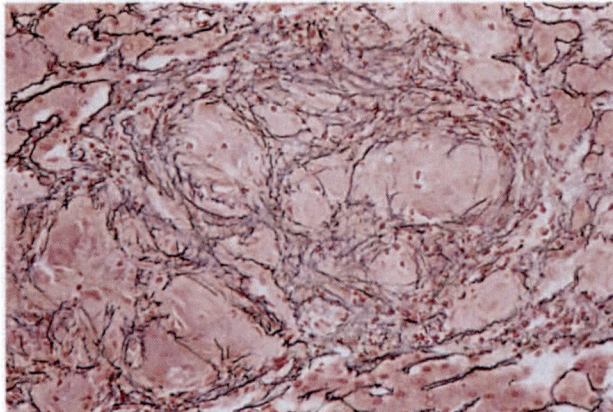

Figure 19.5 Sarcoidosis. Same patient as Figure 19.3. This granuloma is undergoing healing by a process of segmentation, each segment being surrounded by reticulin fibres. Reticulin, neutral red.

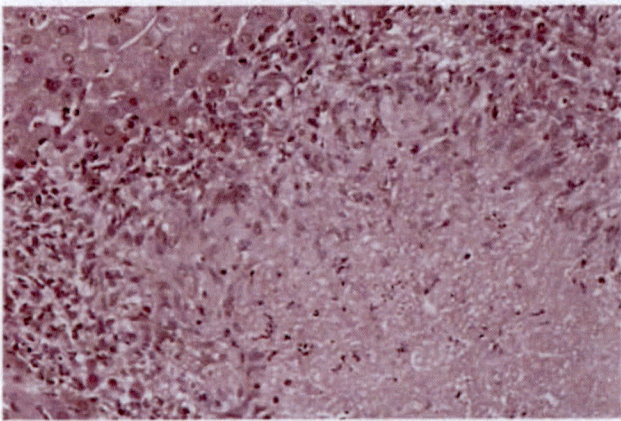

Figure 19.6 Miliary tuberculosis. A 58-year-old male with a pyrexial illness and a past history of pulmonary tuberculosis. Liver biopsy was performed as a diagnostic procedure and revealed multiple granulomas. This section shows a large lesion with a caseous centre surrounded by epithelioid cells. No organisms were seen, but Mycobacterium tuberculosis was subsequently cultured from a part of the biopsy.

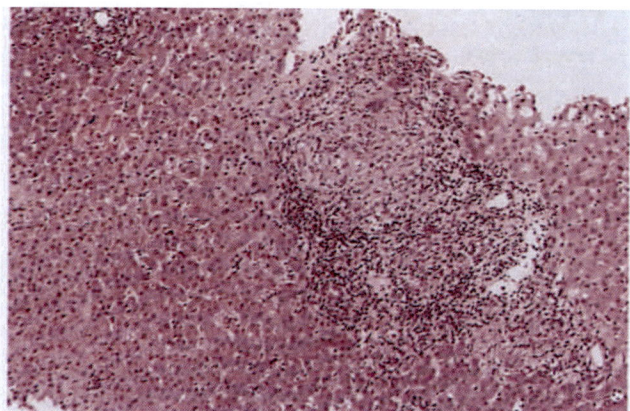

Figure 19.7 Miliary tuberculosis. Same biopsy as Figure 19.6. This granuloma is composed of epithelioid and giant cells and is surrounded by a cuff of lymphocytes. Note that tuberculous granulomas do not always show central caseation and thus this diagnosis should always be entertained when granulomas are found.

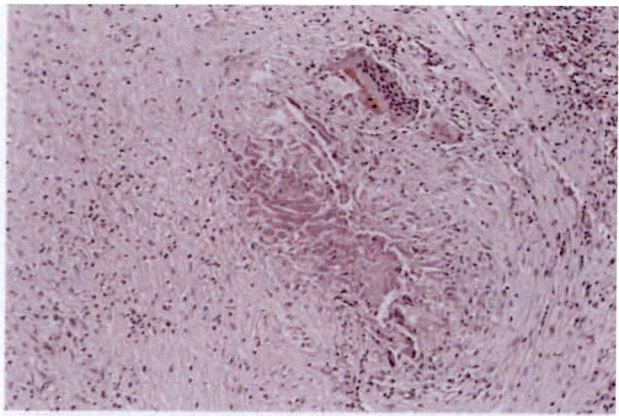

Figure 19.8 Recent biopsy site. A 45-year-old female underwent liver transplantation and a routine wedge biopsy was taken at the conclusion of the procedure. She required a further laparotomy 5 days later and the surgeon took a second biopsy from the same site. The section shows central fibrinoid change surrounded by a palisade of macrophages. A foreign body giant cell containing brown foreign material can also be seen (upper right).

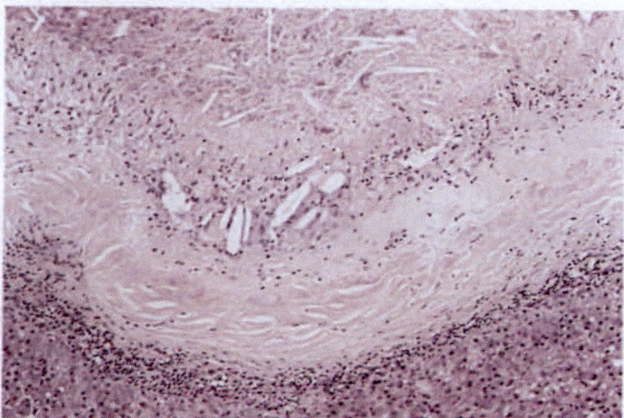

Figure 19.9 Necrotic metastatic carcinoma. A 63-year-old male underwent anterior resection for a carcinoma of the sigmoid colon. A liver nodule was biopsied. The section shows that this is largely hyalinized and contains a number of cholesterol clefts. At the margin there are a few lymphocytes but no true granulomatous response. The true nature of this lesion was revealed by the presence of a few viable tumour cells at one margin.

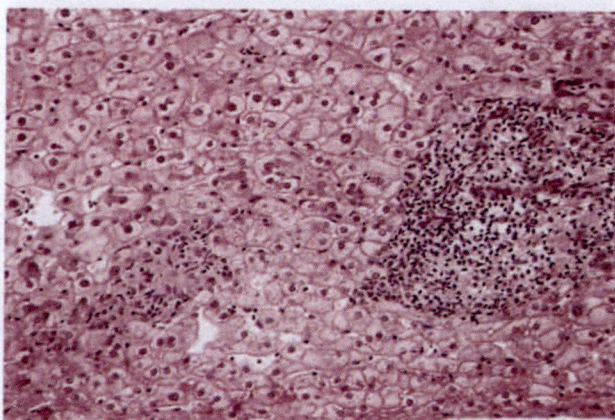

Figure 19.10 Granulomatous hepatitis with pyrexia. A 45-year-old female with recurrent pyrexia. The only definite abnormality discovered amongst very many investigations is shown in this liver biopsy. The portal tract is enlarged and contains a dense collection of lymphocytes and an ill-defined epithelioid granuloma. There is also a small epithelioid and macrophage granuloma in the adjacent parenchyma. There was a good clinical response to corticosteroid drugs.

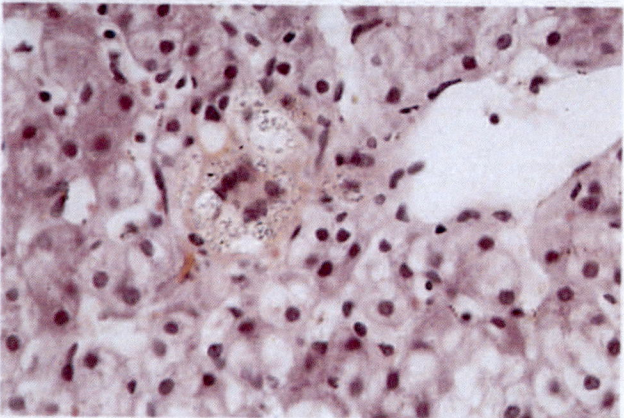

Figure 19.11 Foreign body reaction, long-term haemodialysis. A 40-year-old male patient in chronic renal failure who had been on haemodialysis for 6 years. The liver biopsy shows a large foreign body giant cell, adjacent to a central vein, which contains refractile granules around its periphery.

bile ducts closely resembling the lesions seen in primary biliary cirrhosis. However, in contrast to the latter condition, eosinophils were always a prominent feature of the drug-related cases.

Eosinophils are rarely seen with tuberculous granulomas and in sarcoidosis. Although sometimes quite numerous in the granulomas associated with visceral larva migrans and histoplasmosis, as already stated, these organisms should be readily identified, and similarly Hodgkin's disease too can generally be recognized on other grounds.

Drugs may thus be more commonly associated with granulomatous hepatitis than hitherto realized and so a careful drug history is an obligatory part of the investigation of any patients with otherwise unexplained granulomatous hepatitis.

GRANULOMAS AND PYREXIA

Fever is a prominent feature in many cases of granulomatous hepatitis[1]. Fever is prominent in sarcoidosis and tuberculosis, but there also remains a residue of patients who have granulomatous hepatitis without detectable cause (Figure 19.10), some of whom respond favourably to corticosteroids[21]. In some of these patients at least the underlying disease may be giant cell arteritis polymyalgia rheumatica or other connective tissue disorder[4,22] but in others no cause is found[21].

LONG-TERM HAEMODIALYSIS

There have been several reports of a foreign body giant cell reaction in the livers of patients on long-term haemodialysis[23]. Foreign body giant cells are found singly or in groups, often in periportal regions, but they may affect any part of the lobule (Figure 19.11). They contain cytoplasmic refractile, non-birefringent, non-stainable colourless granules of uncertain origin. Ultrastructurally the material appears to be contained within lysosomal membranes and it may be derived from the interaction of blood with dialysis tubing.

REFERENCES

1. Fauci, A. S. and Wolff, S. M. (1976). Granulomatous hepatitis. In Popper, H. and Schaffner, F. (eds). Progress in Liver Disease. V. pp. 609–621. New York: Grune and Stratton
2. Leading article. (1975). Granulomas of the liver. Lancet, 2, 1079–1080
3. Scheuer, P. J. (1988). The Liver in Systemic Disease, Pregnancy and Organ Transplantation. In Liver Biopsy Interpretation. 4th edn. pp. 218–261. London: Baillière Tindall
4. Holdstock, G., Iredale, J., Millward-Sadler, G. H. and Wright, R. (1992). Hepatic changes in systemic disease. In Millward-Sadler, G. H., Wright, R. and Arthur, M. J. P. (eds). Wright's Liver and Biliary Disease. 3rd edn. pp. 995–1038. London: W B Saunders
5. MacSween, R. N. M. (1987). Liver pathology associated with disease of other organs. In MacSween, R. N. M., Anthony, P. P. and Scheuer, P. J. (eds). Pathology of the Liver. 2nd edn. pp. 646–688. Edinburgh: Churchill Livingstone
6. McMaster, K. R. and Hennigar, G. R. (1981). Drug induced granulomatous hepatitis. Lab. Invest., 44, 61–73
7. Cappell, M. S. (1991). Hepatobiliary manifestations of the acquired immune deficiency syndrome. Am. J. Gastroenterol., 86, 1–15
8. Klatskin, G. (1977). Hepatic granulomata: problems in interpretation. Mt Sinai J. Med., 44, 798–812
9. Reynolds, T. B., Campra, J. L. and Peters, R. L. (1990). Hepatic granulomata. In Zakim, D. and Boyer, T. D. (eds). Hepatology. A Textbook of Liver Disease. 2nd edn. pp. 1098–1114. Philadelphia: W B Saunders
10. Lieberman, J. (1975). Elevation of serum angiotensin-converting enzyme (ACE) level in sarcoidosis. Am. J. Med., 59, 365–372
11. Rudzki, C., Ishak, K. G. and Zimmerman, H. J. (1975). Chronic intrahepatic cholestasis of sarcoid. Am. J. Med., 59, 373–387
12. Maddrey, W. C., Johns, C. J., Boittnott, J. K. and Iber, F. L. (1970). Sarcoidosis and chronic hepatic disease: a clinical and pathological study of 20 patients. Medicine, 49, 375–395
13. Essop, A. R., Posen, J. A., Hodkinson, J. H. and Segal, I. (1984). Tuberculous hepatitis: a clinical review of 96 cases. Quart. J. Med., 77, 465–477
14. Foster, C. S. (1993). Infections and infestations of the liver. In Wight, D. G. D. (ed). Liver, Biliary Tract and Exocrine Pancreas. Vol. 11. Systemic Pathology. Symmers, W. S. C., series ed. 3rd edn. Edinburgh: Churchill Livingstone
15. Lebovics, E., Dworkin, B. M., Heier, S. K. and Rosenthal, W. S. (1988). The hepato-biliary manifestations of immunodeficiency virus infection. Am. J. Gastroenterol., 83, 1–7
16. Schneiderman, D. J., Arenson, D. M., Cello, J. P., Margaretten, W. and Weber, T. (1987). Hepatic disease in patients with the acquired immunodeficiency syndrome. Hepatology, 7, 925–930
17. Pellegrin, M., Delsol, G., Auvergnat, J. C., Familiades, J., Faure, H., Guiu, M. and Voigt, J. J. (1980). Granulomatous hepatitis in Q fever. Hum. Pathol., 11, 51–57
18. Marazuela, M., Moreno, A., Yebra, M., Cerezo, E., Gomez, G. C. and Vargas, J. A. (1991). Hepatic fibrin-ring granulomas: a clinicopathologic study of 23 patients. Hum. Pathol., 22, 607–613
19. Weinbren, K. (1978). The liver. In Symmers, W. S. C. (ed). Systemic Pathology. Vol 3. 2nd edn. pp. 1200–1301. Edinburgh: Churchill Livingstone
20. Spink, W. W., Hoffbaue, F. W., Walker, W. W. and Green, R. A. (1949). Histopathology of the liver in human brucellosis. J. Lab. Clin. Med., 34, 40–58
21. Zoutman, D. E., Ralph, E. D. and Frei, J. V. (1991). Granulomatous hepatitis and fever of unknown origin: an 11 year experience of 23 cases with three years' follow-up. J. Clin. Gastroenterol., 13, 69–75
22. Litwack, K. D., Bohan, A. and Silverman, L. (1977). Granulomatous liver disease and giant cell arteritis. Case report and literature review. J. Rheumatol., 4, 307–312
23. Krempien, B., Bommer, J. and Ritz, E. (1981). Foreign body giant cell reaction in lungs, liver and spleen. A complication of long-term haemodialysis. Virchows Archiv. [A], 392, 73–80

LIVER CHANGES ASSOCIATED WITH INFLAMMATORY BOWEL DISEASE

Abnormalities of liver function have been associated with ulcerative colitis for many years. More recently it has been appreciated that Crohn's disease, especially when it affects the large bowel, probably has a very similar range and incidence of liver complications[1]. The precise incidence of liver involvement is almost impossible to assess because of the difficulties associated with comparisons between different series, patient selection and needle versus wedge biopsy amongst others. It is generally accepted that up to 50% of patients will show minor abnormalities of function (5-nucleotidase, alkaline phosphatase, BSP retention). Less than 10%, however, will have significant clinical disease[2]. Jaundice is uncommon.

There are the same difficulties over assessment of the incidence of morphological abnormalities, and Perrett and his colleagues[3,4] showed a poor correlation of biopsy findings with biochemistry. Similarly, there appears to be no clear association of either morphological or biochemical features with severity, duration or extent of disease. The range of conditions encountered is shown in Table 20.1.

Table 20.1 Liver and biliary abnormalities in inflammatory bowel disease*

	Ulcerative colitis	Crohn's disease
Fatty Liver	Common	Common
Chronic active hepatitis	Unusual	Unusual
Primary sclerosing cholangitis	Common	Uncommon
Cryptogenic cirrhosis	Unusual	Unusual
Granulomatous hepatitis	–	Rare
Amyloidosis	Very rare	Rare
Bile duct carcinoma	Rare	–
Cholelithiasis	Normal prevalence	Increased

* Based on Holdstock, G., Iredale, J., Millward-Sadler, G. H. and Wight R. (1992). Hepatic changes in systemic disease. In Millward-Sadler, G. H., Wright, R. and Arthur M. J. P. (eds). *Wright's Liver and Biliary Disease*, 3rd edn. pp. 995–1038. London: W B Saunders

Fatty liver is the commonest abnormality. It is of variable degree, may be diffuse or focal and, unlike the other liver changes, it may well correlate to some extent with severity of disease[5]. Morphologically the fat is indistinguishable from that due to other causes except that here it is occasionally periportal in distribution (Figure 20.1).

The other liver abnormalities seen in ulcerative colitis and Crohn's disease are morphologically identical to those seen without IBD. Both *chronic active hepatitis* and *cryptogenic cirrhosis* are found more frequently than expected in patients with IBD and each occurs in about 1% of patients. Their pathogenesis remains obscure.

PRIMARY SCLEROSING CHOLANGITIS

Primary sclerosing cholangitis (PSC) is a chronic cholestatic liver disease characterized by an unexplained fibrosing inflammation of segments of the extrahepatic biliary tree, with or without involvement of intrahepatic ducts. Ultimately, the condition leads to portal hypertension, biliary cirrhosis and hepatic failure. Introduction of endo-

Table 20.2 Sclerosing cholangitis*

Secondary to	Infection	Bacterial
		Parasitic infestation
		Opportunist
	Immunological Disorder	Genetic
		AIDS
		Graft vs host disease
	Vascular	Trauma
		Arterial 5-FUDR
	Drugs and chemicals	Hydatid caustics
		Thiabendazole
	Miscellaneous	Langerhans' histiocytosis
Primary	No predisposing cause	

* Based on Wight, D. G. D. (1993). Cholestasis and extrahepatic bile ducts. In Wight, D. G. D. (ed.) *Liver, Biliary Tract and Exocrine Pancreas*, 3rd edn. Edinburgh: Churchill Livingstone

scopic retrograde cholangiography in the 1970s resulted in a dramatic increase in the number of cases diagnosed, together with considerable enhancement of our understanding of the disease process. Despite these advances, the cause remains unknown and no fully effective therapy short of liver transplantation has been identified.

PSC must be distinguished from other conditions associated with sclerosis of bile ducts (Table 20.2). As with all conditions where the term *primary* is used to denote an unknown aetiology, the distinction between primary and secondary becomes more and more blurred as the condition becomes better understood. It is unclear, for example, whether the sclerosing cholangitis seen in association with cryptosporidiosis (Figure 20.2)[6] is PSC in which the cause is known, or whether it is a similar endpoint arrived at from a different route.

Prospective and retrospective studies of the liver in patients with inflammatory bowel disease have frequently shown chronic inflammatory lesions of the portal tracts, a lesion termed *pericholangitis*[7], reviewed by Vierling[8]. With the increased use of cholangiography, it clear that at least some of these patients actually have otherwise typical PSC, perhaps with greater emphasis on small bile ducts[9]. Pathologists have been advised that they should no longer use the term pericholangitis as a morphological diagnosis[10].

Inflammatory bowel disease occurs in 50 to 75% of patients with primary sclerosing cholangitis[11,12]. The great majority have ulcerative colitis, whilst occasional patients have Crohn's disease. Conversely, the prevalence of PSC in patients with ulcerative colitis ranges between 1% and 5.6%[13]. The pancreatic duct may be involved in the same process, giving rise to chronic pancreatitis[14]. PSC has also been linked with a great range of other conditions. These include other idiopathic fibrosing conditions such as Riedel's thyroiditis, retroperitoneal and mediastinal fibrosis, orbital pseudotumour and Peyronie's disease. More recently, a link with childhood immunodeficiency has been described[6]. Nevertheless 25 to 50% of cases occur in otherwise healthy individuals. The disease is probably identical in those patients with inflammatory bowel disease and those without[15]. Nevertheless, inflammatory bowel disease is an adverse prognostic factor[15].

Approximately 70% of patients are male and two-thirds are under 45 years at the time of diagnosis. Although it has been described in infancy and in childhood, most cases occur in adults. Patients generally present with persistent or intermittent signs of cholestatic liver disease, which have often been present for two years or more before diagnosis[16]. They include intermittent fluctuating jaundice, pruritus, nausea, abdominal pain and fatigue. Bacterial cholangitis is most unusual prior to surgical intervention. Occasionally, established cirrhosis with portal hypertension is already present at the time of presentation. An increasing number of patients is being diagnosed with asymptomatic disease, with, for example, persistent elevation of serum alkaline phosphatase,[15] particularly in patients with chronic ulcerative colitis, some 4% of whom have PSC on cholangiography[17]. The colitis may be diagnosed after PSC as well as before.

Diagnosis is nearly always made primarily or confirmed by cholangiography[18], which shows a distinctive picture of strictures alternating with normal or dilated segments. This imparts a beaded appearance to the larger ducts, whilst disappearance of small ducts gives a pruned tree appearance.

The pathogenesis of PSC remains uncertain. Various aetiological factors which have been considered include infective agents such as bacteria and viruses, various toxins, and immunological factors[19].

Treatment is essentially symptomatic. The role of immunosuppressive drugs such as cyclosporin remains to be established[1]. Many patients with PSC progress to end-stage liver disease and thus this is one of the commonest indications for liver transplantation[20]. Previously undiagnosed cholangiocarcinoma (Chapter 24) may be found in up to 10% of livers excised at the time of transplantation[21].

Pathology

PSC may involve bile ducts of all sizes. The large extrahepatic ducts, which are frequently involved radiologically, are only usually seen by pathologists when bile duct carcinoma is suspected, or at transplantation. However, biopsy specimens tend to show a thickened fibrous wall with mixed inflammatory infiltrates often concentrated around the wall glands.[22] These changes are in no way specific and cannot be distinguished from benign post-operative stricture.

The most specific histological features are periductal fibrosis and fibro-obliterative duct lesions[23]. Saccular dilatations of the large ducts, or cholangiectases,[24] are also highly distinctive features of PSC, although rarely seen in biopsy material.

Fibro-obliterative lesions

Bile ducts with normal internal diameters but thickened fibrous walls are found most commonly in the medium-sized intrahepatic ducts, mainly the interlobular and smaller septal ducts, although also occasionally in hilar segmental ducts. This periductal fibrosis (Figure 20.4) is sometimes referred to as of 'onion-skin' type because the concentric lamellae may be recognizable as individual fibres. The biliary epithelium within the collars may show focal degenerative changes. Step sections of such ducts may show transition to complete loss of the epithelium[25] and of the lumen to become a solid fibrous cord (Figure 20.4)[23]. These fibrous cords, or fibro-obliterative lesions, are almost pathognomonic of PSC and may be recognized on biopsy. Small portal tracts may show reduced numbers of interlobular ducts, recognizable because arteries are unaccompanied by ducts, but no fibrous scar.

Cholangiectases

The changes in the larger intrahepatic ducts are similar to those seen in the extrahepatic ducts. Fibrosed segments alternate with dilatations or *cholangiectases* which may be either tubular or saccular (Figure 20.5)[23,24], corresponding with the beading seen radiologically. They are generally lined by intact epithelium and have thin fibrous walls with little inflammation. Some are surrounded by a collar of dense fibrous tissue. Cholangiectases range up to 0.6 cm in diameter and most are between 1 and 2 cm in length[24]. They affect mainly the segmental and occasionally the septal bile ducts.

Portal tracts may show a variety of non-specific changes. Inflammation is rarely conspicuous, but consists of diffuse or focal collections of chronic inflammatory cells, mainly lymphocytes but also including macrophages, plasma cells and neutrophils. The inflammation may be concentrated around bile ducts (Figure 20.6) or, in the case of the large bile ducts, around the glands in the wall. In the smaller portal tracts these are the changes previously called *pericholangitis*[7]. Involvement of the gall-bladder and pancreas[14] have both been described, although the changes are not specific. Canalicular cholestasis of varying severity is found in all cases[23].

Ultimately, as with other forms of persistent cholestasis, secondary changes come to dominate the picture. There is increasing portal fibrosis, with focal bile ductular proliferation, although this is rarely prominent. Initially, fibrous septa tend to link adjacent portal tracts before ultimately a true biliary cirrhosis develops. Parenchymal changes are initially slight, but eventually there is biliary piecemeal necrosis with periportal cholestasis, Mallory's hyalin and accumulation of copper-associated protein (Figure 20.7). The fully developed cirrhosis may be difficult to distinguish from other forms of biliary cirrhosis (Figure 20.8) (Chapters 16 and 17). Ludwig[22] has described four stages of PSC, which correspond to the four stages of PBC, namely portal, periportal, septal and cirrhotic. As with the stages of PBC these represent stages in the natural history of the disease and are in no way diagnostic. There is also an increased risk of cholangiocarcinoma in PSC (Chapter 24).

COELIAC DISEASE

Minor abnormalities of liver function occur in a significant proportion of patients with coeliac disease[26-28]. There have been few systematic studies of liver histopathology, but two retrospective series[27,29] showed that chronic active hepatitis, which had progressed to cirrhosis in a few instances, was more common than would be expected by chance. Both series also included one case of hepatocellular carcinoma. In addition, non-specific changes such as portal fibrosis and chronic inflammatory cell infiltration are common. There is an increased risk of gastrointestinal malignancy in coeliac disease, particularly epithelial tumours of the small bowel and oesophagus, and lymphomas. It has recently been recognized that many of the latter belong to a distinct subgroup, originally called malignant histiocytosis of the intestine[30], but now recognized to be a high-grade T cell lymphoma[31] (see Chapter 25).

CYSTIC FIBROSIS OF THE PANCREAS

Cystic fibrosis is inherited as an autosomal recessive condition, recently localized to a region of approximately 250 000 base pairs[32] on the long arm of human chromosome 7. In approximately 70 per cent of cystic fibrosis patients there is a single common gene defect that consists of a specific deletion of three base pairs, the delta 508 mutation[33,34]. It usually presents in the new-born period

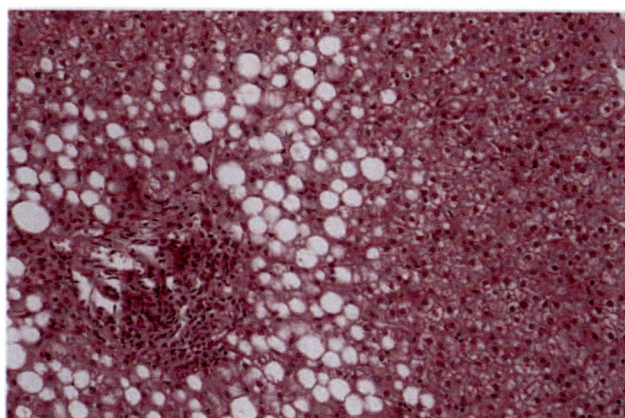

Figure 20.1 Ulcerative colitis, fatty change. A 45-year-old female with panproctocolitis. Liver biopsy performed at the time of colectomy, at which time there were no symptoms or signs referable to the liver. The biopsy shows periportal fatty change of moderate degree. Note that the portal tract contains a few chronic inflammatory cells but is otherwise normal.

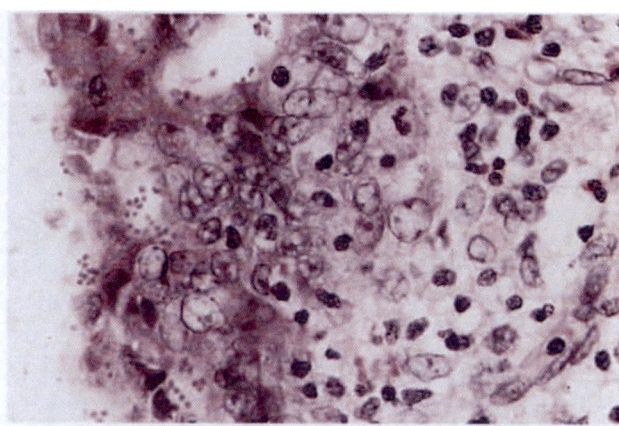

Figure 20.2 Sclerosing cholangitis associated with cryptosporidiosis. A six year-old child with immunodeficiency required a liver transplant for radiologically typical PSC. Note the inflammation in the wall of this major hilar bile duct, the hyperplasia of the epithelium and the numerous cryptosporidia, visible only as tiny blue dots on the epithelial surface.

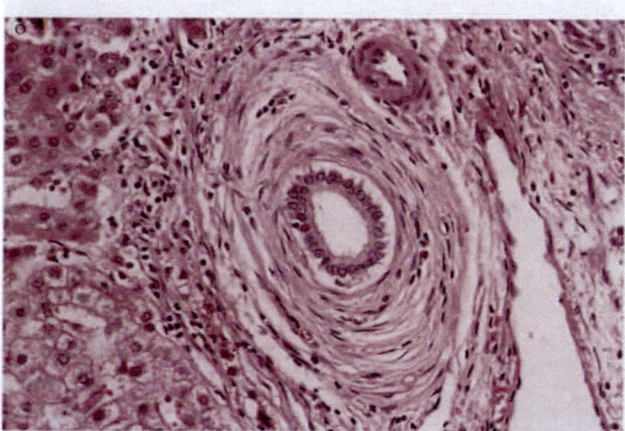

Figure 20.3 Primary sclerosing cholangitis. Note the concentric fibrosis around this interlobular bile duct from a small peripheral portal tract. Note also that there is some vacuolation of the biliary epithelium.

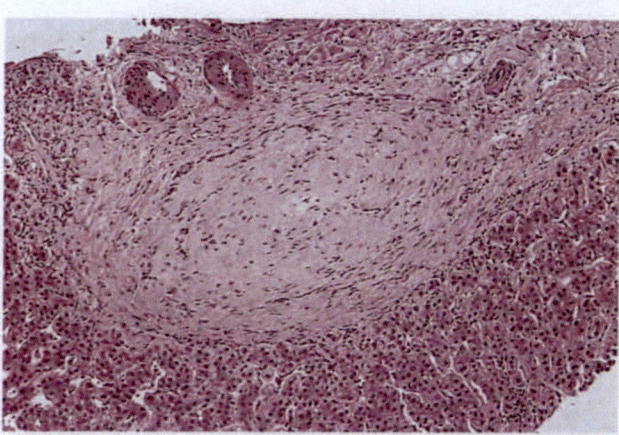

Figure 20.4 Primary sclerosing cholangitis-fibro-obliterative lesion. A 24-year-old male with a similar history to the patient illustrated in Figure 20.3. Radiological changes were pathognomonic. The only abnormality in a needle biopsy is illustrated here. This portal tract contains a hyaline scar in which the collagen fibres are faintly concentric, but there is no central bile duct. The latter has been totally obliterated.

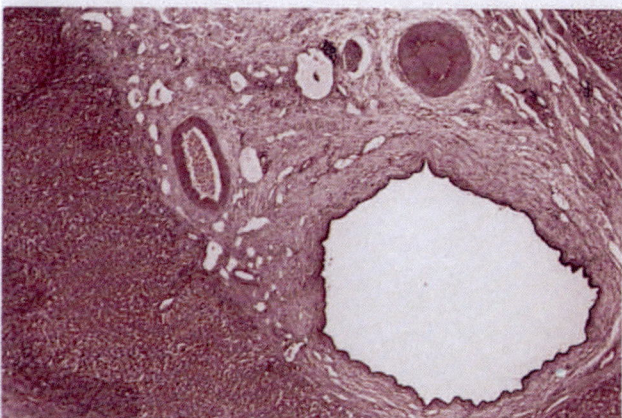

Figure 20.5 Primary sclerosing cholangitis-cholangiectasis. Note the greatly distended bile duct, which should normally have roughly the same diameter as the accompanying arteries.

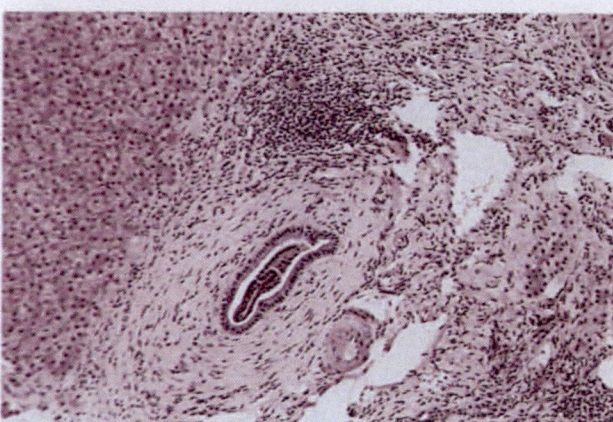

Figure 20.6 Ulcerative colitis, pericholangitis. A 30-year-old male with a 4-year history of chronic ulcerative colitis which was moderately well controlled. No hepatic symptoms, but there was a slight elevation of serum alkaline phosphatase. Biopsy shows an expanded portal tract in which an interlobular bile duct is surrounded by concentric fibrosis. There is also a lymphoid aggregate adjacent to a portal venule.

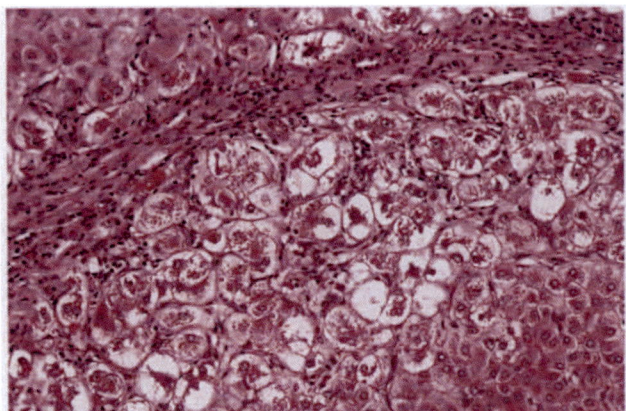

Figure 20.7 Primary sclerosing cholangitis. Late disease showing typical biliary-type piecemeal necrosis at the margin of a nodule, with ballooned hepatocytes containing bile and Mallory's hyalin. These changes are non-specific and indistinguishable from those seen in other cholestatic conditions such as PBC.

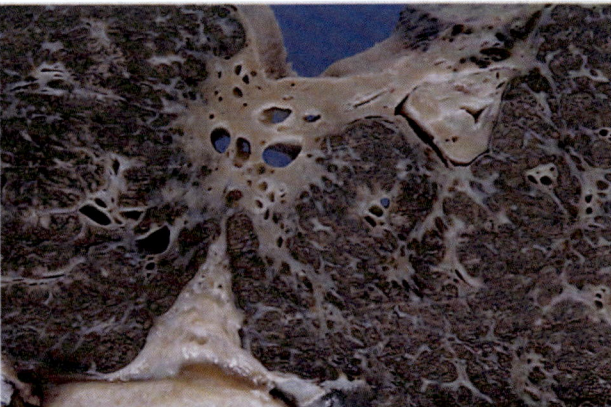

Figure 20.8 Primary sclerosing cholangitis. A 29-year-old patient with a long history of mild ulcerative colitis with gradual onset of jaundice and pruritis, which was progressive. Cholangiography showed the classic beaded appearance of the intrahepatic biliary tree. This section of liver removed at transplantation shows marked fibrous thickening of the portal tracts at the hilum. Stellate scars can also be seen radiating from the smaller portal tracts, amounting at this stage to a full biliary-type cirrhosis.

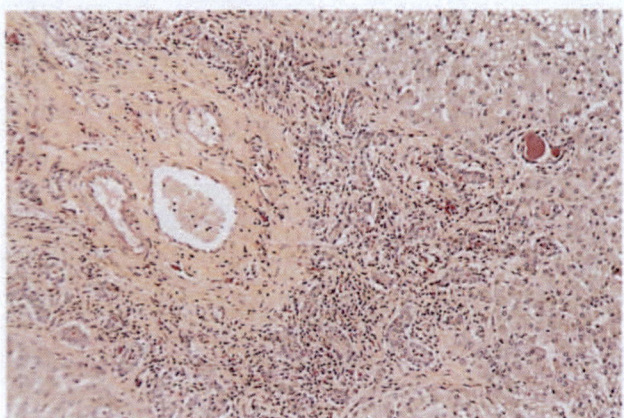

Figure 20.9 Cystic fibrosis, focal biliary fibrosis. A 4-year-old male child who died of pulmonary complications of cystic fibrosis. A number of stellate scars were visible on the cut surface of the liver. The section shows a portal tract from one of these. There is marked peripheral bile ductular proliferation, together with a light chronic inflammatory cell infiltrate. One of the ductules has a dilated lumen filled with PAS-positive secretion. PAS diastase.

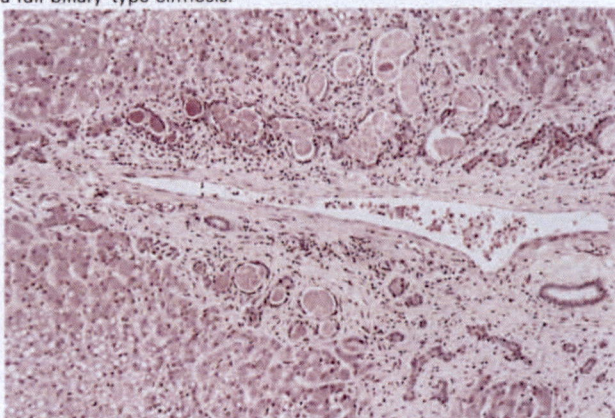

Figure 20.10 Cystic fibrosis, focal biliary fibrosis. Same patient as Figure 20.9. Another portal tract again shows peripheral bile ductular proliferation, but now all have a distended lumen filled with granular eosinophilic secretion.

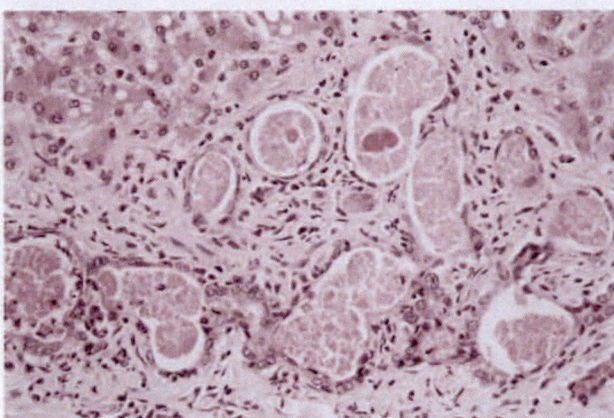

Figure 20.11 Cystic fibrosis, focal biliary fibrosis. Same patient as Figures 20.9 and 20.10. Higher magnification shows the distended ductules in more detail. Other portal tracts in the same liver were entirely normal, an important diagnostic point.

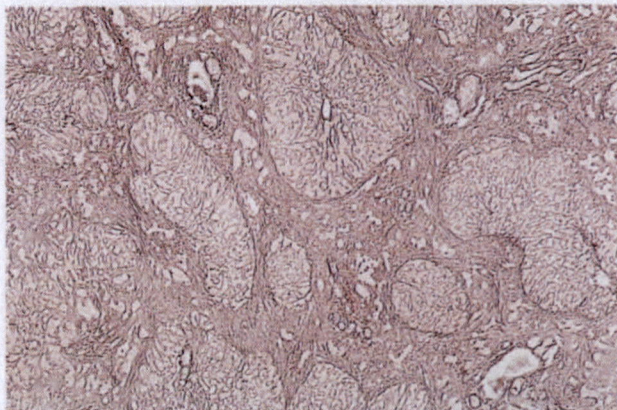

Figure 20.12 Cystic fibrosis, focal cirrhosis. Same patient as Figures 20.9–20.11. Another field shows localized biliary cirrhosis. Although this has morphological similarities with focal nodular hyperplasia (Chapter 22), the clinical context is totally different and thus confusion is unlikely to arise. Reticulin, neutral red.

with meconium ileus or in early childhood with recurrent respiratory infections. As the latter can now be managed so skilfully, more and more affected children reach adult life and thus the chronic hepatic disease is becoming more important. Biochemical changes, particularly elevation of the alkaline phosphatase, and hepatomegaly are common and overt liver disease occurs in about 5% of patients overall, although this increases with increasing age[35]. Histological abnormalities are seen in about half of all cases, even in the presence of normal liver function tests. However, liver biopsy is not a reliable method of assessing serious disease because of its essentially focal distribution, at least in the early stages. Fatty change is common, and is most often periportal in distribution, but focal biliary fibrosis (FBF) is the most distinctive lesion and is found in at least 25% of cases, increasing in incidence with survival[36,37]. Macroscopically the affected liver contains a number of depressed triangular or stellate scars, distributed randomly throughout the parenchyma. Microscopically these are centred upon portal tracts which show a variable degree of fibrosis and peripheral ductular proliferation (Figures 20.9 and 20.10). The ductules are sometimes dilated, rounded and filled with inspissated secretion which is intensely PAS-positive and diastase-resistant (Figures 20.9–20.12). With the passage of time these lesions of FBF become more numerous and may eventually involve the whole liver, leading to portal hypertension, which is much the most important clinical problem[38]. At this late stage it may be difficult to distinguish from a true cirrhosis, although the irregularity of involvement, with deep clefts between nodules, has been likened to the traditional hepar lobatum[36].

OTHER GASTROINTESTINAL DISORDERS

Abnormalities may be found in the liver in Whipple's disease[39], in morbid obesity, and after total parenteral nutrition and jejuno-ileal bypass surgery (Chapter 12).

REFERENCES

1. Holdstock, G., Iredale, J., Millward-Sadler, G. H. and Wright, R. (1992). Hepatic changes in systemic disease. In Millward-Sadler, G. H., Wright, R. and Arthur, M. J. P. (eds). Wright's Liver and Biliary Disease. 3rd edn. pp. 995–1038. London: W B Saunders
2. Greenstein, A. J., Jarowitz, H. and Sachar, D. (1976). Extraintestinal complications of Crohn's disease and ulcerative colitis: a study of 700 patients. Medicine, 55, 401–412
3. Perrett, A. D., Higgins, G., Johnston, H. H., Massarella, G. R., Truelove, S. C. and Wright, R. (1971). The liver in Crohn's disease. Quart. J. Med., 40, 187–209
4. Perrett, A. D., Higgins, G., Johnston, H. H., Massarella, G. R., Truelove, S. C. and Wright, R. (1971). The liver in ulcerative colitis. Quart. J. Med., 40, 211–238
5. Eade, M. N. (1970). Liver disease in ulcerative colitis. 1. Analysis of operative biopsy in 138 consecutive patients having colectomy. Ann. Intern. Med., 72, 475–487
6. Davis, J. J., Heyman, M. B., Ferrell, L., Kerner, J., Kerlan, R. and Thaler, M. M. (1987). Sclerosing cholangitis associated with chronic cryptosporidiosis in a child with congenital immunodeficiency disorder. Am. J. Gastroenterol., 82, 1196–1202
7. Mistilis, S. P. (1965). Pericholangitis and ulcerative colitis. 1. Pathology, aetiology and pathogenesis. Ann. Intern. Med., 63, 1–16
8. Vierling, J. M. (1990). Hepatobiliary complications of inflammatory bowel disease. In Zakim, D. and Boyer, T. D. (eds). Hepatology. A textbook of liver disease. pp. 1126–1158. Philadelphia: Saunders
9. Wee, A. and Ludwig, J. (1985). Pericholangitis in chronic ulcerative colitis: Primary sclerosing cholangitis of the small bile ducts? Ann. Intern. Med., 102, 581–587
10. MacSween, R. N. M. (1984). Primary sclerosing cholangitis. In Anthony, P. and MacSween, R. N. M. (eds). Recent Advances in Histopathology. Number 12. pp. 158–167. Edinburgh: Churchill Livingstone
11. Chapman, R. W. G., Arborgh, B. Å. M., Rhodes, J. M., Summerfield, J. A., Dick, R., Scheuer, P. J. and Sherlock, S. (1980). Primary sclerosing cholangitis: a review of its clinical features. Gut, 21, 870–877
12. Wiesner, R. H. and La Russo, N. F. (1980). Clinicopathological features of the syndrome of primary sclerosing cholangitis. Gastroenterology, 79, 200–206
13. Olsson, R., Danielsson, A., Jarnerot, G., Lindstrom, E., Loof, L.,
14. Rolny, P., Bengt-Olof, R., Ryden, B. O., Tysk, C. and Wallerstedt, S. (1991). Prevalence of primary sclerosing colangitis in patients with ulcerative colitis. Gastroenterology, 100, 1319–1323
15. Epstein, O., Chapman, R. W. G., Lake-Bakaar, G., Foo, A. Y., Rosalki, S. B. and Sherlock, S. (1982). The pancreas in primary biliary cirrhosis and primary sclerosing cholangitis. Gastroenterology, 83, 1177–1182
16. Wiesner, R. H., Grambsch, P. M., Dickson, E. R., Ludwig, J., MacCarty, R. L., Hunter, E. B., Fleming, T. R., Fisher, L. D., Beaver, S. J. and LaRusso, N. F. (1989). Primary sclerosing cholangitis: natural history, prognostic factors and survival analysis. Hepatology, 10, 430–436
17. Wiesner, R. H., LaRusso, N. F., Ludwig, J. and Dickson, E. R. (1985). Comparison of the clinicopathologic features of primary sclerosing cholangitis and primary biliary cirrhosis. Gastroenterology, 88, 108–114
18. Shepherd, H. A., Selby, W. S., Chapman, R. W. G., Nolan, D., Barbatis, C., McGee, J. O. and Jewell, D. P. (1983). Ulcerative colitis and persistent liver dysfunction. Quart. J. Med., 52, 508–513
19. Dickson, E. R., LaRusso, N. F. and Wiesner, R. H. (1984). Primary sclerosing cholangitis. Hepatology, 4, 33S–35S
20. Wight, D. G. D. (1993). Cholestasis and extrahepatic bile ducts. In Wight, D. G. D. (ed.). Liver, Biliary Tract and Exocrine Pancreas. Vol. 11. Systemic Pathology. Symmers, W. S. C., series ed. 3rd edn. Edinburgh: Churchill Livingstone
21. Wight, D. G. D. (1993). The pathology of liver transplantation. In Wight, D. G. D. (ed.). Liver, Biliary Tract and Exocrine Pancreas. Vol. 11. Systemic Pathology. Symmers, W. S. C., series ed. 3rd edn. Edinburgh: Churchill Livingstone
22. Marsh, J. W., Iwatsuki, S., Makowka, I. et al. (1988). Orthotopic liver transplantation for primary sclerosing cholangitis. Ann. Surg., 207, 21–25
23. Ludwig, J., LaRusso, N. F. and Wiesner, R. H. (1990). The syndrome of primary sclerosing cholangitis. Progr. Liver Dis., 9, 555–566
24. Harrison, R. F. and Hübscher, S. G. (1991). The spectrum of bile duct lesions in end-stage primary sclerosing cholangitis. Histopathology, 19, 321–327
25. Ludwig, J., MacCarty, R. L., LaRusso, N. F., Krom, R. A. F. and Wiesner, R. H. (1986). Intrahepatic cholangiectases and large-duct obliteration in primary sclerosing cholangitis. Hepatology, 6, 560–568
26. Nakanuma, Y., Hirai, N., Kono, N. and Ohta, G. (1986). Histological and ultrastructural examination of the intrahepatic biliary tree in primary sclerosing cholangitis. Liver, 6, 317–325
27. Lindberg, T., Berg, N. O., Borulf, S. and Jakobsson, I. (1978). Liver damage in coeliac disease or other food intolerance in childhood. Lancet., 1, 390–391
28. Hagander, B., Berg, N. O., Brandt, L., Norden, A., K, S. and Stenstam, M. (1977). Hepatic injury in adult coeliac disease. Lancet., 2, 270–272
29. Jacobsen, M. B., Fausa, O., Elgjo, K. et al. (1990). Hepatic lesions in adult coeliac disease. Scand. J. Gastroenterol., 25, 656–662
30. Pollock, D. J. (1977). The liver in coeliac disease. Histopathology, 1, 421–430
31. Isaacson, P., Wright, D. H., Judd, M. A. and Mepham, B. L. (1979). Primary gastrointestinal lymphomas. A classification of 66 cases. Cancer, 43, 1805–1819
32. Isaacson, P. G., O'Connor, N. T. J., Spencer, J., Bevan, D. H., Connolly, C. E., Kirkham, N., Pollock, D. J., Wainscoat, J. S., Stein, H. and Wright, D. H. (1985). Malignant histiocytosis of the intestine: a T cell lymphoma. Lancet, 2, 688–690
33. Rommens, J. M., Iannuzzi, M. C., Kerem, B.-S. et al. (1989). Identification of the cystic fibrosis gene: chromosome walking and jumping. Science, 245, 1059–1065
34. Kerem, B.-S., Rommens, J. M. and Buchanan, J. A. (1989). Identification of the cystic fibrosis gene: genetic analysis. Science, 245, 1073–1080
35. McMahon, C. J., Genet, S. A., Middleton, P. H., Rutland, P., Pembrey, M. E. and Malcolm, S. (1990). The major cystic fibrosis mutation in a British population. Hum. Genet., 86, 236–237
36. Scott-Jupp, R., Lama, M. and Tanner, M. S. (1991). Prevalence of liver disease in cystic fibrosis. Arch. Dis. Child., 66, 698–701
37. Di Sant'Agnese, P. A. and Blanc, W. A. (1956). A distinctive type of biliary cirrhosis of the liver associated with cystic fibrosis of the pancreas. Pediatrics, 18, 387–409
38. Oppenheimer, E. H. and Esterly, J. R. (1975). Hepatic changes in young infants with cystic fibrosis: possible relation to focal biliary cirrhosis. J. Pediatr., 86, 683–689
39. Psacharopoulos, H. T., Howard, E. R., Portmann, B., Mowat, A. P. and Williams, R. (1981). Hepatic complications of cystic fibrosis. Lancet, 2, 78–80
40. Girardin, M., Zafrani, E. S., Chaumette, M. and et al. (1984). Hepatic granulomas in Whipple's disease. Gastroenterology, 86, 753–756

Systemic Disease

21

NON-SPECIFIC REACTIVE HEPATITIS

Unexplained pyrexia, hepatomegaly and minor abnormalities of liver function tests are amongst the most common indications for liver biopsy. All may be associated with non-specific reactive hepatitis (NSRH), which represents the hepatic consequences of systemic infection or inflammatory disease[1,2]. Identical changes may also be found in the neighbourhood of focal hepatic lesions.

Both portal tracts and the parenchyma can be affected, but involvement is always patchy and variable. Thus, of adjacent portal tracts, one may be severely inflamed, the other normal (Figure 21.1). This is an important distinction from chronic persistent hepatitis where involvement is much more uniform, particularly of the small portal tracts (see Chapter 7). Involved portal tracts contain variable numbers of chronic inflammatory cells, predominantly lymphocytes (Figure 21.2), with only very occasional plasma cells and rarely, or never, neutrophils. Very occasionally well-formed lymphoid follicles are seen, particularly in older age groups. There is no piecemeal necrosis at the limiting plates (Figure 21.2). In the parenchyma scattered focal necroses of hepatocytes are surrounded by aggregates of lymphocytes and macrophages (Figure 21.3). These often have a faintly granulomatous appearance, although they are not truly epithelioid and giant cells are not seen. There may also be a more general Kupffer cell prominence throughout the lobules, which is much more uniform than that seen following viral hepatitis. Focal fatty change and increased variability of size and staining of liver cell nuclei may also be noted (Figure 21.2).

This is a frequent diagnosis in routine practice and it is important that NSRH should be distinguished from chronic persistent hepatitis and residual viral hepatitis (Chapter 7). Occasionally portal tract infiltration may even be sufficiently intense to mimic malignant lymphoma.

CONNECTIVE TISSUE DISEASES

Clinically overt liver disease is unusual in the connective tissue diseases, but minor abnormalities in liver function tests are quite common. Non-specific abnormalities such as fat or non-specific reactive hepatitis are also regularly seen in liver biopsies. However, it may be difficult or impossible to distinguish changes directly due to the primary condition from those merely secondary to debility or to therapy (e.g. corticosteroid drugs). In the *rheumatic disorders* (rheumatoid arthritis, Still's disease and Felty's syndrome), in addition to non-specific changes[3], an occasional patient has concomitant primary biliary cirrhosis, chronic active hepatitis, nodular regenerative hyperplasia or amyloidosis[4]. Changes are more common and, in general, livers contain more inflammatory cells in both portal tracts and sinusoids in Felty's syndrome than in the other conditions[5]. The incidence of liver disease in *systemic sclerosis* is very low, but again there may be a link with primary biliary cirrhosis[6], especially when associated with the CREST syndrome (Calcinosis cutis, Raynaud's, Oesophageal involvement, Sclerodactyly and Telangiectasis)[7]. There is no clear link between *systemic lupus erythematosus* (SLE) and the lupoid form of chronic active hepatitis, despite a number of common symptoms and laboratory findings. Minor hepatomegaly is not uncommon, but jaundice is more often secondary to haemolysis than to liver disease. A recent review found clear evidence of liver disease in 43 of 238 patients with SLE[8]. The spectrum of disease included cirrhosis, chronic active hepatitis, granulomatous hepatitis, chronic persistent hepatitis and fatty change.

PREGNANCY

Pregnant patients are no more or less susceptible to the common liver diseases than non-pregnant patients[2,9]. Thus jaundice may be due to viral hepatitis, pre-existing chronic liver disease or other conditions. There are, however, several diseases peculiar to pregnancy.

Idiopathic recurrent cholestasis of pregnancy is the commonest of these[10]. It usually presents with pruritus followed by jaundice in the early part of the third trimester. On biopsy the only changes are those of centrilobular canalicular cholestasis (Chapter 16). The course is benign, but it is liable to recur in subsequent pregnancies and on exposure to oral contraceptive drugs[11].

In *pre-eclampsia* jaundice is rare, although biochemical abnormalities are quite common. In *eclampsia* jaundice may be deep and secondary to disseminated intravascular coagulation (DIC), which is often fatal. Histologically there is fibrin deposition in portal vessels associated with irregular islands of periportal liver cell necrosis (Figures 21.4 and 21.5)[12]. Very similar appearances are found in DIC from any other cause; for example, in paroxysmal nocturnal haemoglobinuria.

Acute fatty liver of pregnancy has been described in Chapter 12.

AMYLOIDOSIS

In this condition there is extracellular deposition of an abnormal protein in various tissues of the body. Its presence is generally silent, except in the kidney, where it interferes with the efficiency of the glomerular filter, and in blood vessel walls, especially of the gut, where its rigidity may interfere with normal haemostasis. All amyloids have the same physical β-pleated sheet conformation, but chemically there are two major classes[13]. The first, designated AL amyloid *(primary)*, is found in association with multiple myeloma and other plasma cell dyscrasias, and has an amino acid sequence identical to that found in the variable part of the light chain component of immunoglobulin. The second, designated AA amyloid *(secondary)*, is deposited in various inflammatory conditions such as chronic infection and connective tissue diseases. This has a unique structure and is derived by proteolytic cleavage from serum amyloid A protein, an acute phase reactant synthesized in the liver[14]. Synthesis in the liver is stimulated by interleukin 1, interleukin 6 and tumour necrosis factor, accounting for the association of this form of amyloidosis with inflammatory conditions[15]. Other rarer forms of amyloid include those associated with familial Mediterranean fever (AA amyloid secondary to recurrent bouts of inflammation that characterize this disease); the familial neuropathies where amyloid is primarily deposited in peripheral nerves (AF amyloid due to deposition of mutant prealbumin); some endocrine tumours (e.g. calcitonin in medullary carcinoma of the

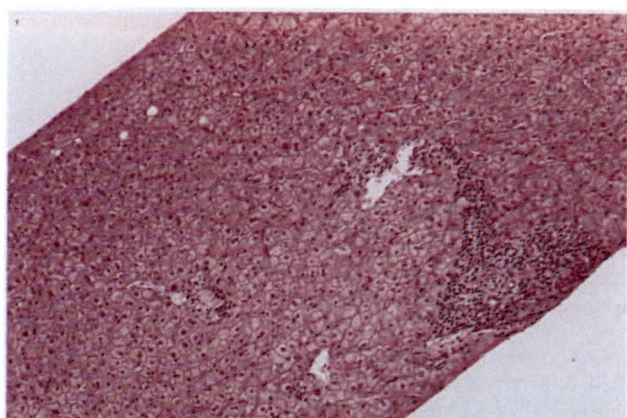

Figure 21.1 Non-specific reactive hepatitis. A 43-year-old female with a pyrexial illness and minor abnormalities of liver function tests. Liver biopsy reveals a patchy non-specific inflammation. The large portal tract (right) contains a fairly dense mononuclear cell infiltrate whilst the smaller portal tracts below centre are normal.

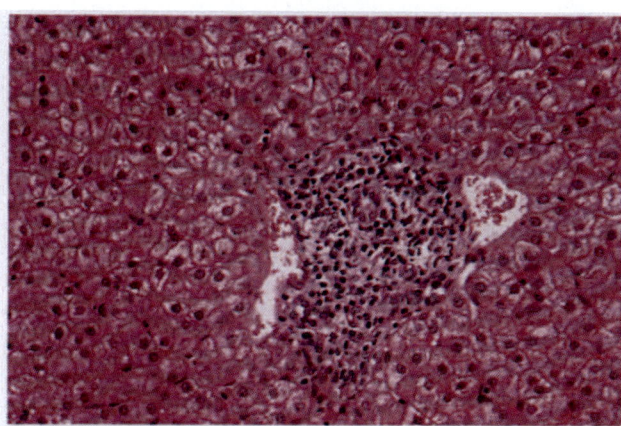

Figure 21.2 Non-specific reactive hepatitis. Another patient with a similar clinical history to Figure 21.1. Higher magnification of a portal tract reveals that the infiltrate is composed almost entirely of lymphocytes. Note that the limiting plates are intact.

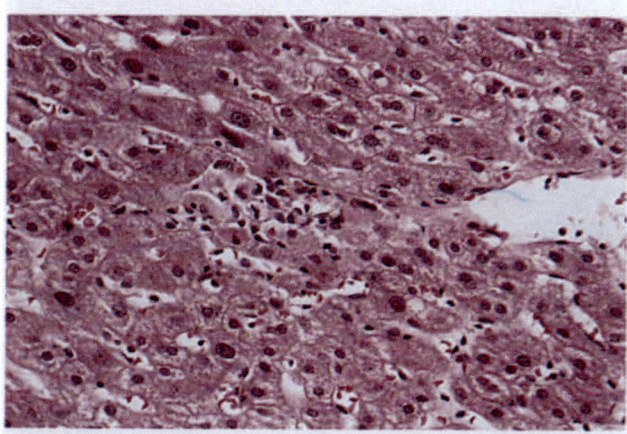

Figure 21.3 Non-specific reactive hepatitis. Same case as Figure 21.1. This section shows a small focal necrosis with an acidophil body and an aggregate of lymphocytes and macrophages (a 'macrophage granuloma') near to a central vein. Note also the hepatocyte pleomorphism. This patient was subsequently shown to have a staphylococcal septicaemia.

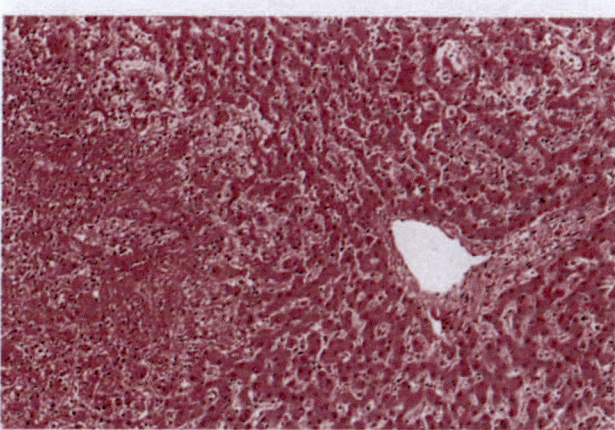

Figure 21.4 Eclampsia. A 25-year-old patient in her first pregnancy developed severe pre-eclamptic toxaemia at about 36 weeks. This progressed to eclampsia with convulsions despite termination of the pregnancy, and she subsequently died. A section of liver shows the distinctive portal and periportal necrosis (left).

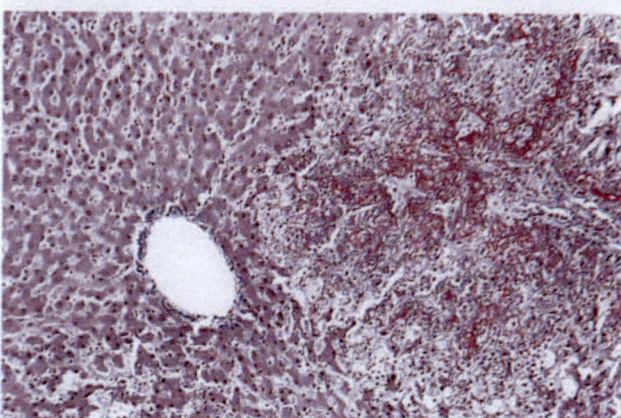

Figure 21.5 Eclampsia. Same patient as Figure 21.4. This section shows that the areas of necrosis contain a significant quantity of fibrin, stained red. Lendrum's picro Mallory.

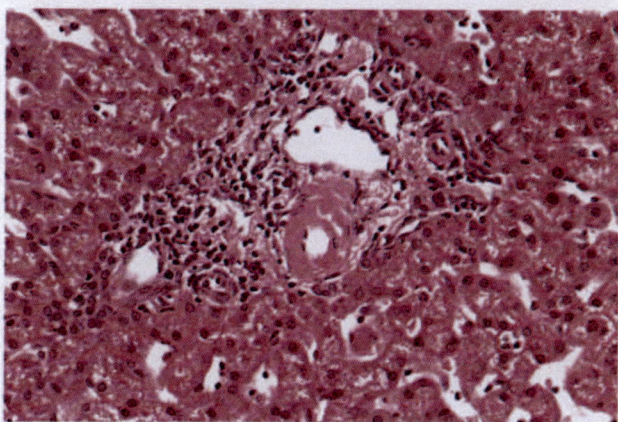

Figure 21.6 Amyloidosis. A 75-year-old patient with chronic rheumatoid arthritis who developed proteinuria terminally. At autopsy, amyloid was found in the renal glomeruli and in the liver. This section of a portal tract shows hyaline thickening of a hepatic artery branch. Amyloid stains were strongly positive. Amyloid was not present elsewhere in the liver, thus this appearance could easily be attributed to hypertension (Figure 18.20) without the use of special stains.

thyroid); and senile plaques in Alzheimer's disease ($\beta4$ amyloid). In each case the soluble precursor protein must be converted into insoluble fibrillar form possibly as a result of defective proteolysis by the monocyte macrophage system[16]. Only AL and AA amyloid are found in the liver. Although AA amyloid is more likely to be associated with extensive systemic involvement, including the parenchymal organs, the distinction from AL amyloid purely on the grounds of distribution is unreliable.

Liver involvement may be both parenchymal and vascular. Even when extensive, hepatomegaly may be the only clinical manifestation of liver involvement. Macroscopically, a severely affected organ has a firm consistency and a translucent waxy appearance on section. Histologically the amyloid takes the form of homogeneous eosinophilic deposits in the space of Disse where it appears to cause compression atrophy of liver cell plates (Figures 21.7 and 21.8). Not all acini are equally affected, but there is usually no difficulty in recognizing its presence. In contrast, when confined to the vessels, mainly the hepatic artery (Figure 21.6), it may be very inconspicuous and indistinguishable from arterial hyalinization (Chapter 18). For this reason amyloid should be specifically considered every time a biopsy is examined and, if there is the smallest suspicion, a special stain can then be applied. The most reliable results are usually obtained with Congo red (Figure 21.8). AL and AA amyloid cannot reliably be distinguished on the basis of their distribution, but AA amyloid loses its affinity for Congo red after prior treatment with potassium permanganate and dilute sulphuric acid[17]. Immunoperoxidase staining with specific antisera is also now a useful technique in the identification of the different forms of amyloid[18].

PORPHYRIAS

The porphyrias are disorders of the biosynthesis of porphyrins and haem. Haem synthesis is normally highly efficient and only small amounts of intermediates escape the pathway and enter the circulation. In porphyria, these amounts are substantially increased. Their distribution within tissues and pattern of excretion reflect to a large extent their physical properties. The earlier precursors are ionized and soluble and thus can be excreted in the urine, whilst the last precursor, protoporphyrin, is lipophilic and non-ionized and thus excreted solely in the bile and thus in the faeces. Coproporphyrin is intermediate and thus is excreted by both routes[19]. All tissues synthesize haem, which is required not only for haemoglobin but also for cytochrome formation. In the liver, cytochrome P450 is the most significant cytochrome, and one of its important characteristics is its inducibility by its substrates (such as administered drugs). In some porphyrias, such as *acute intermittent porphyria*, the effect of cytochrome induction is to cause acute haem depletion and accumulation of the precursors prior to the enzymic block–the haem-deficient porphyrias. In others, the capacity for haem synthesis is normal, for example *protoprophyria*, and are therefore unaffected by inducers of cytochrome P450– the haem-compensated porphyrias. Porphyrins (but not ∂-aminolaevulinic acid or porphobilinogen) are red-purple in colour and are fluorescent. The fluorescence reflects the fact that porphyrins undergo excitation by light. When the excitation occurs *in vivo*, for example in skin capillaries, the relaxation to unexcited state results in the release of active molecules–possibly free radicals–which cause inflammation and tissue damage.

Porphyrias are usually divided into hepatic and erythropoietic types depending on the major site of porphyrin accumulation. However, although the liver and the bone marrow are significant sites of synthesis, it is important to realize that all tissues synthesize haem and thus all may potentially be affected by a genetic defect in the haem pathway[19]. Most porphyrias are inherited as autosomal dominant conditions, but porphyria cutanea tarda is generally considered to be acquired and associated with alcoholism (see below). The diagnosis rests upon the detection of the porphyrins or their precursors in urine, faeces or blood.

Acute intermittent porphyria (AIP)

The basic defect is a 50% reduction of hepatic porphobilinogen deaminase activity[19], which results in accumulation of porphobilinogen and ∂-aminolaevulinic acid. AIP is characterized clinically by attacks of severe colicky abdominal pain, constipation, neuropsychiatric disturbance and protean neurological lesions including peripheral neuropathy, which may last for 48 hours. These are frequently precipitated by cytochrome P450 inducing drugs, such as barbiturates, oestrogens and possibly alcohol. It is not clear whether the neurological changes (the abdominal pain is probably also neurological in nature) are due to intrinsic deficiency of haem or whether the nerve cells require exogenous haem. Classically the urine contains an excess of porphobilinogen, detectable by the generation of a pink complex with Ehrlich's reagent[20], and darkens on standing as this becomes converted non-enzymatically to porphyrins. Histologically the liver may be normal or show minor changes, such as an increase in iron and focal fatty change[21]. Hereditary coproporphyria and variegate porphyria are related conditions which are very similar to AIP with, in addition, a photosensitive rash.

Porphyria cutanea tarda (PCT)

This condition is usually diagnosed by its characteristic clinical picture of a photosensitive blistering rash and by the demonstration of uroporphyrin I in the urine or faeces. This is a haem-compensated porphyria and thus is not associated with neurological disturbances and is unaffected by enzyme inducers. It is generally seen in men with underlying liver disease, generally related to excessive alcohol consumption, and in some way is associated with the accumulation of iron in the liver[22]. It has traditionally been regarded as an acquired condition, but there is recent evidence suggesting that there may be both genetic and acquired types[23]. Further support for this view comes from the large series from Madrid[24], where half the patients consumed little or no alcohol. The enzyme uroporphyrin decarboxylase from patients with familial PCT is more sensitive in vitro to inhibition by iron than that from normal individuals[25]. HLA markers of haemochromatosis are often present in patients with PCT, and it has been suggested that, in addition to deficiency of uroporphyrin decarboxylase, a single 'dose' of the gene for haemochromatosis may be necessary for the expression of clinical disease[26]. Removal of the iron by venesection has a markedly beneficial effect upon the course of the disease.

Histologically, needle-shaped cytoplasmic inclusions in liver cells are the hallmark of the disease (Figure 21.9)[24]. They are birefringent and give a characteristic red fluorescence in ultraviolet light. However, in routine preparations this material is likely to be removed, since it is water-soluble, and thus it is best demonstrated in unfixed cryostat sections allowed to dry in air. The other changes regularly seen include siderosis, although this is often slight, excess lipofuscin, focal fatty change, regenerative activity, focal hepatocyte necroses and portal inflammation. There is a close correlation between the age of the patient and the presence of architectural disturbance and cirrhosis, suggesting that the disease

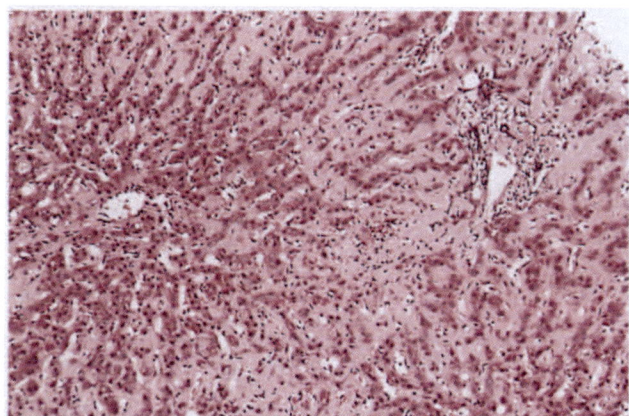

Figure 21.7 Amyloidosis. A 45-year-old male with severe ankylosing spondylitis developed proteinuria followed by chronic renal failure. Liver biopsy shows very extensive deposition of amyloid in the space of Disse, particularly severe periportally where there is atrophy of liver cell plates. Despite this, hepatomegaly was the only clinical sign of liver involvement.

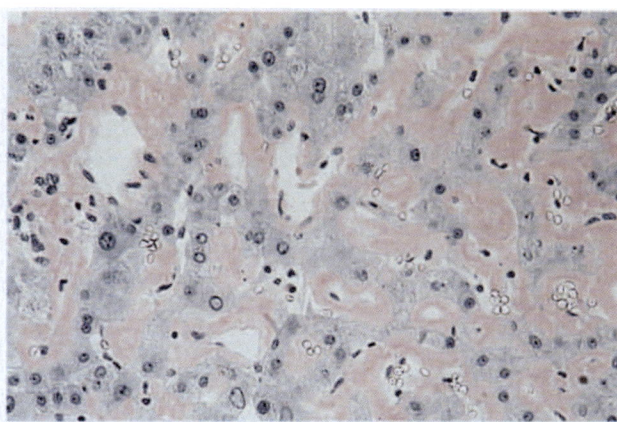

Figure 21.8 Amyloidosis. Same case as Figure 21.7. This stain shows the amyloid as pale red hyaline material between liver cell plates and it gave brilliant apple green birefringence when viewed in polarized light. Congo red.

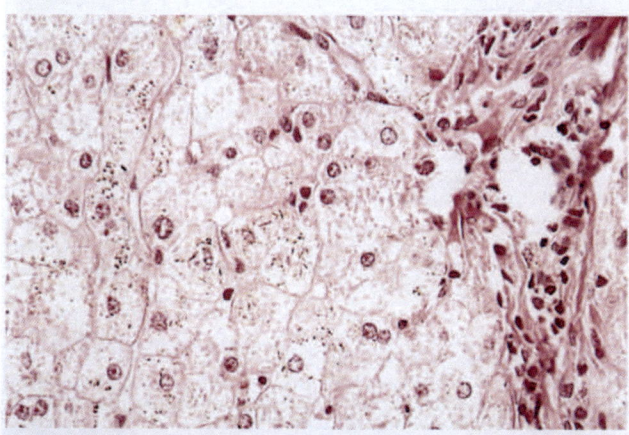

Figure 21.9 Porphyria cutanea tarda. A 61-year-old male with typical disease. This section shows a cluster of needle-shaped inclusions in the liver cells at the centre of the field. Note also the excess lipofuscin and a slight excess of lymphocytes in the portal tract (right). Although this was a routine paraffin section, cryostat sections are much more reliable, since many of the crystals will be removed during processing.
The author is deeply indebted to Dr F. J. Paradinas who kindly supplied the section from which this figure was prepared.

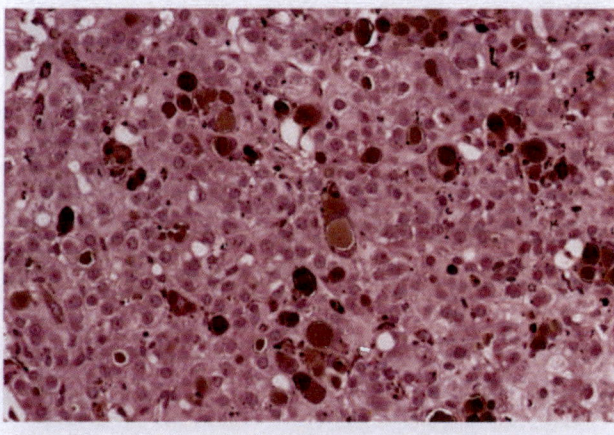

Figure 21.10 Protoporphyria. Eighteen-year-old girl with severe photosensitivity and established cirrhosis. This section shows diffuse brown pigmentation, localized in bile canaliculi and Kupffer cells.

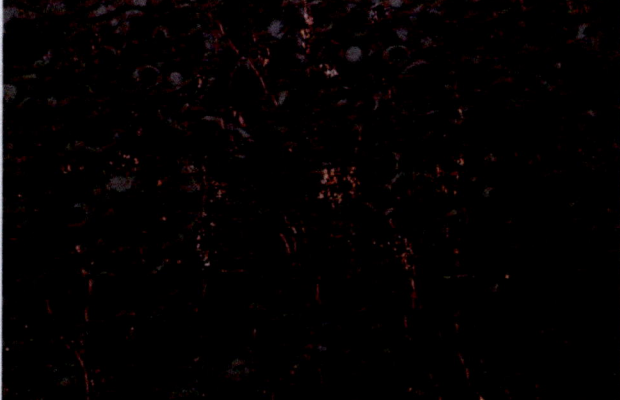

Figure 21.11 Protoporphyria. A section from another case viewed in polarized light showing that the pigment is brilliantly birefringent.

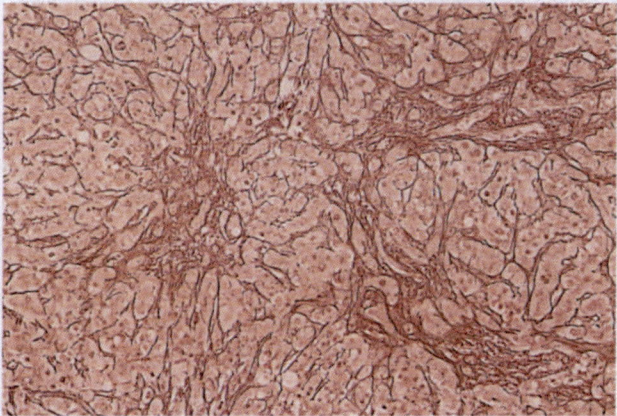

Figure 21.12 Protoporphyria. Same case as Figure 21.11. This section shows that there is disturbance of the lobular architecture due to the presence of thin fibrous septa radiating from both portal tracts and central veins. Reticulin, neutral red.

is progressive. Contrary to expectation, alcoholic liver disease is rarely seen.

Protoporphyria

This relatively common condition, also known as erythropoietic protoporphyria, is usually characterized by a mild cutaneous photosensitivity largely due to leakage of protoporphyrins from erythrocytes[19]. There is a deficiency of the enzyme ferrochelatase in red cells, and diagnosis depends upon demonstration of increased amounts of protoporphyrin in red cells, plasma and faeces. Haemoglobin synthesis does not appear to be affected, suggesting that protoporphyrin is produced in excess of that required for haem formation[27]. In a few individuals there is a significant liver component[28]. In these patients there is focal accumulation of dense dark brown pigment (Figures 21.10 and 21.11) in bile canaliculi, interlobular bile ducts, Kupffer cells and even portal tract connective tissue. The pigment has an intense red autofluorescence in cryostat sections, but it can also be demonstrated more easily in paraffin sections by polarization microscopy. Here the pigment is bright red and granular with a central Maltese cross (Figure 21.11). There is no doubt that in a few patients the liver disease is progressive, increasing liver damage further interfering with protoporphyrin excretion, and can lead to death from acute liver failure or cirrhosis (Figure 21.12)[29].

REFERENCES

1. Popper, H. and Schaffner, F. (1957). Liver. Structure and Function. New York: McGraw-Hill
2. Millward-Sadler, G. H. (1993). The liver in systemic disease. In Wight, D. G. D. (ed.). Liver, Biliary Tract and Exocrine Pancreas. Vol. 11. Systemic Pathology. Symmers, W. S. C., series ed. 3rd edn. Edinburgh: Churchill Livingstone
3. Mills, P. R. and Sturrock, R. D. (1982). Clinical associations between arthritis and liver disease. Ann. Rheum. Dis., 41, 295–307
4. Whaley, K. and Webb, J. (1977). Liver and kidney disease in rheumatoid arthritis. Clin. Rheum. Dis., 3, 527–547
5. Sullivan, S., Hamilton, E. B. D. and Williams, R. (1978). Rheumatoid arthritis and liver involvement. J. R. Coll. Phys. Lond, 12, 416–422
6. Murray-Lyon, I. M., Thompson, R. P. H., Ansell, I. D. and Williams, R. (1970). Scleroderma and primary biliary cirrhosis. Br. Med. J., 3, 258–259
7. Holdstock, G., Iredale, J., Millward-Sadler, G. H. and Wright, R. (1992). Hepatic changes in systemic disease. In Millward-Sadler, G. H., Wright, R. and Arthur, M. J. P. (eds). Wright's Liver and Biliary Disease. 3rd edn. pp. 995–1038. London: W B Saunders
8. Runyon, B. A., Labrecque, D. R. and Anuras, S. (1980). The spectrum of liver disease in SLE. Report of 33 histologically proved cases and review of the literature. Am. J. Med., 69, 187–194
9. Gitlin, N. (1992). Liver disease in pregnancy. In Millward-Sadler, G. H., Wright, R. and Arthur, M. J. P. (eds). Wright's Liver and Biliary Disease. 3rd edn. pp. 1155–1169. London: W B Saunders
10. Reyes, H. (1982). The enigma of intrahepatic cholestasis of pregnancy; lesson from Chile. Hepatology, 2, 87–96
11. Dalen, E. and Westerholme, B. (1974). Occurrence of hepatic impairment in women jaundiced by oral contraceptives and in their mothers and sisters. Acta Med. Scand., 195, 349–463
12. Rolfes, D. B. and Ishak, K. G. (1986). Liver disease in toxaemia of pregnancy. Am. J. Gastroenterol., 81, 1218–1219
13. Pepys, M. B. (1988). Amyloidosis: some recent developments. Quart. J. Med., 252, 283–298
14. McAdam, K. P. W. J., Elin, R. J., Sipe, J. D. and Wolff, S. M. (1978). Changes in human serum amyloid A and C-reactive protein after etiocholanolone-induced inflammation. J. Clin. Invest., 61, 390–394
15. Woo, P., Sipe, J., Dinarello, C. A. and Colten, H. R. (1987). Structure of human serum amyloid A gene and modulation of its expression in transfected L cells. J. Biol. Chem., 262, 15790–15795
16. Cotran, R. S., Kumar, V. and Robbins, S. L. (1989). Diseases of immunity. In Robbins Pathological Basis of Disease. 4th edn. pp. 210–220. Philadelphia: W B Saunders
17. Wright, J. R., Calkins, E. and Humphrey, R. L. (1977). Potassium permanganate reaction in amyloidosis. A histologic method to assist in differentiating forms of this disease. Lab. Invest., 36, 274–281
18. Chastonay, P. and Hurlimann, J. (1986). Characterization of different amyloids with immunologic techniques. Pathol. Res. Pract., 181, 657–663
19. Bissell, D. M. (1992). Haem metabolism and the porphyrias. In Millward-Sadler, G. H., R., W. and Arthur, M. J. P. (eds). Wright's Liver and Biliary Disease. 3rd edn. pp. 397–422. London: W. B. Saunders
20. Watson, C. J. and Schwartz, S. (1941). A simple test for urinary porphobilinogen. Proc. Soc. Exp. Biol. Med., 47, 393–394
21. Biempica, L., Kosower, N., Ma, M. H. and Goldfischer, S. (1974). Hepatic porphyrias. Cytochemical and ultrastructural studies of liver in acute intermittent porphyria and porphyria cutanea tarda. Arch. Pathol., 98, 336–343
22. Turnbull, A., Baker, H., Vernon-Roberts, B. and Magnus, I. A. (1973). Iron metabolism in porphyria cutanea tarda and in erythropoietic protoporphyria. Quart. J. Med., 42, 341–355
23. de Verneuil, H., Nordmann, Y., Phung, N. et al. (1978). Familial and sporadic porphyria cutanea: two different diseases. Int. J. Biochem., 9, 927–931
24. Cortes, J. M., Oliva, H., Paradinas, F. J. and Hernandez-Guio, C. (1980). The pathology of the liver in porphyria cutanea tarda. Histopathology., 4, 471–485
25. Mukerji, S. K., Pimstone, N. R. and Tan, K. T. (1985). A potential biochemical explanation for the genesis of porphyria cutanea tarda. Fed. Eur. Biochem. Soc. Lett., 189, 217–220
26. Edwards, C. Q., Griffen, L. M., Goldgar, D. E., Skolnick, M. H. and Kushner, J. P. (1989). HLA-linked hemochromatosis alleles in sporadic porphyria cutanea tarda. Gastroenterology, 97, 972–981
27. DeLeo, V. A., Poh-Fitzpatrick, M., Matthews-Roth, M. and Harber, L. C. (1976). Erythropoietic protoporphyria: ten years' experience. Am. J. Med., 60, 8–22
28. Bloomer, J. R. (1988). The liver in protoporphyria. Hepatology, 8, 402–407
29. Cripps, D. J., Gilbert, L. A. and Goldfarb, S. S. (1977). Erythropoietic protoporphyria. Juvenile protoporphyrin hepatopathy, cirrhosis and death. J. Pediatr., 91, 744–748

Benign Tumours and Tumour-like Conditions

22

Tumour-like conditions may arise from any of the component cells of the liver, including hepatocytes, bile ducts and endothelium. They are classified in Table 22.1.

Table 22.1 Classification of benign hepatic nodules

	Tumour-like conditions	Benign tumours
Hepatocytes	FNH* NRH Adenomatous hyperplasia Partial nodular transformation	LCA Multiple adenomatosis
Bile Duct	von Myenburg complex Simple cysts (Chapter 8)	Bile duct adenoma Cystadenoma Bile duct papilloma (Chapter 24)
Endothelium		Haemangioma Infantile haemangioendothelioma
Mesenchyme	Mesenchymal hamartoma	
Connective tissue	Lipoma, Angiomyolipoma, Fibroma, Leiomyoma	

* For abbreviations see text.

FOCAL NODULAR HYPERPLASIA (FNH)

Synonyms include hamartoma, cholangiohepatoma and focal cirrhosis. These lesions are usually firm and macroscopically nodular. They are most often less than 5 cm in diameter, but sometimes reach as much as 24 cm. On section they are distinctly lighter than the surrounding liver (Figures 22.1 and 22.2) and typically contain one or more central depressed stellate scars (Figure 22.1) with septa radiating out and surrounding or partly surrounding nodules of liver which may closely resemble those seen in cirrhosis (Figure 22.3). There is usually no capsule but there may be compression of the adjacent liver, which is otherwise normal. Most examples of FNH are found near the free edge of the liver and occasionally they may even be extruded on a stalk. Multiple lesions are also sometimes found.

Microscopically the liver cells appear normal and of the same size as the surrounding parenchymal cells (Figure 22.4). Mitoses are not seen. At times it may be difficult on microscopy alone to detect a discrete junction between FNH and normal liver. Septal fibrous tissue or parenchymal fat or glycogen may make the distinction easier (Figure 22.5). Liver cell plates are often irregular and contain two or more layers of cells. Distended bile canaliculi containing inspissated bile are an occasional finding. The fibrous septa invariably contain proliferating bile duct-like structures which are most numerous at the interface with liver cells (Figure 22.4). These are thought to arise from hepatocyte metaplasia rather than from pre-existing bile ducts[1]. Collections of similar bile ductules may be found within the nodules where they merge imperceptibly with the surrounding liver cells[2]. Inflammatory cells, mostly lymphocytes but also neutrophils and plasma cells, are sometimes seen in the septa, often between the bile ductules. Some septa contain numerous thin-walled blood vessels, others larger vessels with asymmetrical nodular thickening of their walls. Thus the key features of FNH are its localized nature and the radiating fibrous septa containing bile ductules. Although there may be some morphological features in common, cirrhotic nodules, partial nodular transformation, nodular regenerative hyperplasia and hepatocellular adenomatosis should all be clearly distinguished from FNH, providing that enough information is available.

FNH is found in all age groups, including children[3], but is most common in women in the 20–40 age group[4]. Most cases are incidental findings at laparotomy or autopsy. However, there is some evidence (see below) that in recent years they have become more likely to present as a result of pain or spontaneous haemorrhage, and this has been linked with oral contraceptive use[5]. If clinically evident, diagnosis is usually suggested by isotope scanning and a fairly characteristic vascular pattern on angiography. Apart from causing considerable problems of interpretation, needle biopsy is possibly contraindicated because of the risk of haemorrhage. This is even more true of liver cell adenoma (see below). It is not clear whether the entity represents a neoplasm, a hamartoma, a reparative or regenerative process, or even whether it might be primarily a blood vessel anomaly[6]. Wanless et al.[7] showed, with serial sections, an abnormal arterial supply unaccompanied by portal vein branches and suggested that this might be a congenital abnormality. The occasional association with haemangiomas in the liver (Figure 22.6)[8] and vascular abnormalities in other organs such as the brain[9] would support this theory. Despite a superficial resemblance between FNH and fibrolamellar hepatocellular carcinoma (Chapter 23), there is no evidence to suggest that FNH is premalignant[4,10]. Nevertheless, the two lesions may co-exist[11].

LIVER CELL ADENOMA (LCA)

Synonyms include benign hepatoma. These are soft, usually solitary, nodules, often lighter in colour than the normal liver from which they are clearly demarcated. They tend to be larger than FNH and are usually more than 5 cm in diameter and occasionally are very large measuring as much as 30 cm. The cut surface may include areas of haemorrhage (Figure 22.7) and occasionally the tumours are bile-stained, but there is no nodularity. The capsule when present is often incomplete (Figure 22.8). They are occasionally multiple, and if more than four are present the term *Adenomatosis* has been used[12]. Microscopically they are composed of morphologically normal hepatocytes which may be a little larger than those in the adjacent parenchyma. As in FNH they are arranged in rather irregular plates, often two or more cells thick, and, especially at the periphery of the nodules, may form rosettes or pseudoducts, some containing bile (Figure 22.9). Bile plugs may also be seen elsewhere. Some liver cells, again particularly at the periphery, contain an excess of glycogen which may cause marked pallor of the cytoplasm, and fatty change is also sometimes seen. In

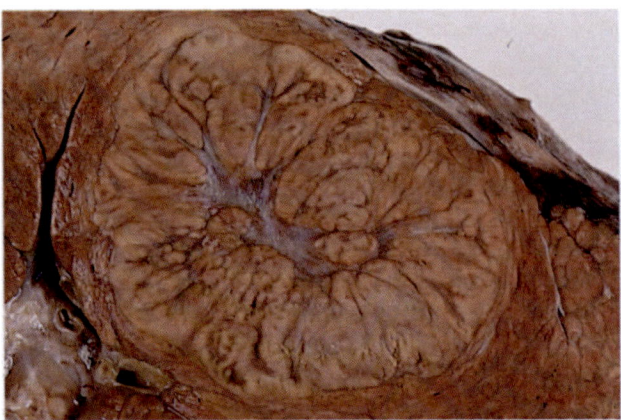

Figure 22.1 Focal nodular hyperplasia. An incidental finding in the liver of a patient who underwent transplantation for α_1-antitrypsin deficiency. The photograph shows that this lesion is about 3 cm in diameter and has a striking stellate scar at its centre, and a scalloped margin.

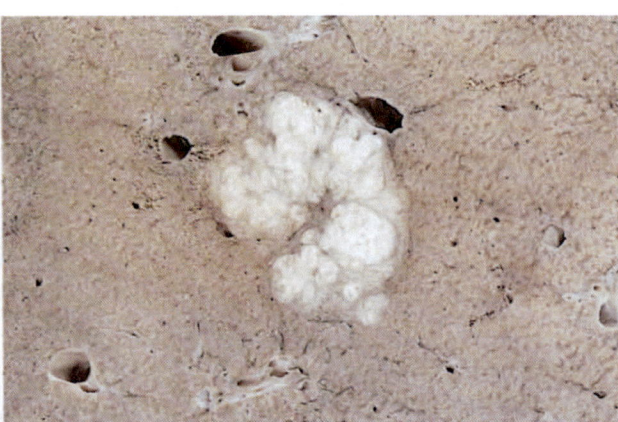

Figure 22.2 Focal nodular hyperplasia. An incidental finding at autopsy in a 64-year-old man with disseminated malignancy. This section shows a pale multinodular lesion which was about 2 cm in diameter.

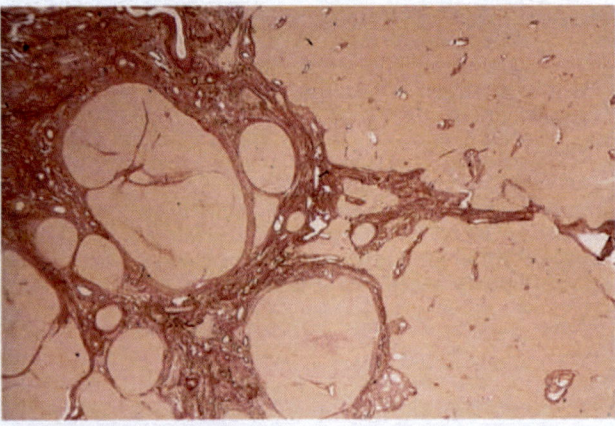

Figure 22.3 Focal nodular hyperplasia. Same case as Figure 22.2. This section shows the abrupt transition between the nodules surrounded by fibrous tissue septa on the right and the normal liver on the left. Elastic van Gieson.

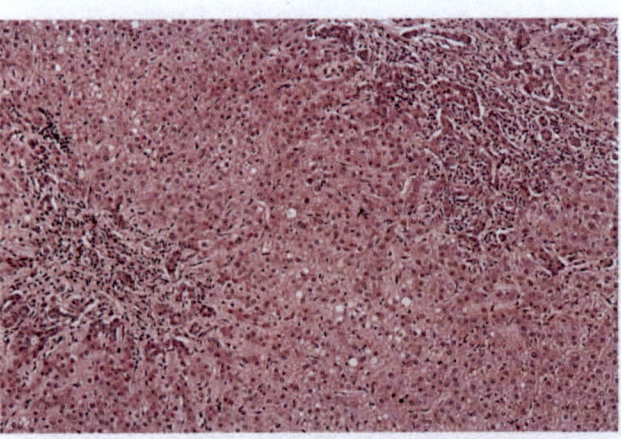

Figure 22.4 Focal nodular hyperplasia. A 35-year-old female in whom a partially pedunculated 4 cm nodule was found in the right lobe of the liver at laparotomy. The section shows rather crowded but otherwise normal hepatocytes with focal scars containing proliferating bile ductules.

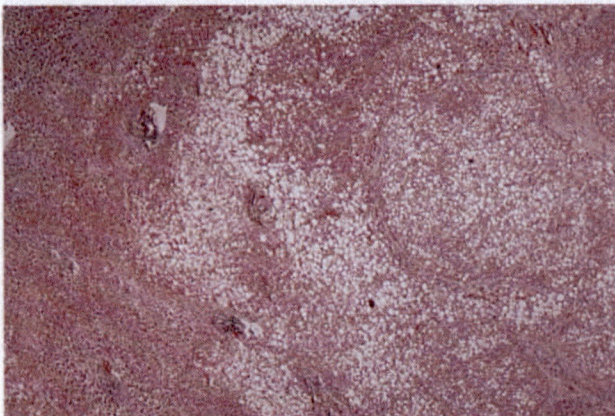

Figure 22.5 Focal nodular hyperplasia. Another lesion found at autopsy. This section shows a generally similar architecture, but in this case there is extensive fatty change confined to the hepatocytes of the nodule.

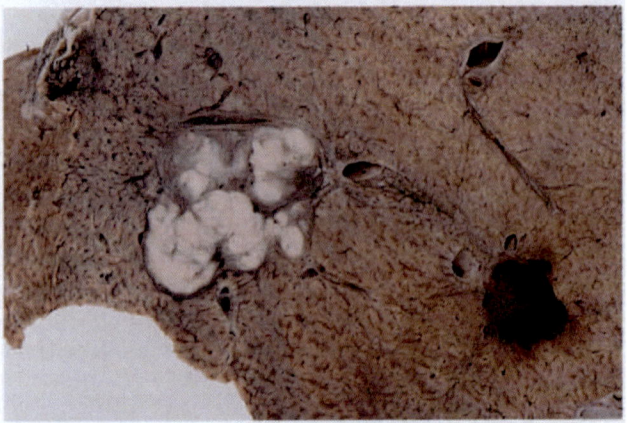

Figure 22.6 Focal nodular hyperplasia with coincidental haemangioma. Same case as Figure 22.2. This is a second lesion in the same liver.

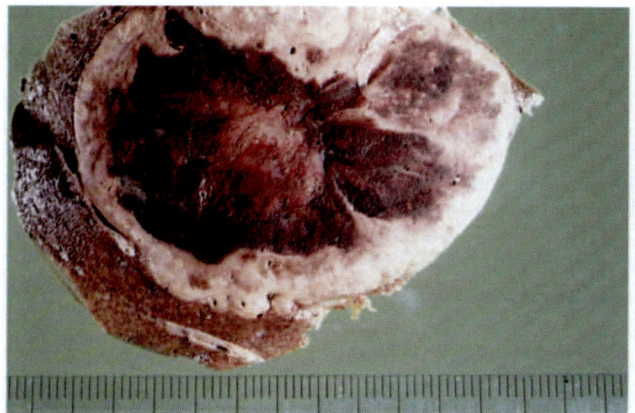

Figure 22.7 Liver cell adenoma. A 34-year-old woman presented with an acute abdomen and subsequently died following haemorrhage from this 10 cm LCA.
The author is deeply indebted to Dr I. D. Ansell who kindly supplied this photograph

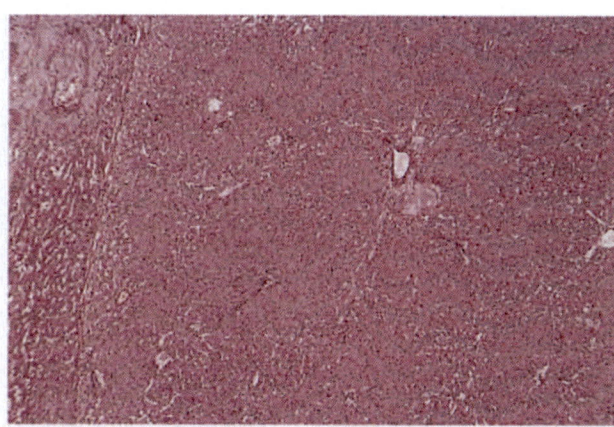

Figure 22.8 Liver cell adenoma. A 38-year-old female who presented as an acute abdominal emergency. Laparotomy revealed a 5 cm nodule at the surface of the liver which had ruptured causing peritoneal haemorrhage. The patient was taking oral contraceptives. The section shows compression of the normal liver (left margin) and that the lesion contains a number of vascular structures.

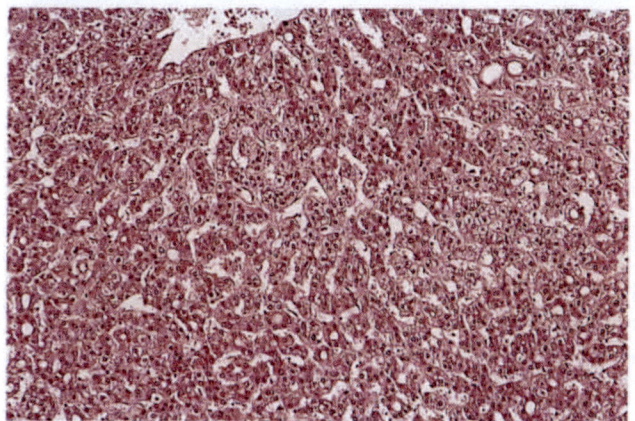

Figure 22.9 Liver cell adenoma. A 31-year-old female with a liver nodule found at laparotomy for recurrent abdominal pain. This section shows that the architecture of the liver cell plates closely resembles that of normal liver, although there is some irregularity in the form of thicker plates and a few rosette-like structures. No portal tract-like structures are visible.

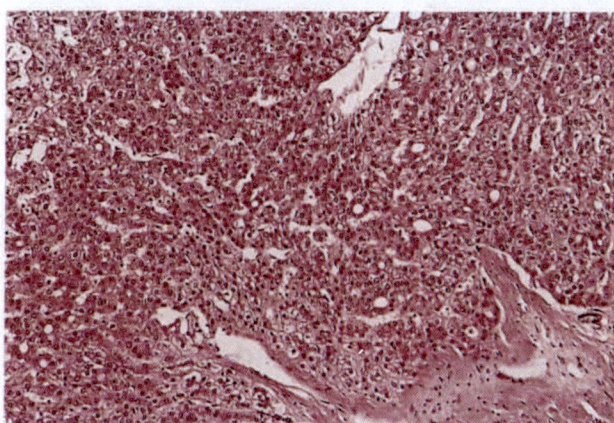

Figure 22.10 Liver cell adenoma. Same case as Figure 22.7. This section shows an area of scarring. Note, in contrast to focal nodular hyperplasia, that there are no bile ductules associated with this.

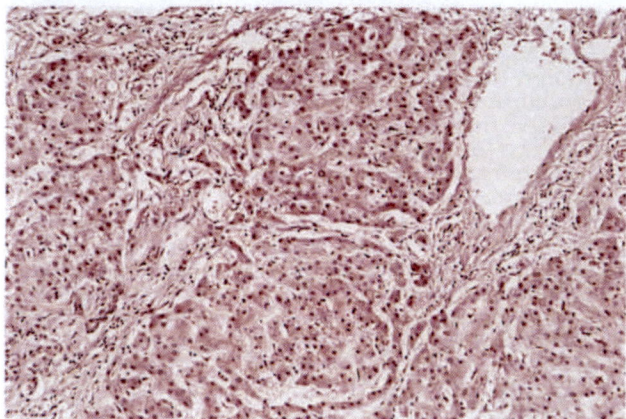

Figure 22.11 Nodular hyperplasia (adenomatous hyperplasia), anabolic steroids. A 17-year-old male with Fanconi's anaemia, treated for many years with anabolic steroids, developed a space-occupying lesion in the liver. Laparotomy was performed and this was subsequently shown to be an adenoma. The section is from the adjacent liver and this shows an irregular nodular hyperplasia. Compare nodular regenerative hyperplasia, Figure 22.12.

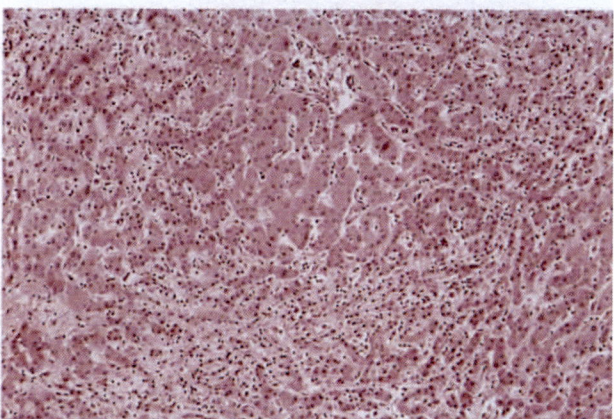

Figure 22.12 Nodular regenerative hyperplasia. A 75-year-old patient who died of haemorrhage from bleeding oesophageal varices. At post-mortem the liver was considered to be cirrhotic. Section, however, shows that the nodularity is non-cirrhotic. There is hyperplasia of periportal liver cells, with twin liver cell plates, and relative atrophy of the centrilobular hepatocytes.

contrast to FNH, the hepatocytes show some ultrastructural abnormalities which are mainly quantitative[13]. Mitochondria are of variable shape and reduced in number. SER is reduced and RER is distended. Bile canaliculi and junctional complexes are markedly reduced. Lipofuscin is absent.

Scattered throughout the nodules are numerous thin-walled vessels resembling terminal hepatic venules (Figure 22.10). Peliosis hepatis-like sinusoidal dilatation is seen occasionally within the tumours[14]. They sometimes contain a few areas of fibrosis, but these are never stellate or encircle nodules of liver and do not contain proliferating bile ductules or portal tract-like structures (Figure 22.10). Extramedullary haemopoiesis is sometimes seen in sinusoids. Like FNH, it can be difficult microscopically to detect the transition from LCA to normal liver at the border, particularly in biopsies.

LCA is occasionally found in children, but the great majority occur in women in the reproductive age group. There seems to be no doubt that there has been a definite increase in their incidence in the last 20–30 years and this has been linked with use of oral contraceptive and other steroid hormones (see below). Unlike FNH, adenomas are commonly symptomatic and abdominal pain and spontaneous rupture leading to haemoperitoneum are the commonest modes of presentation. Isotope scans and arteriography usually show a characteristic picture, but LCA cannot be distinguished from FNH with these techniques. Needle biopsy here too may be dangerous and once detected the treatment of choice is complete resection where possible because of the risk of malignant transformation[15] or that the lesion is malignant *ab initio*. There may be some problems in distinguishing LCA from well-differentiated hepatocellular carcinoma, a difficulty that seems to be particularly acute in the tumours related to anabolic steroids where a number of diagnoses have had to be revised.

The link between benign tumours and oral contraceptives

Since 1973, when Baum and her colleagues[16] first drew attention to a possible link with oral contraceptives, there has been an avalanche of reports and series all pursuing this possible relationship. Initially, both FNH and LCA appeared to be more frequent and also to be linked with oral contraceptive (OC) use. In pursuit of this link, there has been a distinct tendency for authors to publish cases in OC users only, without control data, and thus the figures may be misleading. Furthermore, the proportion of women in this age group in the USA, where most reports originate, who are taking contraceptive pills is very high and this may also lead to bias. Finally, not all authors have applied diagnostic criteria rigidly and so it is not always possible, in some of the earlier papers, to determine whether the description refers to FNH or to LCA[17]. Understandably there have been few large controlled trials – nevertheless, the following conclusions would appear to be justified:

1. Focal nodular hyperplasia was as common before the OC era as it is now[17]. There is, however, evidence that the tumours are larger and more likely to present with acute haemorrhage in OC users than non-users[18,19].

2. Adenomas of the liver were rare before the OC era but are now significantly more common[17,20]. Furthermore, there is a definite association between length of exposure to OC and development of adenoma[20]. This last group also found that adenomas were heavily loaded in favour of mestranol as the oestrogen

component. However, this may be no more than an expression of increased length of exposure, since mestranol was the oestrogen in the first pills to be marketed. The tumours are also larger and more likely to bleed in the pill-users than non-pill-users[17,18]. This had led several authors to suggest that one of the prime actions of the pill may be upon blood vessels and vascularity of the tumours, increasing the risk of rupture and haemorrhage (Figure 22.7)[17–19]. Additional evidence includes the fact that haemorrhage is occasionally associated with menstruation, pregnancy or the post-partum period and that sinusoidal dilatation, mostly periportal, has been observed in non-tumorous liver in a few patients taking these hormones[20,21].

3. HCC has been reported in users of oral contraceptives[22–24]. More significantly, apparently unequivocal evidence of malignant transformation has been seen in a number of benign tumours[18,25], but only in contraceptive-users. Foci of dysplasia, regarded as possibly pre-malignant, have also been seen in adenomas[26,27].

4. If OCs do increase the incidence of these tumours, the risk must be very low. Vessey and his colleagues have only found one case of FNH amongst their data covering over 300 000 woman-years in two contraceptive studies and all the hospital admission and death statistics over 5 years from two areas with a total population of over 6 million[28].

5. The results of animal experiments are generally inconclusive[29].

Male hormones and liver tumours

Anabolic/androgenic steroids give rise to cholestatic jaundice (Chapter 10), peliosis hepatis and liver cell tumours[30]. Peliosis hepatis, or cystic transformation of the liver parenchyma (Chapter 18) in this context, has been reviewed by Paradinas et al.[31]. These authors added 11 new cases of their own in which they noted sinusoidal dilatation affecting any part of the lobule, cyst formation, occasional liver cell acini and in nine cases, liver cells were observed within the lumina of central veins. The pathogenesis of peliosis is quite unknown, but Paradinas and his colleagues wondered whether this prolapse of hepatocytes into central veins and partial obliteration of their lumina might be causative.

Liver tumours associated with androgenic hormones were also reviewed by Paradinas et al.[31], who found 25 cases reported since 1965 in addition to their own. Most of these patients received steroids in the course of treatment of Fanconi's anaemia or aplastic anaemia. Although most of the reported tumours have been regarded as malignant, doubt has been cast upon this conclusion by several authors[31–33], since metastasis has only occurred in one case and several tumours have regressed after withdrawal of the drug. Furthermore, most of the supposedly malignant tumours do not produce alpha-fetoprotein[11]. They thus appear to be very similar to the liver cell adenomas discussed above. Sweeney and Evans[34] have described a diffuse nodular hyperplasia (*Adenomatous Hyperplasia*) in three patients receiving anabolic steroids which they felt was a precursor lesion of the adenoma comparable to the sequence induced in some experimental animals by carcinogens (Figure 22.11).

NODULAR REGENERATIVE HYPERPLASIA (NRH)

This term was coined by Steiner[35], who described a diffuse nodularity of the hepatic parenchyma resembling cirrhosis but without fibrous septa. The condition is often mistaken for cirrhosis macroscopically, but microscopically the nodules, usually smaller than the liver lobules, are surrounded by compressed liver cells rather than fibrous tissue. Within the nodules the liver cells appear morphologically normal, although they are usually arranged in plates two or more cells thick (Figure 22.12). In contrast, the liver cells between the nodules are smaller than normal and arranged in plates one cell thick with crowding of reticulin fibres (Figure 22.13). The nodules usually contain no vascular structures, but occasionally a small portal tract is found at the centre. Efferent venules are confined to the atrophic areas between nodules[36]. Portal tract fibrosis is common and the number of portal vein branches may be reduced or some may be replaced by telangiectatic vessels[36]. Most patients present with portal hypertension, often with oesophageal varices, and thus cirrhosis is suspected clinically. Needle biopsy may be confusing, since the nodules may not be evident[37], and thus the diagnosis is usually made by surgical biopsy or at autopsy. NRH is uncommon, but probably not as rare as the small number of reports in the literature would seem to suggest. Wanless et al.[38] found an incidence of 2.6% in a series of 2500 consecutive general hospital autopsies, many having been unsuspected in life. The commonest associated conditions are systemic vasculitis, polymyalgia rheumatica, massive tumour infiltration and mineral oil deposition[38]. Rheumatoid arthritis or Felty's syndrome, tuberculosis, and haematological disorders, particularly polycythaemia rubra vera are also regular associations. The pathogenesis of NRH is unknown, but Wanless and his colleagues suggest that it may follow reduced portal blood flow, which also causes both the portal hypertension and the splenomegaly. These authors provide morphometric evidence of a reduction in size and number of portal venous radicals within the liver, which they called obliterative portal venopathy, and suggest that in their cases this is most probably a consequence of multiple platelet emboli within the liver[36]. They further propose that the exact liver lesion may be determined by the site of the portal vein obstruction. Thus obstruction of the main portal vein might be the cause of partial nodular transformation (rather than a consequence) and obstruction of a small vessel might be the cause of FNH. Experimental portacaval anastomosis in rats produces a lesion very similar to NRH[39], providing support for this general hypothesis that deprivation of portal blood can lead to nodularity of the liver. However, others[40] take the view that the nodules might represent preneoplastic change that might potentially develop into adenomas and carcinomas (see *Micronodular Transformation* below).

PARTIAL NODULAR TRANSFORMATION (PNT)

Sherlock et al.[41] first used this term to describe four cases which presented with portal hypertension and a hepatic lesion characterized by non-cirrhotic nodules found grouped around the portal vessels at the hilum of the liver. Overall the liver was normal or reduced in size and the nodules were multiple. Several contained a central stellate scar, but there was no fibrous capsule and the margin was recognized histologically by compression of the adjacent liver cells. Within the lesions there was nodularity of liver cells with twinning of liver cell plates often centred upon portal tracts giving rise to an apparent reversed lobulation effect, closely resembling that seen in NRH. Although distinct macroscopically (Figure 22.14) the nodules were much less obvious microscopically and the relatively slight architectural disturbance might be undetectable in needle biopsy. A number of similar cases has subsequently been described[42], all having in common portal hypertension and nodularity of the liver, stopping short of total involvement. Several authors have suggested that the nodules caused the portal hypertension. However, where it was known, the liver weight in most cases was below normal and it seems at least as probable that the nodules might be a consequence of deprivation of portal blood as proposed in NRH. Indeed, the distinction from NRH appears to be principally one of degree, with partial nodular transformation apparently a localized form of NRH (Figure 22.15), and thus the two disorders may well represent different points on a spectrum, as proposed by Shedlofsky et al.[43] and more recently by Wanless[38].

MICRONODULAR TRANSFORMATION

Wanless has introduced a new classification of hepatic nodules together with a unifying hypothesis embracing all types of hepatic nodule, which in a very large autopsy study he found formed a continuous spectrum rather than being discrete entities[38]. His four major subdivisions are *Focal Atrophy Without Nodules* (Infarct of Zahn); *Nodular Transformation, Type 1 (ischaemic)* (which includes Nodular regenerative hyperplasia, partial nodular transformation/or macronodular transformation/adenomatous changes in incomplete septal cirrhosis and cirrhotic nodules); *Nodular Transformation, Type 2 (hyperaemic)* (which includes solitary and multiple focal nodular hyperplasia) and *Nodular Transformation, Type 3 (Neoplastic)* (which includes adenomatosis). This classification is important since it recognizes five major points: a) a spectrum of nodular transformation exists in which NRH is the most severe histological manifestation, b) Nodular transformation in NRH, incomplete cirrhosis and cirrhosis differ only in the amount of fibrosis, c) most cases can be divided into one of two groups depending on the size of the nodules, d) in some cases with large nodules the vascular abnormality may cause focal hyperaemia rather than ischaemia, e) some otherwise identical nodules may have a quite different mechanism, namely neoplasia. Distinction of the various types of nodule may be impossible in small biopsies[38].

VON MEYENBURG COMPLEXES

These are small (usually less than 0.5 cm in diameter), multiple, portal or periportal collections of bile ducts set in a fibrous stroma (Figure 22.16). The ducts usually have a dilated lumen, often with bile stained contents and are lined by cuboidal epithelium. They have variously been regarded as hamartomas, part of the spectrum of adult polycystic disease or a consequence of hepatic ischaemia[44].

BILE DUCT ADENOMA (CHOLANGIOMA, CHOLANGIOADENOMA)

These are rare tumours which invariably are incidental findings at laparotomy or necropsy[4]. They are more common in men and are usually less than 1 cm in diameter. Typically they are white in colour and are composed of branching bile duct-like structures which may be set in a dense fibrous stroma (Figure 22.17)[45] or the stroma may be relatively scanty. The lining cells are flat or low cuboidal and mitoses are not seen. Normal portal areas may be recognisable within the lesion. Associated inflammatory cells are often present. Intraluminal mucin secretion may be seen, but they do not contain bile, in contrast to von Meyenburg complexes (see below). It is not always possible to distinguish bile duct adenoma from metastatic adenocarcinoma or cholangiocarcinoma[14] with complete confidence, although in most cases the absence of pleomorphism and mitoses should indicate its benign nature.

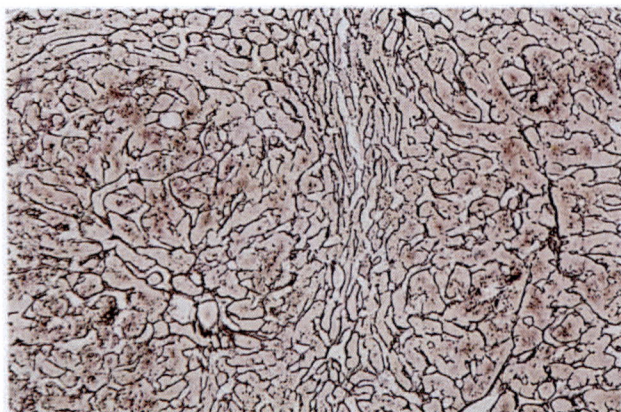

Figure 22.13 Nodular regenerative hyperplasia. Same case as Figure 22.12. Reticulin staining shows these features more clearly, demonstrating apparent compression of the centrilobular cells. Reticulin.

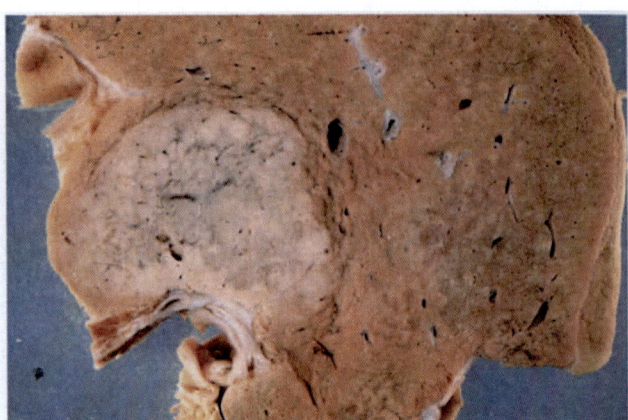

Figure 22.14 Partial nodular transformation. A 45-year-old female who presented with ascites. At autopsy, this 5 cm nodule was situated posteriorly at the hilum of the liver.

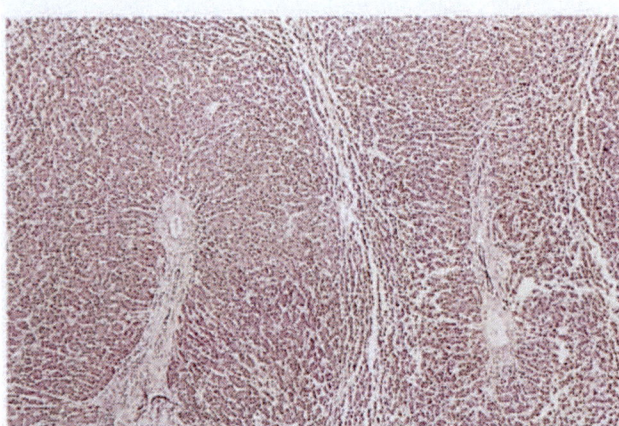

Figure 22.15 Partial nodular transformation. Same case as Figure 22.14. The section shows an appearance indistinguishable from that of nodular regenerative hyperplasia (compare Figures 22.12 and 22.13), but in this case the major part of the liver was histologically normal.

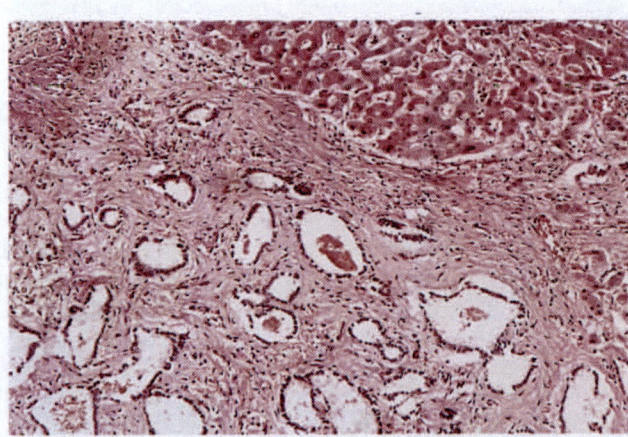

Figure 22.16 Von Meyenburg complex. Tiny miliary nodules were noted in the liver at autopsy in a patient with no other findings than myocardial infarction. The section shows a group of distended bile ducts, some containing bile, lined by attenuated epithelium and set in a fibrous stroma. Note the close resemblance to the liver lesion seen in some cases of adult polycystic disease of the kidney (Chapter 8).

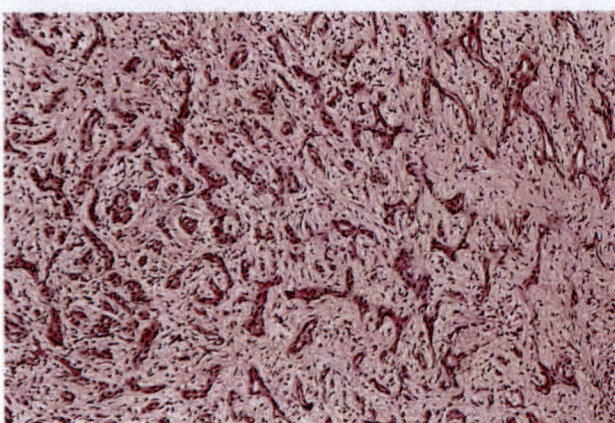

Figure 22.17 Bile duct adenoma. A 1 cm nodule noted in the liver during the course of an anterior resection operation for sigmoid colon adenocarcinoma, thought to be a metastasis. The section shows an anastomosing network of small bile ductules, set in a fibrous stroma. They are reminiscent of the atypical ductules seen in primary biliary cirrhosis. The patient is alive and well 8 years later and thus metastasis can be confidently discounted.

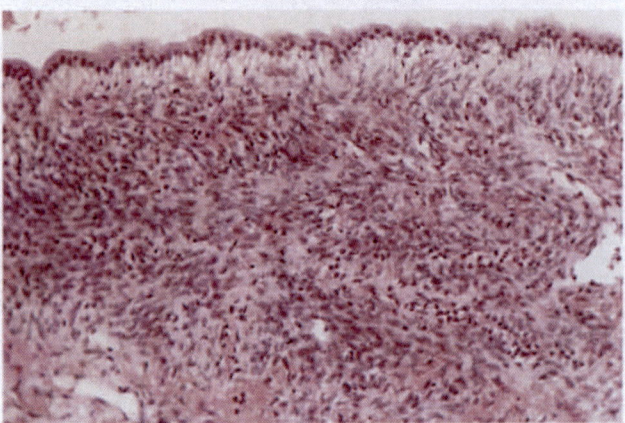

Figure 22.18 Bile duct cystadenoma with mesenchymal stroma. A 52-year-old female presented with abdominal pain and hepatomegaly. A 20 cm unilocular cyst was excised. Note the tall columnar epithelial lining and the mesenchymal stroma.

CYSTADENOMA

This tumour is considerably less common than bile duct adenoma, but is much more likely to present clinically, usually with vague symptoms of discomfort or abdominal pain[4]. Isotope and ultrasonic scans may reveal a filling defect, most often in the right lobe. The tumours are well defined and multilocular on section, ranging up to 20 cm in diameter. Microscopically there are two types of cystadenoma. One, called Cystadenoma with Mesenchymal Stroma[46], is found only in women has a cellular mesenchymal stroma resembling that in ovarian mucinous cystadenomas (Figure 22.19). Cystadenomas in men lack the distinctive stroma (Figures 22.20 and 22.21). Both types are lined by a mucin-producing cuboidal or columnar epithelium which may show papillary projections (Figures 22.19 and 22.21). Solid areas, dysplasia or capsular invasion all indicate malignant transformation[47].

HAEMANGIOMA

This is much the most common benign tumour of the liver[4] with a post mortem incidence of about 5%. It is found at all ages and in both sexes an is usually wholly asymptomatic/the majority being incidental findings are laparotomy or necropsy. They do, however, seem to be more likely to present clinically in females, suggesting a possible role of female hormones. Abdominal swelling, severe pain due to thrombosis or haemoperitoneum due to rupture, may all be encountered.

Most haemangiomas are solitary and less than 5 cm in diameter (Figures 22.6 and 22.21), although those which present clinically may be 30 cm or more in diameter (Figure 22.22). The latter are best demonstrated preoperatively by angiography. Macroscopically they are reddish-purple or black in colour and are well circumscribed but usually not encapsulated (Figures 22.6, 22.21 and 22.22). Microscopically they are composed of vascular spaces of varying size lined by endothelium and separated from one another by varying quantities of fibrous stroma, but no smooth muscle (Figure 22.23). Thrombosis, fibrosis and calcification are all commonly seen.

INFANTILE HAEMANGIOENDOTHELIOMA

This is another rare tumour but is probably the most common of the mesenchymal tumours of the liver in childhood[48]. About 90% are diagnosed in the first 6 months of life and the most common presentation is with congestive heart failure and hepatomegaly[49]. About half of the affected patients also have multiple cutaneous haemangiomas. The haemodynamic features are those of arteriovenous shunts and there are often associated haematological features such as anaemia, thrombocytopenia or leukocytosis.

The tumours may be solitary, when they are usually in the right lobe, or multiple and range in size from a few millimetres to over 15 cm in diameter. They have a spongy red-brown cut surface and the larger tumours may show central scarring with or without calcification and/or haemorrhage. Microscopically they are composed of vascular channels lined by plump endothelial cells supported by a variable amount of fibrous or myxoid stroma. There may be scattered bile ductules and foci of haemopoiesis. The endothelial cells may form a single layer (Type I) or be multilayered (Type II). The latter may show nuclear pleomorphism with occasional mitoses, thus mimicking haemangiosarcoma. In contrast to this entity, however, the margin is always well-defined, although usually not encapsulated.

The prognosis is variable and depends to a great extent on the size of the lesions. Many patients die in congestive heart failure, others of rupture with intraperitoneal haemorrhage. Surgical excision is only practicable if the lesion is solitary, but successes have been claimed with irradiation and hepatic artery ligation. Many of the less severe cases resolve spontaneously with progressive fibrosis from six months onwards[49].

MESENCHYMAL HAMARTOMA

These lesions are rare, only about 50 having been described, and are probably true hamartomas since they consist of elements normally present in the liver. They usually present with gradual abdominal enlargement in the first year of life. Clinically they must be distinguished from the more common retroperitoneal tumours, in contrast to which the prognosis is excellent with no recorded examples of recurrence after excision.

The size ranges from 1 to 25 cm in diameter and most are found in the right lobe. A significant proportion project from the anterior margin, thus facilitating surgical excision[50]. Macroscopically the tumours are gelatinous, almost fluctuant, with a cystic and weeping outer surface. There may be a capsule or the lesion may merge with normal liver.

Microscopically they consist of loose immature mesenchymal connective tissue composed of stellate cells embedded in an abundant mucopolysaccharide matrix[51]. The stroma may accumulate large quantities of fluid in cystic spaces suggestive of lymphangiomatous channels but without an endothelial lining. The fluid accumulation is probably the cause of the very rapid increase in size sometimes seen clinically. Bile duct structures, usually surrounded by a collar of mature collagen which merges with the mesenchyme, are scattered irregularly through the lesion (Figure 22.24). They may be morphologically normal or be branched and tortuous. Occasional small islands of liver cells or haematopoietic cells are also frequently found. Mitoses are not seen. Other Tumours Benign connective tissue tumours, such as fibroma, lipoma and leiomyoma, also occur in the liver. All are uncommon but are indistinguishable from similar tumours at other sites. Adrenal nests are also rarely seen.

REFERENCES

1. Butron Vila, M. M., Haot, J. and Desmet, V. J. (1980). Cholestatic features in nodular hyperplasia of the liver. Hum. Pathol., 11, 181–186

2. Knowles, D. M., Casarella, W. J., Johnson, P. M. and Wolff, M. (1978). The clinical radiologic, and pathologic characterization of benign hepatic neoplasms. Alleged association with oral contraceptives. Medicine (Baltimore), 57, 223–237

3. Stocker, J. T. and Ishak, K. G. (1981). Focal nodular hyperplasia of the liver: a study of 21 pediatric cases. Cancer, 48, 336–345

4. Ishak, K. G. (1988). Benign tumors and pseudotumors of the liver. Appl. Pathol., 6, 82–104

5. Moesner, J. (1977). Focal nodular hyperplasia of the liver. Possible influence of female reproductive steroids on the histological picture. Acta Path Microbiol Scand [A], 85, 113–121

6. Lough, J., Spicer, P. and Kinch, R. (1980). Focal nodular hyperplasia of the liver. EM study of vascular lesions. Hum Pathol, 11, 181–186

7. Wanless, I. R., Mawdsley, C. and Adams, R. (1985). On the pathogenesis of focal nodular hyperplasia of the liver. Hepatology, 5, 1194–1200

8. Mathieu, D., Zafrani, E. S., Anglade, M. C. and Dhumeaux, D. (1989). Association of focal nodular hyperplasia and hepatic hemangioma. Gastroenterology, 97, 154–157

9. Goldin, R. D. and Rose, D. S. (1990). Focal nodular hyperplasia of the liver associated with intracranial vascular malformations. Gut, 31, 554–555

10. Vecchio, F. M. (1988). Fibrolamellar carcinoma of the liver: a distinct entity within the hepatocellular tumors. A review. Appl Pathol, 6, 139–148

11. Paradinas, F. J. (1993). Liver tumours and tumour-like conditions. In Wight, D. G. D. (ed). Liver, Biliary Tract and Exocrine Pancreas.

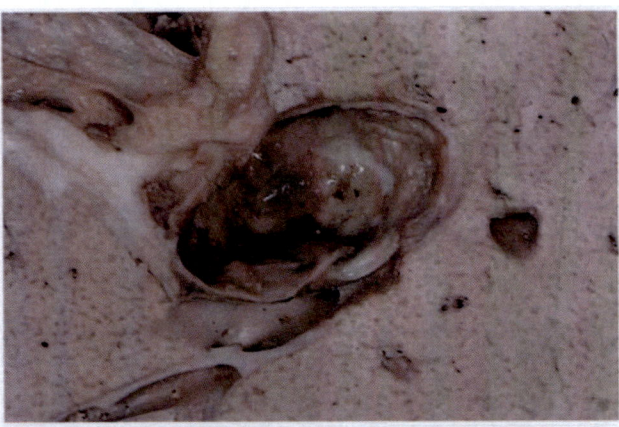

Figure 22.19 Bile duct cystadenoma (without mesenchymal stroma). A 36-year-old man presented with obstructive jaundice. This 5 cm cystic lesion was found at the hilum of the liver.
The author is deeply indebted to Dr Portmann who kindly supplied this photograph, and the slides from which Figure 22.20 was prepared.

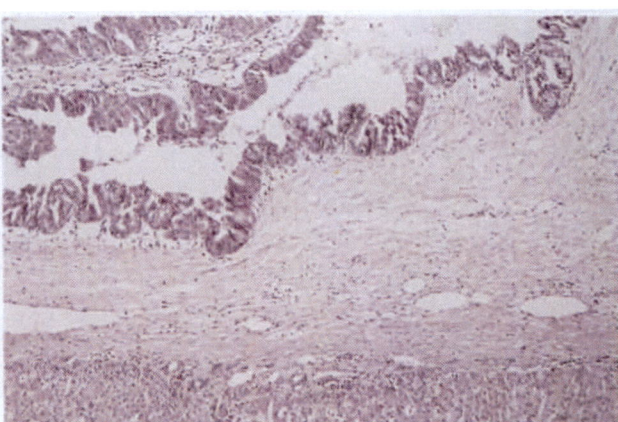

Figure 22.20 Bile duct cystadenoma (without mesenchymal stroma). Same case as Figure 22.19. The cyst is lined by tall columnar mucin-secreting epithelium showing numerous micropapillary projections. Note the plain fibrous stroma in this lesion from a male patient.

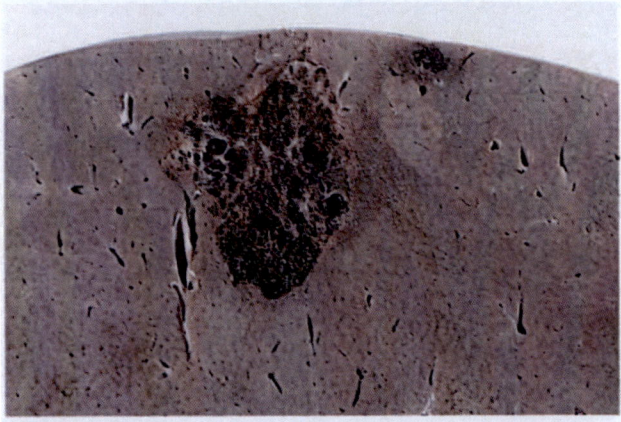

Figure 22.21 Haemangioma. Incidental finding at post-mortem. The liver section shows two subcapsular lesions, the larger about 2.5 cm in diameter, with a typical honeycomb cut surface.

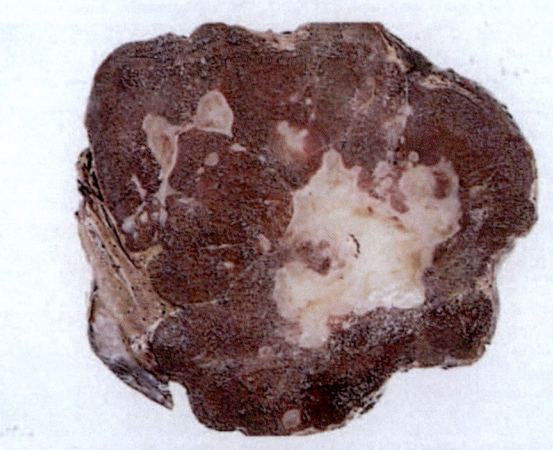

Figure 22.22 Giant haemangioma. A 34-year-old male presented with hepatomegaly. This solitary lesion in the left lobe of the liver measured 18 cm in diameter.

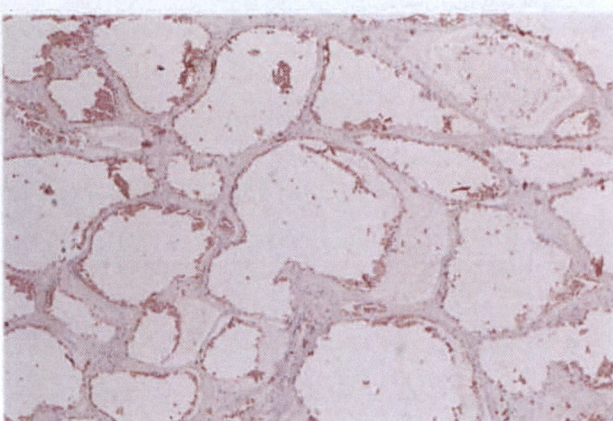

Figure 22.23 Haemangioma. Same case as Figure 22.21. The section shows a network of vascular spaces with a fibrous wall.

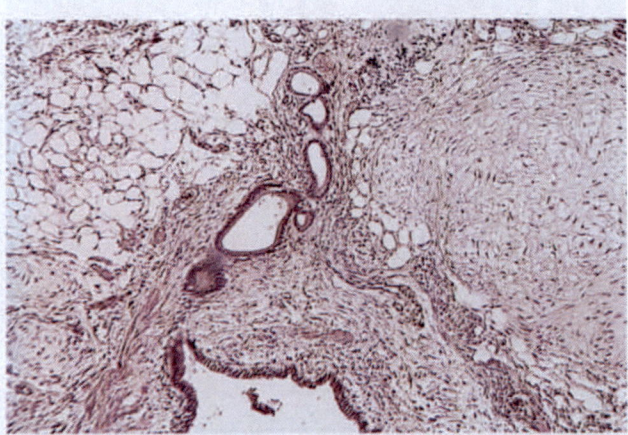

Figure 22.24 Mesenchymal hamartoma. A 1-year-old child presented with an abdominal mass which was found to be projecting from the inferior margin of the liver and measured 8 cm in diameter. Histologically the appearances were very varied, but this section shows the main components found. There are bile duct structures with smooth muscle, adipose tissue and (right) cartilage, all fully mature.

Vol. 11. Systemic Pathology. Symmers, W. S. C. Series ed. 3rd edn. Edinburgh: Churchill Livingstone

12. Brophy, C. M., Bock, J. F., West, A. B. and McKhann, C. F. (1989). Liver cell adenoma: diagnosis and treatment of a rare hepatic neoplastic process. Am J Gastroenterol, 84, 429–432

13. Phillips, M. J., Langer, B., Stone, R., Fisher, M. M. and Ritchie, S. (1973). Benign liver tumours, classification and ultrastructural pathology. Cancer, 32, 463–470

14. Gold, J. H., Guzman, I. J. and Rosai, J. (1978). Benign tumours of the liver. Pathological examination of 45 cases. Am J Clin Pathol, 70, 6–17

15. Craig, J. R., Peters, R. L. and Edmondson, H. A. (1989). Tumors of the liver and intrahepatic bile ducts. In Atlas of Tumour Pathology. Fascicle 26. Second series. Washington DC: AFIP

16. Baum, J. I., Holtz, F., Bookstein, J. J. and Klein, E. W. (1973). Possible association between benign hepatomas and oral contraceptives. Lancet, 1, 926–929

17. Fechner, R. E. (1977). Benign hepatic lesions and orally administered contraceptives. Report of seven cases and analysis of the literature. Hum Pathol, 8, 255–268

18. Klatskin, G. (1977). Hepatic tumours: possible relationship to use of oral contraceptives. Gastroenterology, 73, 386–394

19. Nime, F., Pickren, J. W., Vana, J., Aronoff, B. L., Baker, H. W. and P. M. G. (1979). Histology of liver tumours in oral contraceptive users observed during a national survey by American College of Surgeons Commission on Cancer. Cancer, 44, 1481–1489

20. Edmondson, H. A., Henderson, B. and Benton, B. (1975). Liver cell adenomas associated with use of oral contraceptives. N Engl J Med, 294, 470–472

21. Winkler, K. and Poulson, H. (1975). Liver disease with periportal sinusoidal dilatation. A possible complication to contraceptive steroids. Scand J Gastroenterol, 10, 699–704

22. Mays, E. T., Christofferson, W. M. and Williams, H. C. (1976). Hepatic changes in young women ingesting contraceptive steroids: hepatic haemorrhage and primary hepatic tumours. J Am Med Assoc, 235, 730–732

23. Glassberg, A. B. and Rosenbaum, E. H. (1976). Oral contraceptives and malignant hepatoma. Lancet, 1, 479

24. Tigano, F., Terlazzo, B. and Barrile, A. (1976). Oral contraceptives and malignant hepatoma. Lancet, 2, 196

25. Davis, M., Portmann, B., Searle, M., Wright, R. and Williams, R. (1975). Histological evidence of carcinoma in a hepatic tumour associated with oral contraceptives. Br. Med J, 4, 496–498

26. Galloway, S. J., Casarella, W. J., Lattes, R. and Seaman, W. B. (1975). Minimal deviation hepatoma: a new entity. Am J Roentgenol. Radium Ther Nucl Med, 125, 184–192

27. Goldfarb, S. (1976). Sex hormones and hepatic neoplasia. Cancer Res, 36, 2584–2588

28. Vessey, M. P., Kay, C. R., Baldwin, J. A., Clarke, J. A. and Macleod, I. B. (1977). Oral contraceptives and benign liver tumours. Br. Med. J., 1, 1064–1065

29. Heston, W. E., Vlahakis, G. and Desmukes, B. (1973). Effects of the antifertility drug Enovid in five strains of mice, with particular regard to carcinogenesis. J Natl Cancer Inst, 51, 209–224

30. Anthony, P. P. (1988). Liver tumours. Baillières Clin Gastroenterol, 2, 501–522

31. Paradinas, F. J., Bull, T. B., Westaby, D. and Murray-Lyon, I. M. (1977). Hyperplasia and prolapse of hepatocytes into hepatic veins during long-term methyl testosterone therapy: possible relationships of these changes to the development of peliosis hepatis and liver tumours. Histopathology, 1, 225–246

32. Anthony, P. P. (1975). Hepatoma associated with androgenic steroids. Lancet, 1, 685-686

33. Søe, K. L., Søe, M. and Gluud, C. (1992). Liver pathology associated with the use of anabolic-androgenic steroids. Liver, 12, 73–79

34. Sweeney, E. C. and Evans, D. J. (1976). Hepatic lesions in patients treated with synthetic anabolic steroids. J. Clin. Pathol., 29, 626–633

35. Steiner, P. E. (1959). Nodular regenerative hyperplasia of the liver. Am. J. Pathol., 35, 943–947

36. Wanless, I. R., Goodwin, T. A., Allen, F. and Feder, A. (1980). Nodular regenerative hyperplasia of the liver in haematologic disorders: a possible response to obliterative portal venopathy. A morphometric study of nine cases with an hypothesis on the pathogenesis. Medicine (Baltimore), 59, 367–369

37. Rougier, P., Degott, C., Rueff, B. and Benhamou, J.-P. (1978). Nodular regenerative hyperplasia of the liver. Report of six cases and review of the literature. Gastroenterology, 75, 169–172

38. Wanless, I. R. (1990). Micronodular transformation (nodular regenerative hyperplasia) of the liver: a report of 64 cases among 2,500 autopsies and a new classification of benign hepatocellular nodules. Hepatology, 11, 787–797

39. Weinbren, K. and Washington, S. L. A. (1976). Hyperplastic nodules after portacaval anastomosis in rats. Nature (London), 264, 440–442

40. Stromeyer, F. W. and Ishak, K. G. (1981). Nodular transformation (nodular 'regenerative' hyperplasia) of the liver. A clinicopathological study of 30 cases. Hum. Pathol., 12, 60–71

41. Sherlock, S., Feldman, C. A., Moran, B. and Scheuer, P. J. (1966). Partial nodular transformation of the liver with portal hypertension. Am. J. Med., 40, 195–203

42. Wanless, I. R., Lentz, J. S. and Roberts, E. A. (1985). Partial nodular transformation of the liver in an adult with persistent ductus venosus. Review with hypothesis on pathogenesis. Arch. Pathol. Lab. Med., 109, 427–432

43. Shedlofsky, S., Koehler, R. E., DeSchryver-Keckskemetir, K. and Alpers, D. H. (1980). Non-cirrhotic nodular transformation of the liver with portal hypertension. Clinical, angiographic and pathologic correlation. Gastroenterology, 79, 938–943

44. Popovsky, M. A., Costa, J. C. and Doppman, J. L. (1979). Meyenburg complexes of the liver and bile cysts as a consequence of hepatic ischaemia. Hum. Pathol., 10, 425–432

45. Allaire, G. S., Rabin, L., Ishak, K. G. and Sesterhenn, I. A. (1988). Bile duct adenoma. A study of 152 cases. Am. J. Surg. Pathol., 12, 708–715

46. Wheeler, D. A. and Edmondson, H. A. (1985). Cystadenoma with mesenchymal stroma (CMS) in the liver and bile ducts. A clinicopathologic study of 17 cases, 4 with malignant change. Cancer, 56, 1434–1445

47. Ishak, K. G., Willis, G. W., Cummins, S. D. and Bullock, A. A. (1977). Biliary cystadenoma and cystadeno-carcinoma. Cancer, 39, 322–338

48. Ishak, K. G. (1976). Primary hepatic tumours in childhood. In Popper, H. and Schaffner, F. (eds). Progr. Liver Dis. V. pp. 636–667. New York: Grune and Stratton

49. Holcomb, G. W., O'Neill, J. A., Mahboubi, S. and Bishop, H. C. (1988). Experience with hepatic hemangioendothelioma in infancy and childhood. J. Pediatr. Surg., 23, 661–666

50. Srouji, M. N., Chatten, J., Schulman, W. M., Ziegler, M. M. and Koop, C. E. (1978). Mesenchymal hamartoma of the liver in infants. Cancer, 2483–2489

51. Stocker, J. T. and Ishak, K. G. (1983). Mesenchymal hamartoma of the liver. Pediatr. Pathol., 1, 245–267

SECONDARY CARCINOMA

In Western societies tumour in the non-cirrhotic liver is much more likely to be secondary to primary sites such as breast, colon, stomach and lung than of hepatic origin[1]. Overall some 10% of unselected post-mortem livers contain metastatic tumour and, indeed, the liver is the most frequent site of blood-borne metastatic growths, being affected in up to 50% of all patients dying of malignant disease. Conversely when the liver is cirrhotic, some 10% can be expected to contain primary tumours, whilst metastases are seen with reduced frequency (in only about 1% if biliary cirrhosis is excluded[2]).

Macroscopically, metastases vary from one to two small nodules, barely visible, to massive replacement of one or both lobes of the liver, so that liver weights of 5000 g are not unusual. The tumour deposits are usually well-defined, roughly spherical in shape and white or off-white in colour. Central necrosis is common and it is this feature which gives rise to the characteristic umbilicated profile of tumour deposits at the surface of the liver. Suspected metastatic liver disease is one of the commonest indications for needle biopsies of the liver in general hospital practice. Blind needle biopsy can be expected to yield positive results in up to 75% of cases when there is overt hepatic involvement[3], but this decreases to as little as 20% when there is no clinical evidence of liver disease. The proportion of positive cases can be increased if the needle is aimed at a lesion which is palpable or directly visualized by computerized tomography, scintiscan or laparoscopy. Multiple punctures through a single skin puncture will also improve the yield, although this will certainly also increase the morbidity. Concomitant cytological examination of the aspirated fluid, together with a smear made by gently rubbing the core over a glass slide, may improve the detection rate by 15%, although this technique may have a small false-positive rate[4,5]. Step sections taken routinely will also help.

The interpretation of metastases frequently presents no difficulty. Tumours of the breast and bronchus can often be recognized as such, but secondary adenocarcinomas may be difficult to distinguish from primary tumours of bile duct origin. Occasionally metastatic tumour may mimic hepatocellular carcinoma when confined to liver cell plates[6] (Figures 23.1 and 23.2). Other potential problems in the interpretation of metastatic disease are shown in Figures 23.2–23.4.

Space-occupying lesions may sometimes be suspected even although not present in the biopsy. Samples taken from the vicinity of a tumour may show congestion, sinusoidal dilatation, Zahn's infarct or cholangitis. Morphological cholestasis in a non-jaundiced patient is particularly suggestive of a tumour elsewhere.

HEPATOCELLULAR CARCINOMA (HCC)

The term hepatoma, although well entrenched in everyday usage, is ambiguous since it is also applied (more correctly) to benign tumours and thus should always be qualified by a 'benign' or 'malignant' prefix, or better, not used at all. HCC is a malignant tumour of hepatocytes and accounts for some 70–85% of primary liver tumours in all parts of the world. Conversely, HCC is one of the commonest of all primary neoplasms in the world amongst men[7]. There is, however, a wide geographic variation in relative incidence, ranging from about 1% of all malignancies in the USA and western Europe to as much as 50% in parts of Africa. Thus it is 100 times as common in Mozambique as in Canada. There is a distinct male predominance, ranging from two to five times the incidence in females. In the West, older age groups are predominantly affected, but in those parts of the world where the tumour is common the age peak is between 35 and 44 years. The overall incidence in the West appears to be stable but has been increasing over the last 20 years in Japan[8]. There is a number of factors considered to be important in the aetiology of HCC.

(1) *Cirrhosis and chronic liver disease*. In all parts of the world the majority of cases of HCC are associated with cirrhosis, ranging from 65–70% in the West to over 90% in Africa. The percentage of patients with cirrhosis who also have HCC appears to be increasing in all parts of the world, but especially in Japan where it is currently about 80%[9]. Alcoholism is a frequent predisposing cause, but haemochromatosis, although itself rare, seems to have the highest risk, possibly because of the long survival of these patients. This view is supported by the observation that HCC is more likely to occur in the alcoholic who has stopped drinking[10]. The risk of HCC is also high in chronic tyrosinaemia and porphyria cutanea tarda, but low in a number of others such as α_1-antitrypsin deficiency, primary biliary cirrhosis and Wilson's disease[11]. The common feature in all types of cirrhosis is continuing liver cell damage which leads to active cell replication which increases the likelihood of mutational events, themselves probably caused by a variety of different mutagens[12].

(2) *Hepatitis B virus (HBV)*. Hepatitis B and the carrier state are both more common in parts of the world with a high incidence of HCC, where cirrhosis is also common. Up to 100% of patients with HCC in parts of Africa and the Far East have serological markers of HBV infection and there is a strong correlation with HBeAg and antibody to HBcAg, both markers of continuing disease activity[13,14]. Prospective studies have shown as much as a 200-fold increased risk of HCC in HBsAg-positive patients compared to matched negative controls[15]. Even in intermediate and low incidence areas, there seems to be a strong correlation between HCC and HBV. Thus if alcoholics were excluded, 73% of patients with HCC and cirrhosis in Los Angeles were found to be HBsAg-positive[16]. HBV DNA is regularly found integrated into the genome of liver cells[17]. However, the HBV genome does not carry an oncogene and integration is apparently random and often multiple. Recent evidence suggests that the product of the HBV X gene, which acts as a

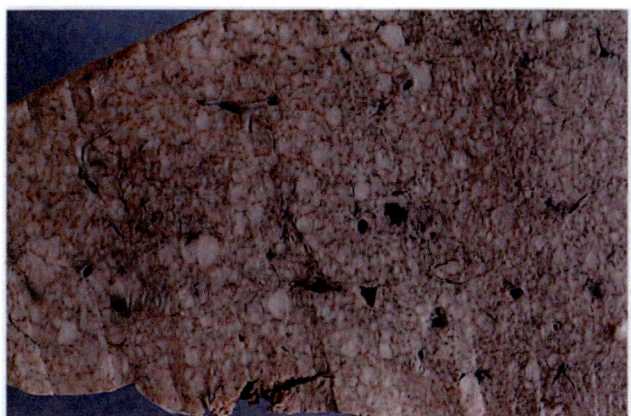

Figure 23.1 Metastatic carcinoma. A 56-year-old man with disseminated oat-cell carcinoma of the bronchus. At autopsy, liver involvement was so diffuse that it resembled a micronodular cirrhosis.

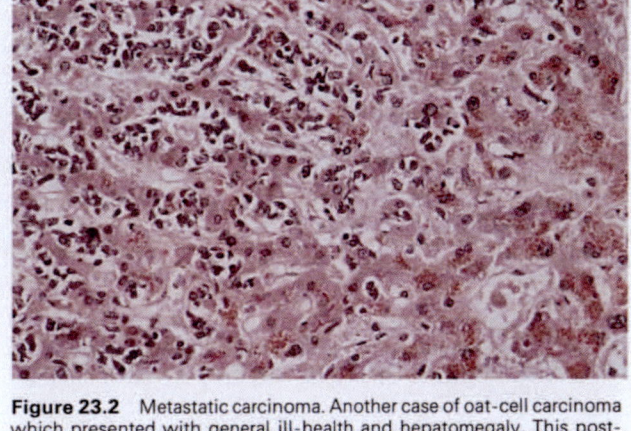

Figure 23.2 Metastatic carcinoma. Another case of oat-cell carcinoma which presented with general ill-health and hepatomegaly. This post-mortem section of liver sows, on the left, diffuse infiltration of sinusoids. Note the resemblance to leukaemia or even infectious mononucleosis, but here the tumour cells are infiltrating liver cell plates as well as sinusoids.

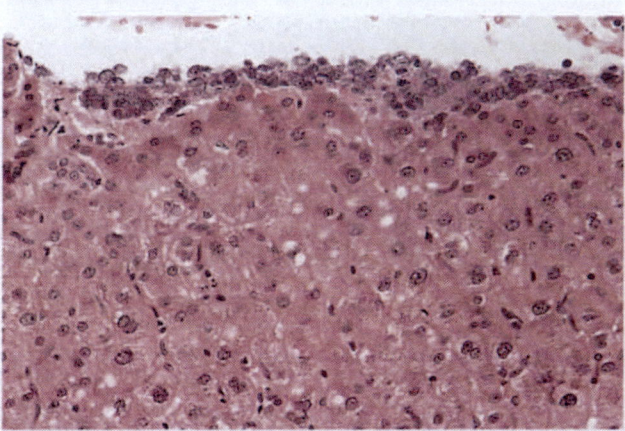

Figure 23.3 Metastatic carcinoma. Liver biopsy was performed as part of the investigation of pyrexia. The sections shows anaplastic carcinoma adherent to one margin of the needle biopsy. This type of appearance should always be interpreted with caution since it could easily represent carry-over from another specimen prior to processing. Deeper levels in this case showed the tumour to be an integral part of the biopsy.

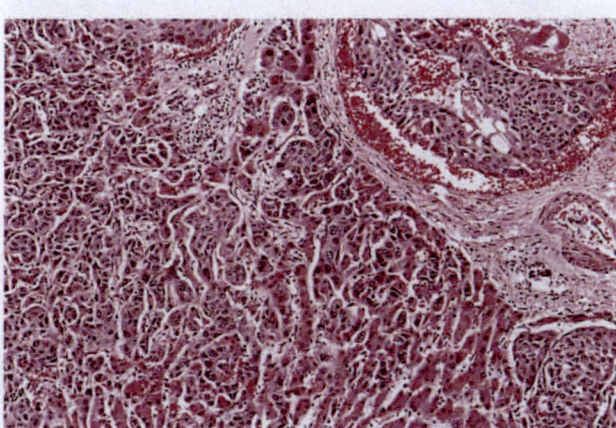

Figure 23.4 Metastatic carcinoma. Metastatic breast carcinoma in a post-mortem section. Although quite obvious in this section, note how in the centre of the field, the tumour cells, which are of similar size and staining properties as hepatocytes, have integrated into the liver cell plates. Infiltration of this kind can be confusing in needle biopsies.

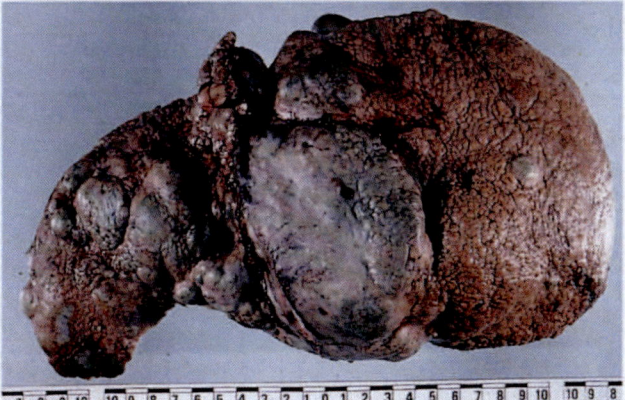

Figure 23.5 Hepatocellular carcinoma (nodular), micronodular cirrhosis. A 45-year-old male alcoholic who deteriorated rapidly. This view of the upper surface of the liver shows a nodular tumour, undoubtedly HCC because of its green colour, superimposed upon an established cirrhosis.

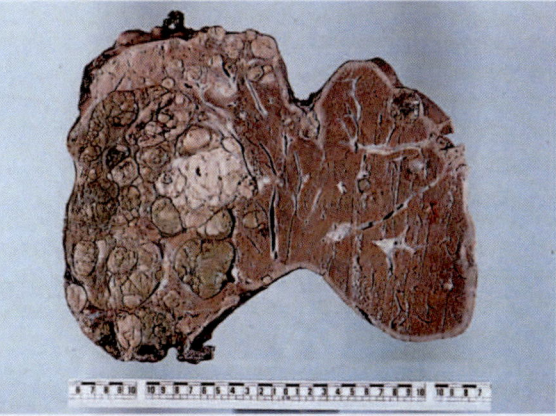

Figure 23.6 Hepatocellular carcinoma (massive). A 30-year-old female who presented with hepatomegaly, eventually treated by transplantation. The excised liver shows a massive tumour in the right lobe. Note that much of the tumour, as in Figure 23.5, is green, indicating the production of bile. The uninvolved liver is non-cirrhotic.

transcriptional transactivator of viral genes, may be the underlying carcinogen[18].

(3) *Hepatitis C virus (HCV)*. Shortly after the development of a method for detecting HCV infection it became apparent that many patients with HCC were positive[9], particularly in southern Europe and Japan. In contrast, HCV positivity amongst patients with HCC is low in those parts of the world where HBV is common (Africa and China). The mean interval between infection and the development of HCC is probably about 30 years[19]. The mechanism whereby hepatitis C might induce malignant transformation remains speculative. It seems unlikely that the virus is directly oncogenic, and thus it seems more probable that by causing chronic hepatitis it is responsible for active replication of hepatocytes and thus increased numbers of mutational events, as outlined above for cirrhosis.

(4) *Mycotoxins*. Aflatoxin, produced by species of the fungus *Aspergillus* is a common contaminant of staple foodstuffs in those parts of the world with a high incidence of HCC. A number of studies have shown an impressive positive correlation between the estimated daily intake of aflatoxin and the crude liver cancer rate in different parts of Africa and Thailand[20]. p53 is recognized as an important tumour suppressor gene, and mutations of the gene are at present the most commonly recognized genetic change in human cancer[21]. Recent work has shown a consistent mutation at the third base of codon 249 in the p53 gene on the short arm of chromosome 17 in 50% of cases of HCC from Chinese and southern African black patients[22]. Codon 249 is the preferred target of aflatoxin in experimental carcinogenesis, and thus mutations at this site may be an important marker of aflatoxin induced HCC.

(5) *Steroid hormones*. There appears to be definite link between synthetic male and female hormone exposure and liver cell tumours (Chapter 22). Most cases are reported as liver cell adenomas, but in a number of the cases of HCC in association with anabolic steroids, doubt has been cast on the diagnosis, in view of the apparently much longer survival than typical HCC and even regression of the tumours after withdrawal of the drug[23]. Of much greater significance, in view of the very large numbers of women taking oral contraceptive (OC) hormones, is the possible link between these and malignant tumours. Although there are a number of isolated case reports of HCC in OC users, a definite association awaits confirmation[24].

(6) *Other* rare associations include previous exposure to thorotrast, the bulk of which becomes localized in the liver[25].

HCC has a uniformly gloomy prognosis with the 5-year survival approaching zero. It is often regarded as having only a limited potential for spread, but lung, lymph node and peritoneal metastases may be found in up to 50% of cases[26]. Invasion of the major vessels and bile ducts within the liver is also common. Although the portal vein is more often invaded, HCC is well known for its occasional capacity to grow by continuity into the hepatic vein and inferior vena cava, even reaching the heart in rare instances.

Pathology

The liver is often vastly increased in size and is cirrhotic in the majority of cases (see above). In contrast to metastases, tumour nodules which bulge through the capsule are not umbilicated and, indeed, may be confused with cirrhotic nodules.

There have been various attempts to classify HCC on the basis of the macroscopic appearance[11,27,28]. Their value is limited since they are purely descriptive, but there are four main macroscopic patterns. The commonest of these is usually called *nodular or spreading* (most cases falling into Peters' *inductive group*[27]). The tumour is composed of multiple nodules of varying size, one of which is often larger than the others and may give the appearance of inducing neoplasia in the adjacent liver (Figure 23.5). Many of the smaller nodules actually represent tumour within vessels. *Massive* or *expanding* tumours show a single very large mass, which may or may not itself be nodular on section, which is well-defined and apparently compressing the surrounding liver (Figure 23.6). There is often a number of much smaller satellite tumours, apparently metastatic in the remaining liver. This is the commonest type observed in non-cirrhotic livers. *Diffuse* involvement of the liver is relatively uncommon and nearly always occurs in cirrhosis (Figures 23.7 and 23.8). Sometimes virtually every liver unit is involved, the tumour apparently arising simultaneously throughout. Neoplasia may even be overlooked because of the close resemblance of tumour nodules to cirrhotic nodules (Figures 23.7 and 23.8). A large proportion of diffuse tumours are attributable to alcohol. *Sclerosing* tumours form the least common group but are probably important to recognize because of their improved prognosis, the majority being *fibrolamellar carcinomas*[29] (see below). This group also may be associated with hypercalcaemia and pseudohyperparathyroidism (see Chapter 24) and the livers are usually not cirrhotic.

Tumour nodules are usually paler than normal liver and are often white or cream-coloured with varying degrees of haemorrhage and opaque foci of necrosis (Figure 23.7). About 10% of HCC are bile-producing and thus, in these cases, the tumour is distinctly yellow or more usually green in colour—a wholly pathognomonic appearance (Figures 23.5 and 23.6).

Microscopically the cells of HCC usually retain some resemblance to normal hepatocytes in the form of abundant cytoplasm, although often denser and more basophilic than normal, and a polyhedral shape (Figures 23.9 and 23.21). Nuclei are large and oval with peripheral condensation of chromatin and usually a large regular nucleolus (Figure 23.9). The degree of differentiation varies considerably, often within the same tumour. In some cases the tumour cells are so like normal liver that they are recognizable as tumour only by virtue of their growth pattern (Figure 23.21). At the other extreme tumour cells may resemble mesenchyme with poorly cohesive, larger, more primitive-looking nuclei and scarce cytoplasm.

Tumour nodules may be very well-defined, even with a capsule, and thus mimic cirrhosis (Figure 23.8). In other cases there is invasion of normal liver at the margin. Growth within portal and hepatic veins is common.

The growth pattern is most often trabecular, the *trabeculae* usually two to four cells thick separated by sinusoids lined by endothelial cells (Figure 23.10a). There are no basement membranes separating the tumour cells from sinusoids, and no Kupffer cells. Sometimes the trabeculae are so broad that the islands of tumour have a cobblestone appearance and may even resemble squamous carcinoma (Figure 23.9).

Acini and *pseudoglandular* formation are quite common. The spaces may be small and resemble bile canaliculi (Figure 23.10b) or much larger, lined by radially orientated cubical or columnar cells and filled with secretion, giving a thyroid-like appearance. Secretion is frequently PAS

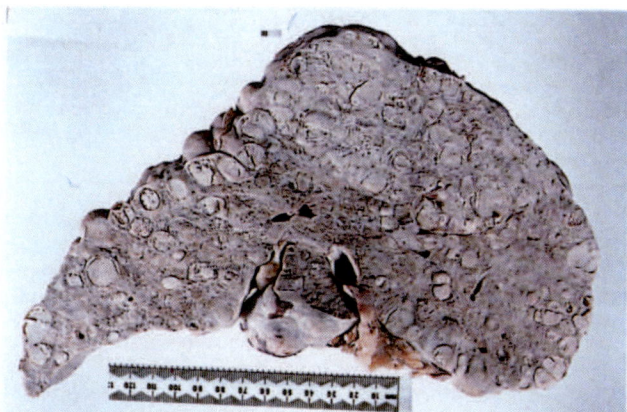

Figure 23.7 Hepatocellular carcinoma (diffuse). A 57-year-old male with known alcoholic cirrhosis died in hepatic failure. At autopsy, the liver was enlarged (4080 g) and had a macronodular capsular surface (lower right in this photograph). The cut surface too is coarsely nodular, but it can be appreciated that the larger white nodules are tumours and the background greenish-brown much smaller nodules represent pre-existing alcoholic cirrhosis. Compare with Figure 23.1.

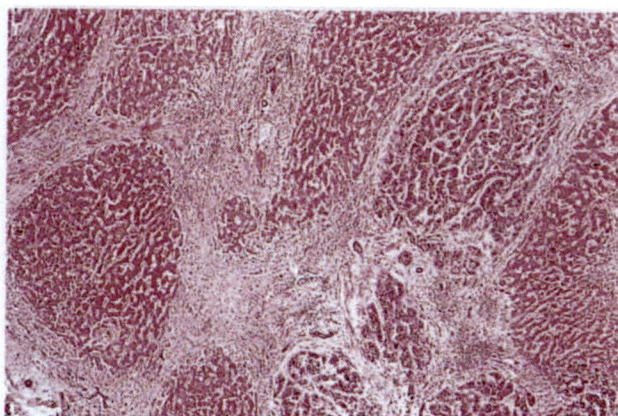

Figure 23.8 Hepatocellular carcinoma (diffuse). A similar case to that in Figure 23.7 showing a uniform micronodular cirrhosis. Closer inspection reveals that several of the nodules are composed of well differentiated HCC (e.g. upper right).

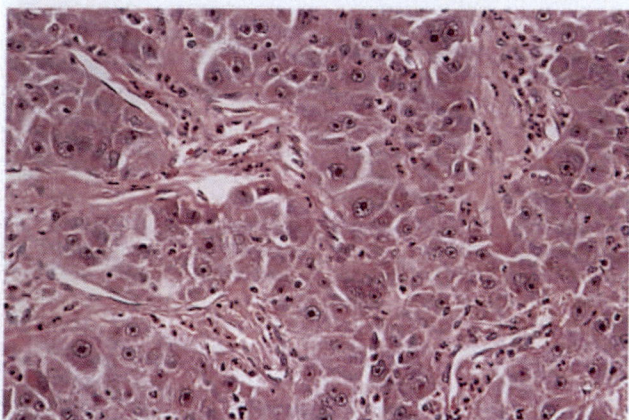

Figure 23.9 Hepatocellular carcinoma. Trabecular growth pattern; the malignant cells retain a general resemblance to hepatocytes. Note the large central nucleoli.

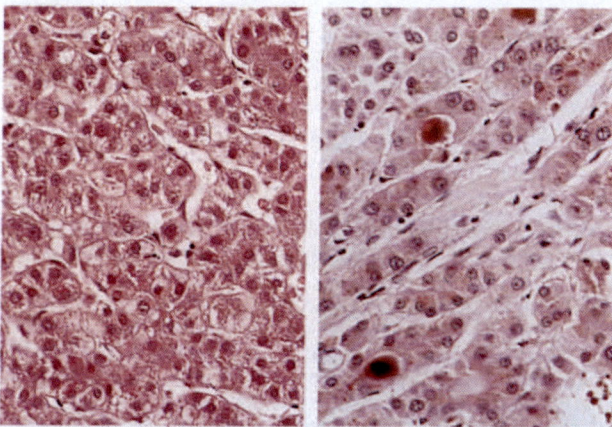

Figure 23.10a (*left*) Hepatocellular carcinoma. Predominantly trabecular growth pattern. Note the lack of pleomorphism and mitoses in this well-differentiated tumour.

Figure 23.10b (*right*) Hepatocellular carcinoma. Another well-differentiated tumour which shows many acini filled with bile.

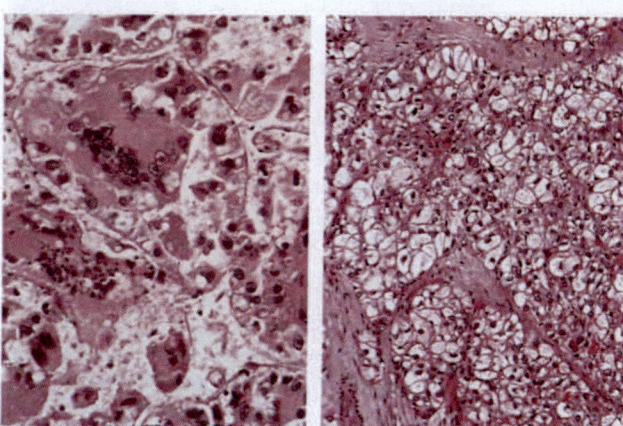

Figure 23.11a (*left*) Hepatocellular carcinoma. Variant with pleomorphic giant cells.

Figure 23.11b (*right*) Hepatocellular carcinoma. Variant with clear cells. Note the close resemblance to renal carcinoma, from which it cannot be distinguished with confidence, when solely of this pattern.

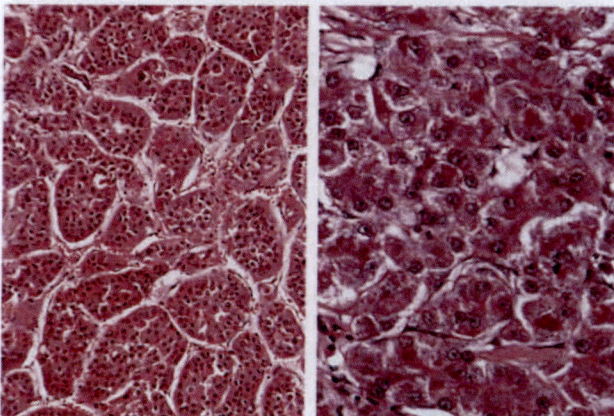

Figure 23.12a (*left*) Hepatocellular carcinoma, pseudopapillae. Note that each is composed of a solid mass of tumour cells and there is no stromal core.

Figure 23.12b (*right*) Hepatocellular carcinoma. Tumour cells containing clumped Mallory's hyaline. This patient was an alcoholic.

positive. Less commonly, bile is seen and it is much more often found in these well-differentiated cases (Figures 23.10b and 23.21), but becomes increasingly rare in the more anaplastic tumours. The presence of bile is pathognomonic of HCC.

Some 10–15% of cases contain one or more *pleomorphic giant cells* (Figure 23.11a). Rarely the tumour is completely composed of these, but in either case they are usually still recognizable as being of liver origin with abundant eosinophilic cytoplasm and the nuclei retain their nucleoli. Some tumours may be composed of spindle cells.

Some tumours contain *clear cells* which contain abundant glycogen and/or lipid (Figure 23.11b). These cells often retain the typical HCC nuclei and they may retain a distinct trabecular pattern of growth. Most tumours contain only focal areas of clear cell change with more typical morphology being seen in other parts, but occasionally it is diffuse, when distinction from metastatic renal carcinoma is difficult or impossible.

Pseudopapillae are found in some tumours (Figure 23.12a), especially the acinar types, but rarely true *papillae* may be seen.

Most tumours contain little or no connective tissue stroma, but, as described below, in a small number, the sclerosing tumours, this is well developed. Here it is composed of fibrillar bands of collagen and fibroblasts arranged in a lamellar and fascicular pattern in delicate bands between nests of tumour cells, a unique appearance which Peters calls fibrolamellar carcinoma (see below), an important variant because of its improved prognosis.

Other cytological features of HCC

Typical *Mallory's hyalin* is an occasional finding in tumour cells (Figure 23.12b), probably most often in association with alcoholism but certainly not confined to alcoholics[27]. Eosinophilic globular *hyaline bodies* of variable size but sometimes occupying most of the cytoplasm of tumour cells are an occasional finding (Figure 23.13a). These closely resemble the hyaline bodies seen in the liver in α_1-anti-trypsin (α_1AT) deficiency and, like these, are PAS-positive and diastase-resistant (Figure 23.13b). Immunocytochemical methods confirm that they are composed of α_1AT. Their presence bears no relationship to the α_1AT phenotype of the patient. Pale homogeneous cytoplasmic inclusions containing *fibrinogen* are found in some fibrolamellar tumours (Figure 23.18)[30]. None of these inclusions is specific for HCC, although they may be useful in diagnosis, and they merely indicate haphazard production or storage of liver proteins[27].

Some tumours contain *fat droplets*. Haemosiderin is distinctly unusual; indeed, new growth in haemochromatosis and in experimental models can be recognized by a relative lack of iron in tumour cells. Blood spaces resembling *peliosis hepatis* (Chapter 18) are occasionally seen within the tumour. As discussed above, hepatitis B Markers are commonly found in the blood and non-neoplastic liver of patients with HCC. Rather less commonly, HBsAg can be demonstrated by orcein staining[31] or immunoperoxidase[32], within tumour cells. Tumour cells do not contain HBcAg. Dark refractile granules of thorotrast may be seen in macrophages and lying extracellularly in the connective tissue stroma of non-neoplastic liver in cases attributable to this agent (Figure 23.14)[25].

Tumour markers

Carcinoembryonic antigen (CEA) and alpha-fetoprotein (AFP), commonly found in the blood, can also be detected immunocytochemically in tumour cells[32]. CEA outlines bile canaliculi in normal liver and HCC, producing a highly characteristic pattern which is unique for HCC[33]. AFP stains malignant cells diffusely, but very variably. Normal hepatocytes and HCC are consistently negative for low molecular weight cytokeratins (including 19), whilst normal bile duct epithelium, cholangiocarcinoma and metastatic adenocarcinomas are positive[34]. However, another study produced less definite results[35].

Preinvasive disease

Liver cell dysplasia may be found in a significant proportion of patients with HCC in Africa. First described by Anthony and colleagues[36] and defined as two- or three-fold cellular enlargement with striking nuclear pleomorphism and multinucleation of liver cells, it occurs in groups or in whole cirrhotic nodules (Figure 23.15). There appeared, in Uganda, to be a strong correlation with hepatitis B, but not all authors have confirmed this relationship[37]. It is also seen occasionally in HCC in non-alcoholic cirrhosis in the West. Since it is found in non-malignant livers at an earlier age than HCC, it is generally regarded as a premalignant condition.

Peters recognized *adenomatous hyperplasia* as a premalignant condition, especially in alcoholic cirrhosis[27]. Bulging nodules of active liver cell growth, composed of more regular cells in broader liver cell plates, may be seen in otherwise quiescent cirrhosis. These may subtly blend with early HCC[38]. This is closely analogous to the diffuse nodular hyperplasia in non-cirrhotic liver in patients treated with anabolic steroids (Chapter 22)[39]. *Macroregenerative nodules* (also called nodules of adenomatous hyperplasia), have been well documented in cirrhotic livers in Japan[40]. They are defined as nodules, usually but not exclusively in cirrhotic livers, which are larger than 1 cm in diameter and internally contain relatively intact architecture, including portal tracts. Their importance lies in the growing evidence that they may be precancerous[41].

Prognosis

Although various grading schemes have been devised for HCC, these seem to be poor predictors of behaviour[42]. There are, however, several clinical and pathological subtypes associated with improved prognosis, namely pedunculated HCC, fibrolamellar carcinoma and small HCC. *Pedunculated HCC* is probably no different from conventional HCC, except that it is more easily resected[11].

Fibrolamellar carcinoma

These are well-defined solitary nodules of tumour, usually in a non-cirrhotic liver, with a firm or hard consistency and often with a central scar resembling that seen in focal nodular hyperplasia (Figure 23.16)[43]. They affect a much younger age group, mean 23 years, and lack the usual male predominance. Berman et al.[29] noted concomitant FNH in a number of their cases and suggested that this tumour might therefore represent an intermediate stage between FNH and the more common malignant variants of HCC, although there is little evidence that this is more than a chance similarity of appearance. The characteristic fibrolamellar pattern, which defines this tumour, may be very focal. When fully developed, trabeculae of well-differentiated eosinophilic hepatocytes are separated from one another by lamellae of fibrous connective tissue (Figure 23.17). Possibly because the tumours are generally well-differentiated the tumour cells often contain inclusions of various types as described above (Figure 23.18)[44]. The prognosis of this group of tumours seems to be substantially better than that of typical HCC.

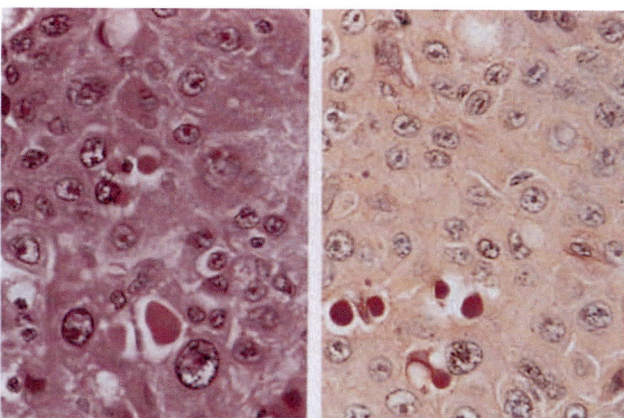

Figure 23.13a (*left*)   Hepatocellular carcinoma. This tumour contains a number of hyaline eosinophilic cytoplasmic globules.

Figure 23.13b (*right*)   Hepatocellular carcinoma. Same case as Figure 23.13a, showing that the globules are strongly PAS-positive. Note the close resemblance to the droplets seen in a₁ anti-trypsin deficiency. PAS diastase.

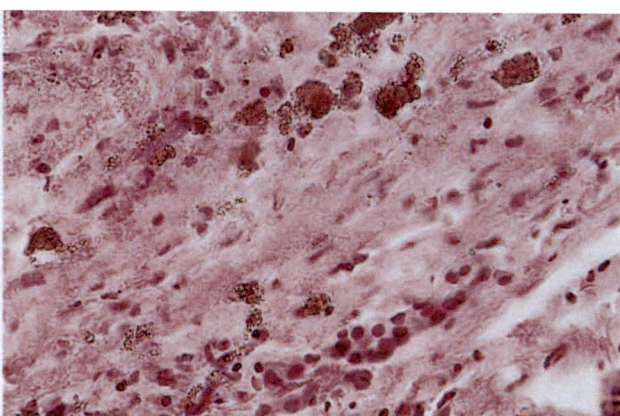

Figure 23.14   Thorotrast. This patient had thorotrast many years previously. The biopsy shows typical refractile granules embedded in fibrous tissue.

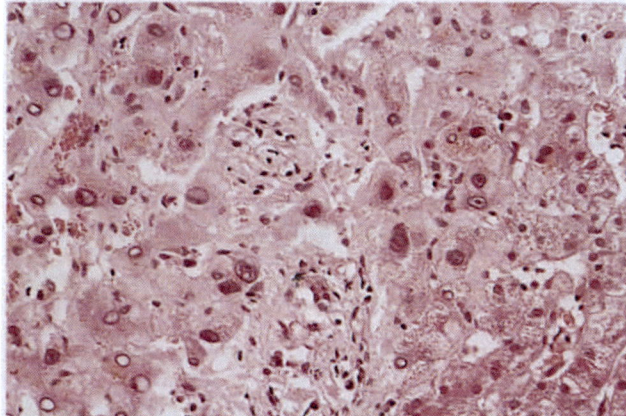

Figure 23.15   Liver cell dysplasia. A 40-year-old male with HBsAg-positive cirrhosis deteriorated, alpha-fetoprotein levels were raised in the blood, needle biopsy revealed HCC. This section shows nuclear and cytoplasmic pleomorphism in the uninvolved liver.

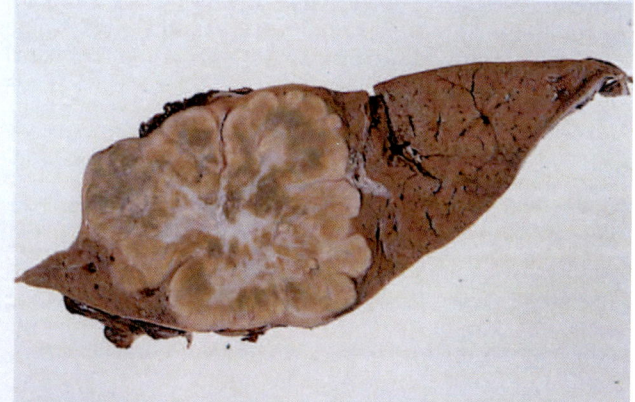

Figure 23.16   Fibrolamellar carcinoma. A 23-year-old female presented with abdominal swelling shown to be due to hepatomegaly. Resection of the left lobe revealed a solitary tumour in a non-cirrhotic liver. Note the central stellate scar and scalloped border resembling focal nodular hyperplasia. Note also the bile-staining, indicating a tumour of hepatocyte origin.

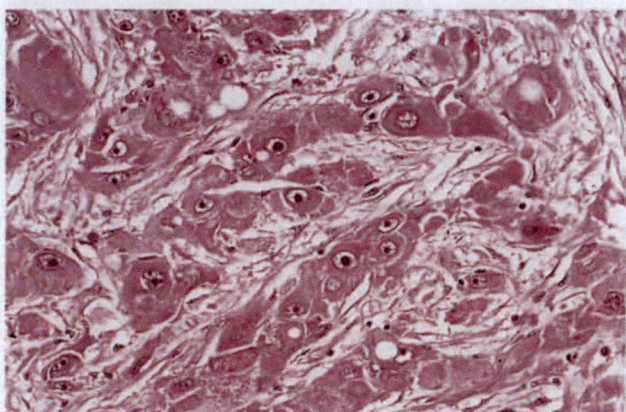

Figure 23.17   Fibrolamellar carcinoma. Another case. Note the distinctive appearance of trabeculae of well-differentiated eosinophilic hepatocyte–like tumour cells separated from one another by lamellae of fibrous tissue.

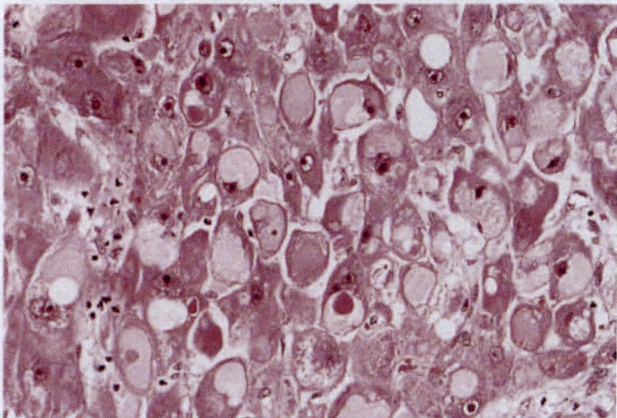

Figure 23.18   Fibrolamellar carcinoma. Same case as Figure 23.16, showing an area with no fibrous tissue. Instead, almost every tumour cell contains an inclusion/either large and pale consisting of fibrinogen, or smaller and eosinophilic and composed of α₁–anti-trypsin.

Small or early HCC

Screening programmes for HCC, especially in Japan, by using a combination of ultrasound examination and serum levels of AFP in patients at risk (i.e. mainly those with cirrhosis) reveal more and more small tumours. These are generally defined as less than 5 cm or 3 cm in diameter (Figure 23.19), and are associated with a better prognosis than typical HCC[9]. It is not clear whether these tumours differ in any other way than their size, but evidence is emerging that, in many cases, they may indeed represent a transitional stage between adenomatous hyperplasia and HCC[9]. Early changes were originally called *small cell dysplasia*[45], but follow-up studies suggest that this is really well differentiated HCC, and has been called *microtrabecular carcinoma*[46]. This can be recognized by the mean cell size and the nuclear cytoplasmic ratio, but this correlates well with the nuclear density as assessed morphometrically[46]; a density greater than 1.3 times normal being regarded as a marker of malignancy. Similar changes were reported by Nakanuma[38] as *atypical adenomatous hyperplasia*.

Diagnosis and differential diagnosis

In life, HCC may be suspected when there is a sudden deterioration in the condition of an otherwise stable cirrhotic patient. This may be associated with an obvious mass or enlargement of the liver. When the diagnosis is considered, confirmation may be obtained by a non-invasive technique such as serum AFP levels, or ultrasound or selenomethionine scintiscan. A tissue diagnosis is by no means always necessary, or indeed possible, in a patient with known chronic liver disease and deteriorating liver function.

The majority of cases of HCC are easily distinguished from other tumours on the basis of the resemblance of the tumour cells to normal hepatocytes, together with a trabecular growth pattern, in at least some part of the specimen. It may sometimes be difficult to distinguish a poorly differentiated tumour from metastases, and pure clear cell tumours can never be distinguished with confidence from metastatic renal carcinoma. HCC trabeculae have no basement membrane separating them from sinusoids. Similarly, acini and pseudoglandular formations have no basement membrane, which should serve to distinguish them from cholangiocarcinoma, metastatic adenocarcinoma or combined tumours. Reticulin stains may be of benefit here, since the trabecular framework in HCC contains little reticulin whilst the tumour cell cytoplasm and nuclei do become stained[47]. Immunostains, particularly antibodies to CEA and AFP as discussed above, may also be useful. It may be difficult or even impossible at times to distinguish between well-differentiated HCC and liver cell adenoma or adenomatous hyperplasia in cirrhosis.

HEPATOCELLULAR CARCINOMA IN CHILDHOOD

HCC is rare in childhood and when it does occur is often associated with pre-existing liver disease[48,49]. Giant cell hepatitis, hereditary tyrosinaemia (Figure 23.20), galactosaemia, glycogen storage disease and biliary atresia have all been implicated. Most affected children are over 5 years of age and the prognosis is very poor, with most being dead within 2 years of presentation. Morphologically, childhood HCC is indistinguishable from that seen in adults (Figure 23.21). Fibrolamellar carcinoma (see above) is occasionally seen in older children as well as young adults[49].

HEPATOBLASTOMA

This is the single most common malignant tumour of the liver in childhood[50], but is nevertheless rare when compared to other childhood neoplasms, accounting for only 0.2–5.8% of the total (excluding leukaemias and lymphomas)[48]. The majority of affected children are less than 2 years of age[51,52] and males exceed females in a ratio of 2.5:1. Most present with hepatomegaly which has to be distinguished clinically from the more common renal and adrenal masses. AFP is present in high titre in the blood in about 85% of cases.

Grossly the tumour is present as a single mass in 80% of cases, with slightly more in the right lobe than the left. It is usually roughly spherical and measures up to 17 cm in diameter (Figure 23.22). There may or may not be a capsule and many tumours have a bulging lobulated cut surface. The colour is usually tan to yellow to greyish-white, but occasional cases are bile-stained (Figure 23.22). A variegated cut surface with areas of necrosis and haemorrhage is particularly characteristic of mixed tumours. Grittiness due to spotty calcification is also occasionally encountered.

Microscopically, hepatoblastoma is generally classified into two groups–the *epithelial type* and the *mixed* epithelial and mesenchymal type. Typically *epithelial tumours*, which account for about half of all cases[11], have a capsule and are divided into irregular lobules by fibrous septa which contain both vascular channels and immature bile ducts. Four epithelial patterns have been described: fetal, embryonal, anaplastic and macrotrabecular[11]. The fetal type is recognizably of hepatic parenchymal origin (Figure 23.23) but the cells are rather smaller than normal liver cells, and have a slightly increased nuclear to cytoplasmic ratio. They tend to be arranged in irregular plates two cells thick with bile canaliculi between cells. The sinusoids are lined by endothelial cells, without Kupffer cells, and the reticulin framework is very poorly developed. The cytoplasm is eosinophilic and granular, or may contain glycogen, fat or bile. Pleomorphism and mitotic figures are rare. Foci of extramedullary haemopoiesis (EMH) in sinusoids are almost invariably found (in contrast to the uninvolved parenchyma where EMH is hardly ever seen)[51]. The second type of cell, seen in about half of the epithelial hepatoblastomas, is termed the embryonal type (Figure 23.23) because of the resemblance to even more primitive hepatocytes. These cells are elongated, smaller and darker with relatively larger nuclei and arranged in ribbons or gland-like formations. Large vascular spaces lined by neoplastic cells are occasionally seen in these areas. Mitotic activity is much more frequent than in fetal type cells. The anaplastic or small-cell pattern is composed of cells with little resemblance to hepatocytes. The last type, macrotrabecular, is impossible to differentiate from HCC in the absence of other patterns.

Mixed hepatoblastomas, which account for the other half of all cases, contain, in addition to the fetal and embryonal type cells described above, mesenchymal elements (Figure 23.24). These include areas of highly cellular primitive mesenchyme, which may merge with the mature connective tissue septa, as well as foci of osteoid and cartilage. Squamous epithelial pearls are also an occasional finding. Both types of hepatoblastoma may show microscopic vascular invasion. Distant metastases are found most often in the lungs and in the abdominal lymph nodes. The metastases, when present, rarely contain mesenchymal elements. Although these tumours often grow rapidly and metastasize early, resection of an affected lobe is occasionally followed by long-term cure, in contrast to the experience in childhood HCC.

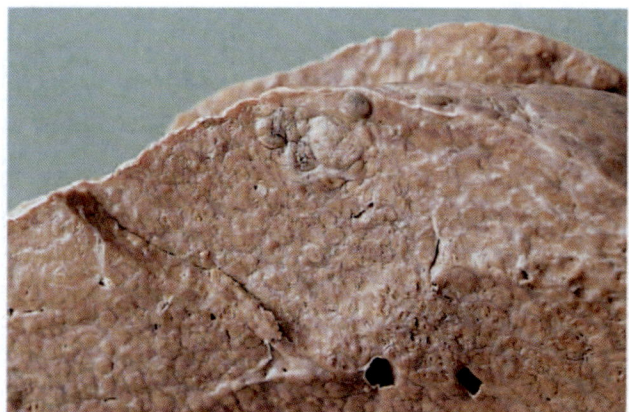

Figure 23.19 Small hepatocellular carcinoma. An incidental finding in a patient with alcoholic cirrhosis who died following haemorrhage from oesophageal varices. Note the tiny green tumour which measured less than 2 cm in diameter.

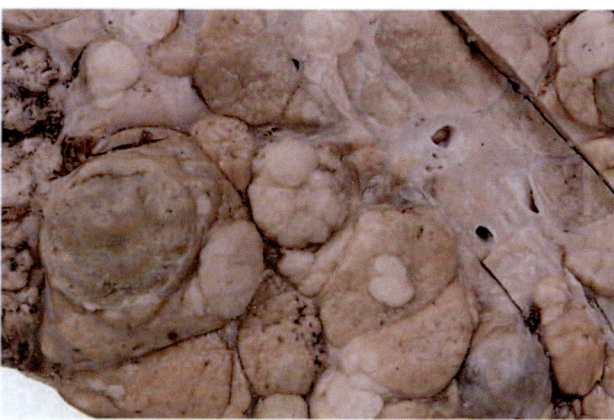

Figure 23.20 Childhood hepatocellular carcinoma. A 4-year-old girl received a liver transplant for hereditary tyrosinaemia. Most of the pale and green nodules represent HCC on a background of cirrhosis.

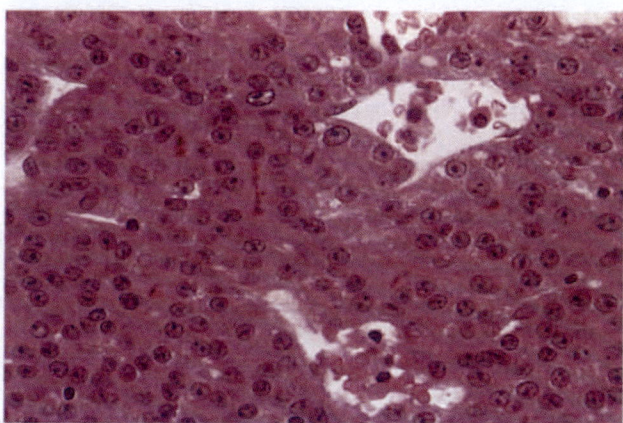

Figure 23.21 Childhood hepatocellular carcinoma. A 4-year-old child who presented with hepatomegaly. Note the very close resemblance of these tumour cells to normal hepatocytes, with bile visible in a number of canaliculi. The arrangement is obviously abnormal with solid masses of cells instead of normal liver cell plates.

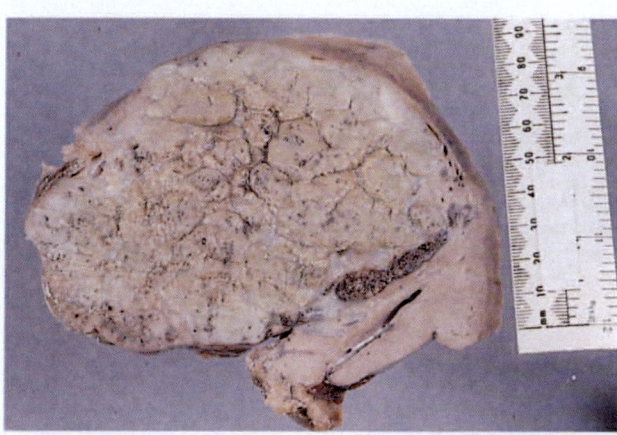

Figure 23.22 Hepatoblastoma. A 1-year-old child who also presented with hepatomegaly. Lobectomy was performed and the tumour can be seen to be occupying much of the lobe. Note the light green colour, indicating the presence of bile and thus its hepatocellular origin.

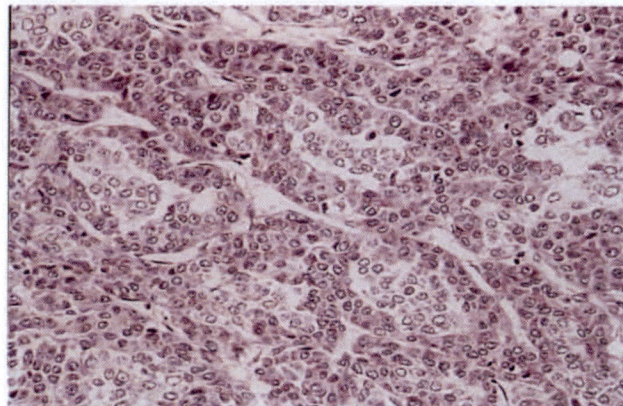

Figure 23.23 Hepatoblastoma (epithelial). Same case as Figure 23.22. The section shows two types of cell present. The larger ones arranged in trabeculae resemble normal fetal liver with a central nucleus and eosinophilic cytoplasm. The smaller embryonal cells in clumps have paler nuclei and little or no cytoplasm.

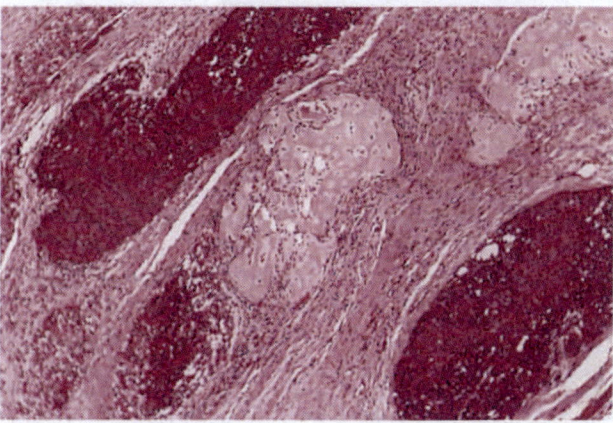

Figure 23.24 Hepatoblastoma, mixed type. Note the central islands of cartilage as well as the darkly-stained epithelial cells in this tumour from a 2-year-old child.

Diagnosis

The main differential diagnosis of hepatoblastoma is from HCC. The presence of more than one cell type, the small size of the neoplastic liver cells, which show little pleomorphism, few mitoses and no tumour giant cells, together with the presence of extramedullary haemopoiesis, should serve to make the distinction quite easy in most cases. Metastases from tumours, such as neuroblastoma, should be readily distinguishable on morphological grounds, as well as by clinical and biochemical parameters

REFERENCES

1. Craig, J. R., Peters, R. L. and Edmondson, H. A. (1989). Tumors of the liver and intrahepatic bile ducts. In Atlas of Tumour Pathology. Fascicle 26. Second series. Washington DC: AFIP
2. Gall, E. A. (1960). Primary and metastatic carcinoma of the liver. Relationship to hepatic cirrhosis. Arch. Pathol., 70, 226–232
3. Fenster, L. F. and Klatskin, G. (1961). Manifestations of metastatic tumours of the liver. A study of 81 patients subjected to needle biopsy. Am. J. Med., 31, 238–248
4. Grossman, E., Goldstein, M. J., Koss, L. G., Winawer, S. J. and Sherlock, P. (1972). Cytological examination as an adjunct to liver biopsy in diagnosis of hepatic metastases. Gastroenterology, 62, 56–60
5. Herbury, C. E. A., Enriquez, R. E., Desuto-Nagy, G. I. and Cann, H. O. (1979). Comparison of histologic and cytologic diagnosis of liver biopsies in hepatic cancer. Gastroenterology, 76, 1352–1357
6. Scheuer, P. J. (1988). Neoplasms and nodules. In Liver Biopsy Interpretation. 4th edn. pp. 147–172. London: Baillière Tindall
7. Parkin, D. M., Stjernsward, J. and Muir, C. S. (1984). Estimates of the worldwide frequency of twelve major cancers. Bull. WHO, 62, 163–182
8. Muñoz, N. and Bosch, X. (1987). Epidemiology of hepatocellular carcinoma. In Okuda, K. and Ishak, K. G. (eds). Neoplasms of the Liver., pp. 3–19. Tokyo: Springer-Verlag
9. Okuda, K. (1992). Hepatocellular carcinoma: recent progress. Hepatology., 15, 948–963
10. Lee, F. I. (1966). Cirrhosis and hepatoma in alcoholics. Gut, 7, 77–85
11. Paradinas, F. J. (1993). Liver tumours and tumour-like conditions. In Wight, D. G. D. (ed.). Liver, Biliary Tract and Exocrine Pancreas. Vol. 11. Systemic Pathology. Symmers, W. S. C., series ed. 3rd edn. Edinburgh: Churchill Livingstone
12. Berman, J. J. (1988). Cell proliferation and the aetiology of hepatocellular carcinoma. J. Hepatol., 7, 305–309
13. Sumithran, E. and MacSween, R. N. M. (1979). An appraisal of the relationship between primary hepatocellular carcinoma and hepatitis B. Histopathology, 3, 447–458
14. Hsu, H. C., Wu, M. Z., Chang, M. H., Su, I. J. and Chen, D. S. (1987). Childhood hepatocellular carcinoma develops exclusively in hepatitis B surface antigen carriers in three decades in Taiwan. Report of 51 cases strongly associated with the rapid development of liver cirrhosis. J. Hepatol., 5, 260–267
15. Beasley, R. P. (1988). Hepatitis B virus. The major etiology of hepatocellular carcinoma. Cancer., 61, 1942–1956
16. Peters, R. L., Afrondakis, A. P. and Tatler, D. (1977). The changing incidence of association of hepatitis B with hepatocellular carcinoma in California. Am. J. Clin. Pathol., 68, 1–7
17. Matsubara, K. (1991). Chromsomal changes associated with hepatitis B virus DNA integration and hepatic carcinogenesis. In McLachlan, A. (ed.). Molecular biology of the hepatitis B virus. pp. 245–261. Boca Raton: CRC Press
18. Kim, C.-M., Koike, K., Saito, I., Miyamura, T. and Jay, G. (1991). HBx gene of hepatitis-B virus induces liver cancer in transgenic mice. Nature, 351, 317–320
19. Kiyosawa, K., Sodeyama, T., Tanaka, E., Gibo, Y., Yoshizawa, K., Nakano, Y., Furuta, S. et al. (1990). Interrelationship of blood transfusion, non-A, non-B hepatitis and hepatocellular carcinoma: analysis by detection of antibody to hepatitis C virus. Hepatology, 12, 671–675
20. Linsell, C. A. and Peers, F. G. (1977). Aflatoxin and liver cell cancer. Trans. R. Soc. Trop. Med. Hyg., 71, 471–473
21. Kew, M. C. (1992). Cancer of the liver. Curr. Opin. Gastroenterol., 8, 474–480
22. Hsu, I. C., Metcalf, R. A., Sun, T., Welsh, J. A., Wang, N. J. and Harris, C. C. (1991). Mutational hotspot in the p53 gene in human hepatocellular carcinoma. Nature, 350, 427–428
23. Anthony, P. P. (1975). Liver tumours and steroid hormones. Lancet, 1, 685–686
24. Goodman, Z. D. and Ishak, K. G. (1982). Hepatocellular carcinoma in women: proable lack of etiologic association with oral contraceptive steroids. Hepatology, 2, 440–444
25. Battifora, H. A. (1976). Thorotrast and tumours of the liver. In Okuda, K. and Peters, R. L. (eds). Hepatocellular carcinoma, pp. 83–93. New York: John Wiley and Sons
26. Mori, W., Machinami, R. and Tanaka, K. (1980). Pathology of hepatocellular carcinoma. Pathol. Res. Pract., 169, 4–20
27. Peters, R. L. (1976). Pathology of hepatocellular carcinoma. In Okuda, K. and Peters, R. L. (eds). Hepatocellular carcinoma, pp. 107–168. New York: John Wiley
28. Okuda, K., Peters, R. L. and Simson, J. W. (1984). Gross anatomic features of hepatocellular carcinoma from three disparate geographic areas. Proposal of new classification. Cancer, 54, 2165–2173
29. Berman, M. M., Libbey, N. P. and Foster, J. H. (1980). Hepatocellular carcinoma. Polygonal cell type with fibrous stroma an atypical variant with a favourable prognosis. Cancer, 46, 1448–1455
30. Stromeyer, F. W., Ishak, K. G., Gerber, M. A. and Mathew, T. (1980). Ground-glass cells in hepatocellular carcinoma. Am. J. Clin. Pathol., 74, 254–258
31. Ilardi, C. F., Ying, Y. Y., Ackerman, L. V. and Elias, J. M. (1980). HBsAg and HCC in the People's Republic of China. Cancer, 46, 1612–1616
32. Thung, S. N., Gerber, M. A., Sarno, E. and Popper, H. (1979). Distribution of five antigens in hepatocellular carcinoma. Lab. Invest., 41, 101–105
33. Christensen, W. N., Boitnott, J. K. and Kuhjada, F. P. (1989). Immunoperoxidase staining as a diagnostic aid for hepatocellular carcinoma. Mod. Pathol., 2, 8–12
34. Johnson, D. E., Herndier, B. G., Medeiros, L. J., Warnke, R. A. and Rouse, R. V. (1988). The diagnostic utility of the keratin profiles of hepatocellular carcinoma and cholangiocarcinoma. Am. J. Surg. Pathol., 12, 187–197
35. van Eyken, P., Sciot, R. A. F., Paterson, A., Callea, F., Kew, M. C. and Desmet, V. J. (1988). Cytokeratin expression in hepatocellular carcinoma: an immunohistochemical study. Hum. Pathol., 19, 562–568
36. Anthony, P. P., Vogel, C. L. and Barker, L. F. (1973). Liver cell dysplasia: a pre-malignant condition. J. Clin. Pathol., 26, 217–223
37. Cohen, C., Berson, S. D. and Geddes, E. W. (1979). Liver cell dysplasia. Association with HCC, cirrhosis and HBAg carrier status. Cancer, 44, 1671–1676
38. Nakanuma, Y., Terada, T. and Terasaki, S. (1990). Atypical adenomatous hyperplasia in liver cirrhosis: low grade hepatocellular carinoma or borderline lesion. Histopathology, 17, 27–35
39. Sweeney, E. C. and Evans, D. J. (1976). Hepatic lesions in patients treated with synthetic anabolic steroids. J. Clin. Pathol., 29, 626–633
40. Furuya, K., Nakamura, M., Yamamoto, Y., Togei, K. and Otsuka, H. (1988). Macroregenerative nodule of the liver: a clinicopathologic study of 345 autopsy cases of chronic liver disease. Cancer, 62, 99–105
41. Theise, N. D., Schwartz, M., Miller, C. and Thung, S. N. (1992). Macroregenerative nodules and hepatocellular carcinoma in forty-four sequential adult liver explants with cirrhosis. Hepatology, 16, 949–955
42. Edmondson, H. A. (1958). Tumors of the liver and intrahepatic bile ducts. In Atlas of Tumour Pathology. Fascicle 25. First series edn. Washington DC: AFIP
43. Craig, J. R., Peters, R. L., Edmondson, H. A. and Omata, M. (1980). Fibrolamellar carcinoma of the liver. A tumour of adolescents and young adults with distinctive clinico-pathologic features. Cancer, 46, 72–379
44. Berman, M. A., Burnham, J. A. and Sheahan, D. G. (1988). Fibrolamellar carcinoma of the liver: an immunohistochemical study of nineteen cases and a review of the literature. Hum. Pathol., 19, 784–794
45. Watanabe, S., Okita, K., Harada, T., Kodama, T., Numa, Y., Takemoto, T. and Takahashi, T. (1983). Morphological studies of the liver cell dysplasia. Cancer, 51, 2197–2205
46. Nagato, Y., Kondo, F., Kondon, Y., Ebara, M. and Ohto, M. (1991). Histological and morphometrical indicators for a biopsy diagnosis of well-differentiated hepatocellular carcinoma. Hepatology, 14, 473–478
47. Nørredam, K. (1977). Primary carcinoma of the liver: histological study of 27 cases from Malawi. Acta. Pathol. Microbiol. Scand. [A], 85, 461–469
48. Ishak, K. G. (1976). Primary hepatic tumours in childhood. In

Popper, H. and Schaffner, F. (eds). Progr. Liver Dis. V. pp. 636–667. New York: Grune and Stratton

49. Weinberg, A. G. and Finegold, M. J. (1983). Primary hepatic tumours of childhood. Hum. Pathol., 14, 512–537

50. Landing, B. H. (1976). Tumours of the liver in childhood. In Okuda, K. and Peters, R. L. (eds). Hepatocellular carcinoma. pp. 205–226.

New York: John Wiley and Sons

51. Ishak, K. G. and Glunz, P. R. (1967). Hepatoblastoma and hepatocarcinoma in infancy and childhood. Cancer, 20, 396–422

52. Lack, E. E., Neave, C. and Vawter, G. F. (1982). Hepatoblastoma. A clinical and pathologic study of 54 cases. Am. J. Surg. Pathol., 6, 693–705

CHOLANGIOCARCINOMA (CCA)

Bile-duct carcinomas may arise peripherally within the liver, at the hilum of the liver, along the course of the extrahepatic biliary tree and at the ampulla of Vater. Only those arising within the liver are normally called cholangiocarcinoma (or cholangiocellular carcinoma), although there is little fundamental difference between hilar tumours and those of the upper part of the extrahepatic biliary tree.

CCA accounts for between 5 and 30% of all cases of primary liver cancer. There appears to be rather less geographic variation than with hepatocellular carcinoma, although the incidence is higher in Hong Kong and other parts of South East Asia where it has been linked with liver fluke infestation[1]. The risk of CCA arising in ulcerative colitis is about thirty times that of the control population and is particularly associated with severe and long-standing disease[2]. It may even follow some years after total colectomy, and is nearly always associated with pre-existing primary sclerosing cholangitis (PSC)[3]. Both PSC and CCA are rare in Crohn's disease[2]. Most series report that gallstones are found slightly more commonly than in the general population[4], although this difference is frequently marginal[5]. There is a definite association with the various forms of cystic disease of the intra- and extrahepatic biliary tree[6–8] and with congenital hepatic fibrosis[9] and cystadenoma[10,11], but in most series these cases form only a small proportion of the whole[12]. In a series of 955 cases of extrahepatic biliary cysts collected from the world literature, bile duct cancer occurred in 23, giving an overall incidence of 2–5%[8]. CCA is one of the commonest primary liver tumours associated with exposure to thorotrast[12], where the aetiological link seems unequivocal. Concomitant cirrhosis is very much less common than in HCC, ranging from 0% to 33% and in at least a proportion of cases is the consequence (as a result of biliary obstruction) rather than the cause of the tumour.

CCA tends to affect rather older age groups than HCC, with maximal involvement in the sixth and seventh decades. It is rare under the age of 40. The frequency is comparable in males and females – most series reporting only a marginal preponderance of males. Most patients present with hepatic enlargement, abdominal pain or obstructive jaundice.

Macroscopically the tumours fall into two quite distinct groups – the peripheral and the hilar tumours[13,14]. *Peripheral* tumours (Figure 24.1), which commonly present with hepatic enlargement, are usually grey-white or yellow-white masses which may be umbilicated at the surface of the liver. On section, they usually have a firm consistency which correlates with the fibrous stroma that is commonly present. This sclerosis is often maximal at the centre of the tumour. The tumour may be quite large, occupying most or all of one lobe of the liver, and is usually composed of a main tumour mass with or without a number of smaller daughter nodules in the adjacent or more distant liver (Figure 24.1), and in this respect may be quite indistinguishable macroscopically from an HCC. Obvious extension within vascular channels is much less common than in HCC.

These peripheral tumours are more likely to metastasize than either hilar cholangiocarcinomas or HCC[14]. The pattern of spread, however, is quite similar, with the lungs and abdominal lymph nodes being the main sites.

In contrast, *hilar (or Klatskin) tumours*[15] tend to be much smaller at the time of presentation and metastasize relatively late (Figure 24.2). They usually present with obstructive jaundice. Most cases macroscopically resemble an annular fibrous collar surrounding the bifurcation of the hepatic ducts, and in this respect may be confused with primary sclerosing cholangitis. Sometimes the tumour may be rather larger, measuring up to 10 cm in diameter, with a firm consistency, often greater at the centre, which again correlates with a fibrous stroma. Occasionally these tumours have a significant polypoid intraductal component. Necrosis and shedding of this may be associated with temporary remission of the jaundice, thus simulating gallstones.

Microscopically, both kinds of CCA are tubular adenocarcinomas in the majority of cases[14], and are frequently well-differentiated (Figure 24.3). The component cells are cubical or columnar with a clear or granular cytoplasm and the acini have a well-defined basement membrane. The tumour cells consistently secrete mucus, possibly more commonly in those cases associated with liver flukes[16], but never bile. The quantity of fibrous stroma is very variable but is usually relatively abundant and desmoplastic, hence the very firm nature of the lesions macroscopically (Figure 24.3). However, not all cholangiocarcinomas have a fibrous stroma, nor does the presence of a fibrous stroma exclude other types of tumour[17].

Some tumours are predominantly *papillary* (Figure 24.4). Others may contain a significant *carcinoid* component (Figure 24.5)[18], the cells of which are Fontana-negative, presumably arising from normal argentaffin cells present in bile duct epithelium. An unusual variant is the tumour called a *cholangiolocellular* carcinoma (Figure 24.6) by Steiner and Higginson[19], which they regarded as arising from the canals of Hering. Microscopically the tumour cells are arranged characteristically in small cords of cuboidal cells which are solid or have a small lumen. The stroma is relatively abundant and may or may not be cellular. Rarely *adenosquamous* and *squamous* carcinomas are found[8,14].

True combined hepatocellular-cholangiocarcinomas do occur, but they are extremely rare (see below, Figure 24.9). Most cases thought to be combined tumours are examples of HCC with pseudo acinus formation.

Diagnosis

A significant proportion of cholangiocarcinomas come to autopsy without a definitive diagnosis. The combined use of ultrasonography and percutaneous transhepatic cholangiography has, however, greatly improved the chances of localizing tumours of the biliary tree. Hilar tumours are then accessible to surgical biopsy and respond relatively well to palliative drainage procedures because of their tendency to metastasize late. The main differential diagnosis is from PSC, in very scirrhous tumours[20], and from benign duct papilloma. The latter is exceedingly rare and in the author's experience even cytologically benign papillomas frequently show invasive carcinoma at the base (Figure 24.4). In some cases it is difficult to differentiate between CCA and proliferating bile ductules or hyperplastic duct wall glands – a search

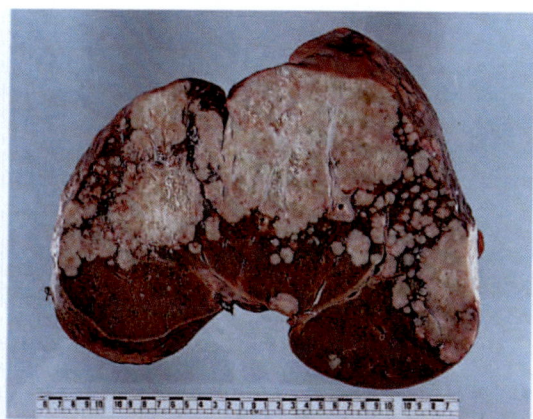

Figure 24.1 Cholangiocarcinoma, peripheral. A 55-year-old male presented with general ill-health and hepatomegaly. Investigations revealed hepatic adenocarcinoma but no evidence of tumour elsewhere so he was treated by liver transplantation. The excised liver shows a large peripheral main tumour-mass with numerous satellites.

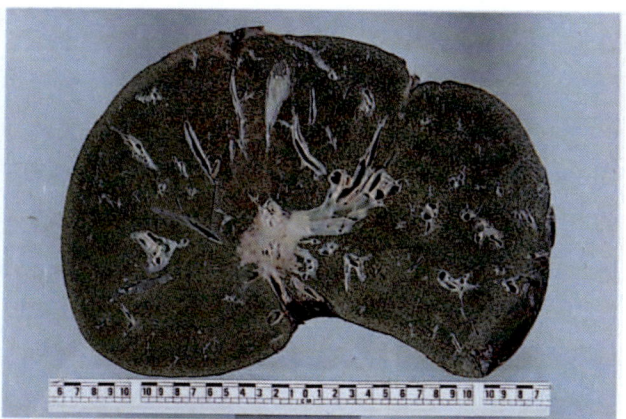

Figure 24.2 Cholangiocarcinoma, hilar (Klatskin tumour). A 48-year-old male who presented insidiously with progressive obstructive jaundice. Investigations revealed a constriction at the point where the hepatic ducts join to form the common bile duct, biopsy of which revealed adenocarcinoma. The excised liver (at transplantation) revealed a 3 cm tumour at this site—the remainder of the liver is dark green because of large duct obstruction. There was no evidence of tumour elsewhere.

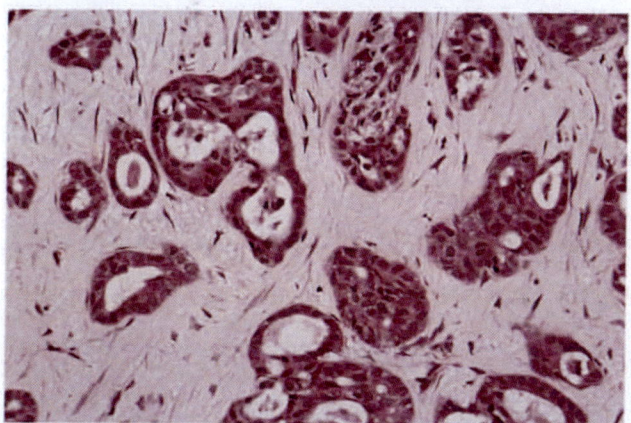

Figure 24.3 Cholangiocarcinoma. A similar case to that in Figure 24.1. Biopsy shows a well-differentiated tubular adenocarcinoma with a relatively abundant fibrous stroma. This could as easily be metastatic as primary and thus diagnosis depends upon the exclusion of other tumours by other investigations.

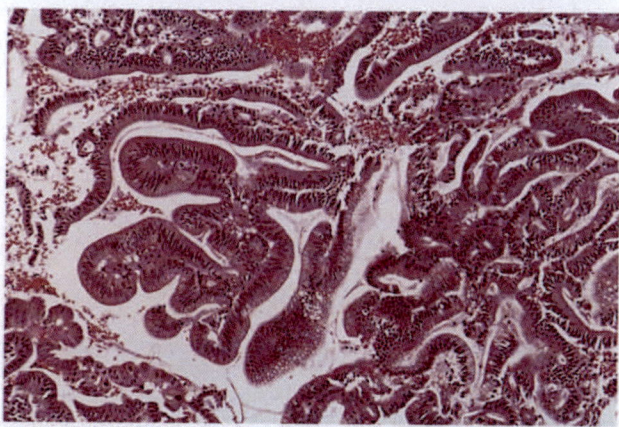

Figure 24.4 Cholangiocarcinoma, papillary. A 43-year-old male who presented with obstructive jaundice. Investigations revealed a filling defect of the hepatic ducts at the hilum of the liver. This was biopsied and shows a well-differentiated papillary tumour composed of tall columnar cells. Subsequent biopsies and the subsequent progress of the patient confirmed that this was part of a cholangiocarcinoma and not a benign tumour.

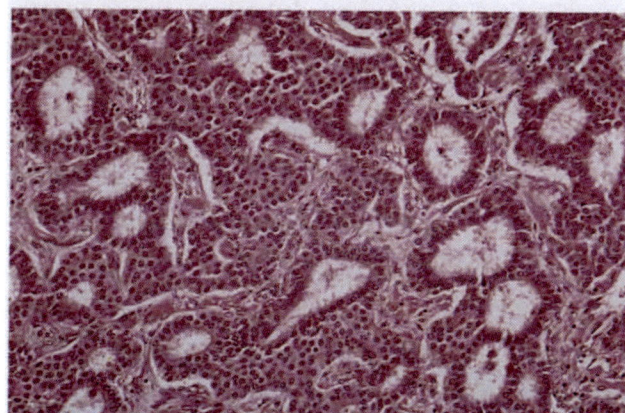

Figure 24.5 Cholangiocarcinoma, carcinoid type. A 43-year-old female who presented with hepatomegaly. Biopsy shows a tumour with the characteristic morphology of a carcinoid tumour with islands of very regular cells and interspersed acini. The cells were Fontana-negative. Laparotomy and subsequent progress confirmed that this tumour was almost certainly of hepatic primary origin.

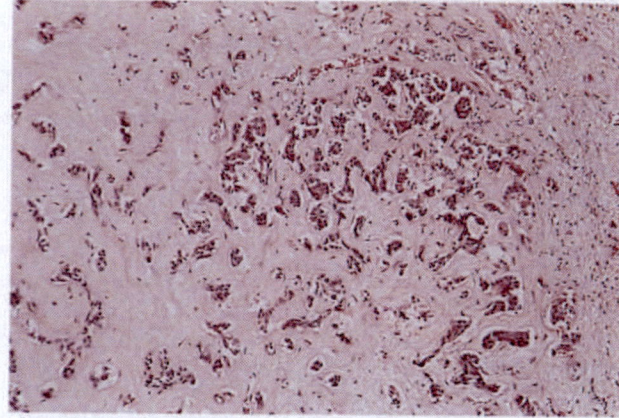

Figure 24.6 Cholangiolocellular carcinoma. A 74-year-old male who died of malignant disease. As autopsy there was a large, very hard tumour replacing much of the right lobe of the liver, but no tumour in any other organ. The section shows a tumour composed of ductule-like elements set in an abundant fibrous stroma.

for perineural invasion may be rewarding in such cases[14]. Variation in nuclear size, cribriform areas and positive staining with antibody to carcinoembryonic antigen may all be helpful, although not absolutely specific, in difficult cases[14].

Peripheral tumours, like HCC, present as space occupying lesions and are much more often encountered in needle biopsy material. Here the main differential diagnosis is from metastatic adenocarcinoma, particularly of the gastrointestinal tract, a distinction which on purely morphological grounds may not be possible. Helpful features include the rather characteristic relationship of tumour acini to the dense collagenous stroma and the relative paucity of mucin in most cases. If electron microscopy is available, the tumour cells will be seen to have small relatively sparse mitochondria, as in normal bile ducts[18]. CCA sometimes spreads along the portal tracts at the periphery of the main tumour mass, both as in situ and invasive tumour. Only the presence of in situ carcinoma can be regarded as a reliable distinguishing feature (Figure 24.7), but even this may be mimicked by adenocarcinoma growing on the endothelial lining of veins and lymphatics[21]. Immunostaining for cytokeratin 19, expressed on normal and neoplastic biliary epithelium, may be useful in distinguishing the true mixed hepatocellular/cholangiocarcinomas[22].

Complications

Hilar tumours especially may be associated with unremitting biliary obstruction, indistinguishable from that due to other causes. Cholangitis, with or without abscess formation, is more likely to complicate cases following surgical intervention.

CYSTADENOCARCINOMA

This is the malignant counterpart of cystadenoma, and most probably arises from pre-existing adenomas[11,23]. They are multilocular tumours with a greater tendency to haemorrhage and necrosis than cystadenomas[21]. Histologically they have greater cellular and architectural atypia, are usually papillary and composed of mucus-secreting cells or tall columnar cells often with foci of squamous metaplasia. In advanced disease solid adenocarcinoma may invade the liver and peritoneum, but initially they may be circumscribed and amenable to surgery[21].

SCLEROSING HEPATOCELLULAR CARCINOMA WITH HYPERCALCAEMIA

Peters[24] drew attention to the association between symptomatic hypercalcaemia and a characteristic sclerosing variant of HCC, in which otherwise characteristic HCC cells are embedded in a fibrous stroma. Although most such tumours are purely hepatocellular, some have both HCC and CCA elements (Figure 24.8)[21,25]. Because of its fibrous stroma, this tumour is macroscopically more like CCA than HCC (Figure 24.9). A parathormone-like substance in tumour cells has been responsible for the hypercalcaemia in some cases[26].

ANGIOSARCOMA

Angiosarcoma was until recently a rare tumour which affected all age groups, including children[27], and showed no sex predilection. However, in 1974, the association of this tumour with industrial exposure to gaseous vinyl chloride was recognized for the first time[28] and this was followed by a rash of subsequent reports[29]. The time between exposure and onset of tumour ranges from 4 to 28 years[30]. Similar tumours have also for long been known

to follow exposure to thorotrast and arsenic, especially amongst vineyard workers. The association with anabolic steroids is more recent[31]. However, no aetiological agent is found in the majority of cases[32]. Although terms such as haemangioendothelial sarcoma, malignant haemangioendothelioma and Kupffer cell sarcoma have all been favoured in the past, these are considered synonymous with, and have generally been superseded by, 'angiosarcoma'.

Now, angiosarcoma is distinctly commoner in males[33] and may present either with non-specific symptoms or with evidence of liver disease, especially hepatomegaly. Occasional cases present with acute haemoperitoneum, due to rupture of a tumour.

Whatever the aetiology, the gross and microscopic appearances of the tumour are indistinguishable (apart from the tell-tale deposits of thorotrast in cases due to this).

Macroscopically the liver may be considerably enlarged due to the presence of usually multiple and often interconnecting purplish haemorrhagic tumours (Figure 24.10). These frequently have a spongy or honeycombed cut surface with larger areas of cystic breakdown and patches of fibrosis. Microscopically the pattern of growth consists of varying combinations of sinusoidal, cavernous and solid foci, but the latter type is not seen alone. The earliest change is the appearance of groups of sinusoidal cells with hypertrophied and hyperchromatic nuclei (Figure 24.11). These may be confined to small areas or found diffusely throughout the liver. With increasing involvement, the sinusoids tend to dilate until eventually there is disruption of the normal pattern of liver cell plates. At this stage groups of liver cells surrounded by malignant endothelial cells often appear suspended in blood spaces. As the tumour cells tend to become multi-layered, the surrounded liver cells atrophy and become replaced by layers of reticulin and then collagen. Eventually cavernous spaces become lined by fronds and strands with a fibrous stroma covered by one or more layers of malignant cells. These are usually elongated with hyperchromatic and often bizarre nuclei. Solid tumour nodules resembling a fibrosarcoma (Figure 24.12), which lack either a sinusoidal or cavernous arrangement, are found in about half the cases. Reticulin is sparse in these areas. Angiosarcoma cells may show erythrophagocytosis[21]. Immunostaining for factor VIII related antigen is usually positive and thus may be diagnostically helpful[34].

Foci of extramedullary haemopoiesis are seen in the majority of cases. Areas of haemorrhage, infarction, thrombosis and fibrosis are also quite commonly seen. Concomitant cirrhosis is rare. Very occasionally angiosarcoma may coexist with HCC or CCA. The spleen, lungs and abdominal lymph nodes are the commonest sites of metastatic spread.

Fibrosis remote from the tumour is a common finding (Figure 24.13). This may take the form of subcapsular and portal tract fibrosis, occasionally dense enough to simulate congenital hepatic fibrosis, and sinusoidal fibrosis associated with disappearance or atrophy of hepatocytes when severe. Proliferation of sinusoid lining cells and patchy sinusoidal dilatation are also commonly seen. All these changes may also be encountered in livers prior to the development of angiosarcoma. Their true predictive or pathogenetic status, however, remains uncertain at this time[35,36].

EPITHELIOID HAEMANGIOENDOTHELIOMA (EH)

Epithelioid haemangioendothelioma was originally described in the lung, and Corrin, on the basis of electron microscopy, recognized its endothelial nature[37]. Ishak described the first series of cases in the liver[38], many of

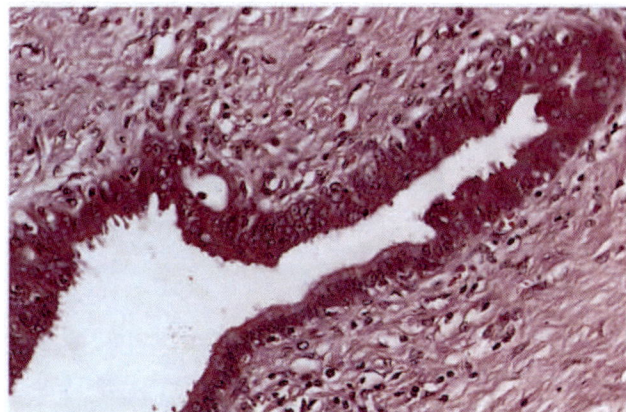

Figure 24.7 Cholangiocarcinoma, dysplastic epithelium. The section shows a transition from normal bile duct epithelium (below centre) to tall columnar dysplastic epithelium resembling that of a large bowel adenoma. This change was observed near to the edge of an infiltrating adenocarcinoma, and provides good evidence that this was of primary bile duct origin.

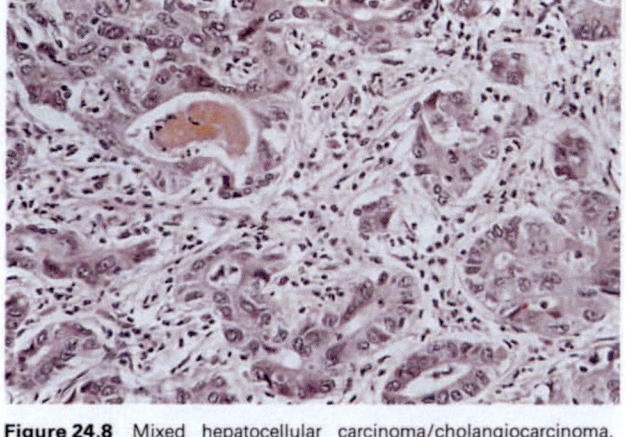

Figure 24.8 Mixed hepatocellular carcinoma/cholangiocarcinoma. This section was from a similar case to that shown in Figure 24.9 and shows a typical tubular adenocarcinoma – indistinguishable from a cholangiocarcinoma – but one of the tubules contains obvious yellow bile which can only have been synthesized by hepatocellular carcinoma cells (more prominent elsewhere in the tumour).

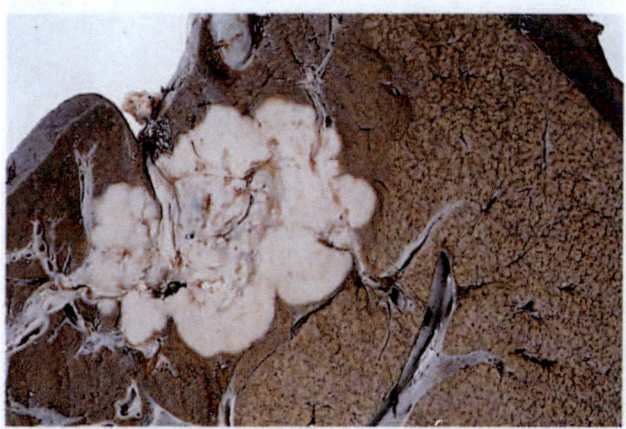

Figure 24.9 Sclerosing carcinoma with hypercalcaemia. A 29-year-old female who presented with hepatomegaly and hypercalcaemia, treated by transplantation. The excised liver contains a 9 cm tumour in the right lobe. This homogeneous white tumour was very hard in consistency and the cut surface shows a scalloped outline.

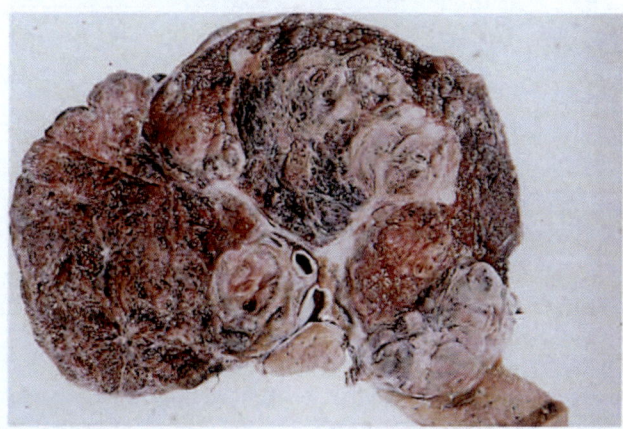

Figure 24.10 Angiosarcoma. The excised liver from a 4-year-old girl (with no known risk factors) which shows multiple nodules of haemorrhagic tumour throughout the liver.

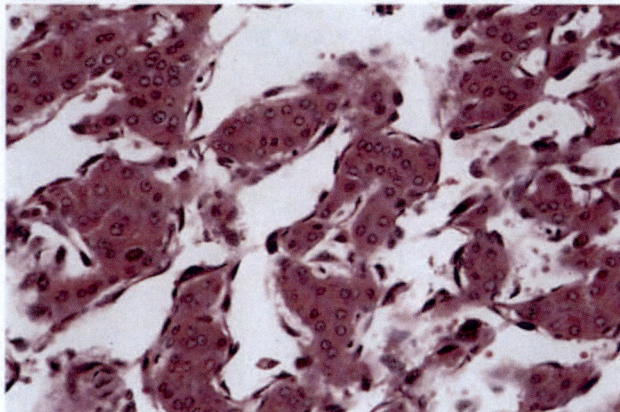

Figure 24.11 Angiosarcoma. A 44-year-old male alcoholic who died suddenly. There was no known exposure to vinyl chloride or other agent known to be associated with this tumour. At autopsy there were multiple nodules of haemorrhagic tumour, largely replacing the liver. The section shows groups of liver cells covered by hyperchromatic and pleomorphic endothelial cells with atrophy of liver cells.

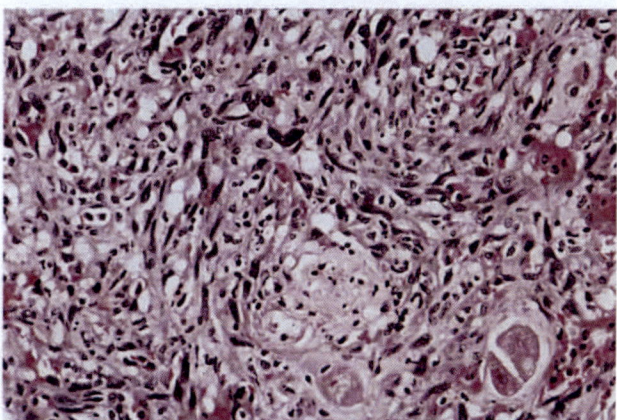

Figure 24.12 Angiosarcoma. Another idiopathic case showing a solid nodule in high magnification. The pleomorphic spindle cells can be clearly seen. Without a sinusoidal component this would be difficult or impossible to distinguish from other mesenchymal neoplasms on morphological grounds alone, although its true nature would be revealed by immunological endothelial cell markers.

which had previously been mistaken for cholangiocarcinoma. EH has been found in adults of all ages, with a mean of 50 years, and a female preponderance[27].

The macroscopic appearance is variable. Tumours may be solitary, multiple or confluent. Early lesions may have a distinctive pink or red blush around the margin (Figure 24.14), whilst older tumours are often hard confluent tumours which may contain areas of calcification. Ishak[38] defined two types of component cell–dendritic and epithelioid. Dendritic cells predominate in areas of fibrosis and may be spindle-shaped or stellate, but the most characteristic feature is the presence of single or multiple lumina within these cells (Figure 24.15). These represent primitive vascular lumina, but may be mistaken for signet-ring adenocarcinoma, unless their endothelial nature is confirmed by immunostaining. Epithelioid cells predominate in less sclerotic areas and may grow into vessels, especially hepatic venules but also portal veins, where they form clusters (Figure 24.16) and may mimic carcinoma. For long periods the overall architecture of the liver is retained in the infiltrated areas which often show a mixture of proliferating bile ductules, sclerosis, residual hepatocytes and obliteration of vessels (Figure 24.17)–a picture which can be very confusing and probably explains why the tumour has often been mistaken for other entities. As the lesion progresses tumour cells may become less and less numerous–the fibrosis and ischaemia 'starve the tumour to death'[38]. The vascular occlusion may cause a superimposed Budd-Chiari-like syndrome (Figure 24.17). Diagnosis depends upon the entity being thought of and at least some of the distinctive tumour cells normally contain factor VIII related antigen or other endothelial markers. The prognosis is said to be intermediate between that of a haemangioma and angiosarcoma[39], although in our own experience death from disseminated tumour is the rule rather than the exception. Liver transplantation may be successful in selected cases.[40]

OTHER MALIGNANT LIVER TUMOURS

Other malignant tumours of the liver are rare and the majority occur in the paediatric age group. Any of the remaining mesenchymal tissues within the liver may give rise to benign or malignant tumours[33], and these are recognized in the liver by the same criteria as those in other organs (Figure 24.18), or may be completely undifferentiated[41]. Primary sarcomas of the liver in adults are very rare, and it is essential to exclude the possibility of metastasis from gastrointestinal and retroperitoneal sites before accepting any sarcoma as primary.

REFERENCES

1. Gibson, J. B. (1971). Parasites, liver disease and liver cancer. In Liver cancer. 1. pp. 42–50. Lyon: IARC Scientific Publication
2. Mir-Madjlessi, S. H., Farmer, R. G. and Sivak, M. V. (1987). Bile duct carcinoma in patients with ulcerative colitis. Relationship to sclerosing colitis: report of six cases and review of the literature. Dig. Dis. Sci., 32, 145–154
3. Wee, A., Ludwig, J., Coffey, R. J., LaRusso, N. F. and Wiesner, R. H. (1985). Hepatobiliary carcinoma associated with primary sclerosing cholangitis and chronic ulcerative colitis. Hum. Pathol., 16, 719–726
4. Murray-Lyon, I. M. (1979). Cholangiocarcinoma. Br. J. Hosp. Med., 21, 478–481
5. Okuda, K., Kubo, Y., Okazaki, N., Arishima, T., Hashimoto, M., Jinnouchi, S., Sawa, Y., Shimokawa, Y., Nakajima, Y., Noguchi, T., Nakano, M., Kojiro, M. and Nakashima, T. (1971). Clinical aspects of intrahepatic bile duct carcinoma including hilar carcinoma. Cancer, 39, 232–246
6. Gallagher, P. J., Millis, R. R. and Mitchinson, M. J. (1972). Congenital dilatation of the intrahepatic bile ducts with cholangiocarcinoma. J. Clin. Pathol., 25, 804–808
7. Ozawa, K. (1980). Carcinoma arising in a choledochocoele. Cancer, 45, 195–197
8. Flanigan, D. P. (1977). Biliary carcinoma associated with biliary cysts. Cancer, 40, 880–883
9. Scott, J. (1980). Bile duct carcinoma: a late complication of congenital hepatic fibrosis. Case report and review of literature. Am. J. Gastroenterol., 73, 113–119
10. Azizah, N. and Paradinas, F. J. (1980). Cholangiocarcinoma coexisting with developmental liver cysts: a distinct entity different from liver cystadenocarcinoma. Histopathology, 4, 391–400
11. Ishak, K. G., Willis, G. W., Cummins, S. D. and Bullock, A. A. (1977). Biliary cystadenoma and cystadeno-carcinoma. Cancer, 39, 322–338
12. Battifora, H. A. (1976). Thorotrast and tumours of the liver. In Okuda, K. and Peters, R. L. (eds). Hepatocellular carcinoma. pp. 83–93. New York: John Wiley and Sons
13. Mori, W. and Nagasako, K. (1976). Cholangiocarcinoma and related lesions. In Okuda, K. and Peters, R. L. (eds). Hepatocellular carcinoma. pp. 227–246. New York: John Wiley and Sons
14. Nakajima, T., Kondo, Y., Miyazaki, M. and Okui, K. (1988). A histopathological study of 102 cases of intrahepatic cholangiocarcinoma: histological classification and modes of spreading. Hum. Pathol., 19, 1228–1234
15. Klatskin, G. (1965). Adenocarcinoma of the hepatic duct at its bifurcation within the portal hepatis. Am J Med, 38, 241–256
16. Chan, S. T. and Chan, C. W. (1976). Mucin-producing cholangiocarcinoma an autopsy study in Hong Kong. Pathology, 8, 321–328
17. Weinbren, K. and Mutum, S. S. (1983). Pathological aspects of cholangiocarcinoma. J. Pathol., 139, 217–238
18. Alpert, L. I., Zak, F. G., Werthamer, S. and Bochetto, J. F. (1974). Cholangiocarcinoma: a clinico-pathological study of five cases with ultrastructural observations. Hum Pathol, 5, 709–728
19. Steiner, P. E. and Higginson, J. (1959). Cholangiolocellular carcinoma of the liver. Cancer, 12, 753–759
20. Qualman, S. J., Haupt, H. M., Bauer, T. W. and Taxy, J. B. (1984). Adenocarcinoma of the hepatic duct junction. A reappraisal of the histologic criteria of malignancy. Cancer, 53, 1545–1551
21. Paradinas, F. J. (1993). Liver tumours and tumour-like conditions. In Wight, D. G. D. (eds). Liver, Biliary Tract and Exocrine Pancreas. Vol. 11. Systemic Pathology. Symmers, W. S. C. Series ed. 3rd edn. Edinburgh: Churchill Livingstone
22. Grigioni, W. F., D'Errico, A., Biagini, G., Villanacci, V., Mazziotti, A., Liotta, L. A., Garbisa, S. and Mancini, A. M. (1987). Primary liver cell carcinoma. New insight for a more correct approach to its classification. Acta Pathol. Jpn., 37, 929–940
23. Craig, J. R., Peters, R. L. and Edmondson, H. A. (1989). Tumors of the liver and intrahepatic bile ducts. In Atlas of Tumour Pathology. Fascicle 26. Second series. Washington DC:
24. Peters, R. L. (1976). Pathology of hepatocellular carcinoma. In Okuda, K. and Peters, R. L. (eds). Hepatocellular carcinoma. pp. 107–168. New York: John Wiley
25. Omata, M., Peters, R. L. and Tatter, D. (1981). Sclerosing hepatic carcinoma: relationship to hypercalcaemia. Liver, 1, 33–49
26. Knill-Jones, R. P., Buckle, R. M., Parsons, V., Calne, R. Y. and Williams, R. (1970). Hypercalcaemia and increased parathyroid hormone activity in primary hepatoma. Studies before and after hepatic transplantation. N. Engl. J. Med., 282, 704–708
27. Noronha, R. and Gonzalez-Crussa, F. (1984). Hepatic angiosacoma in childhood. Am. J. Surg. Pathol., 8, 863–871
28. Creech, J. L. and Johnson, M. N. (1974). Angiosarcoma of the liver in the manufacture of polyvinyl chloride. J. Occupat. Med., 16, 150–151
29. Popper, H., Thomas, L. B., Telles, N. C., Falk, H. and Selikoff, I. J. (1978). Development of hepatic angiosarcoma in man induced by vinyl chloride. thorotrast. arsenic. Comparison with cases of unknown aetiology. Am J Pathol, 92, 349–369
30. Makk, L., Delmore, F., Creech, J. L., Ogden, L. L., Fadell, E. H., Songster, C. L., Clanton, J., Johnson, M. N. and Christopherson, W. M. (1976). Clinical and morphological features of hepatic angiosarcoma in vinyl chloride workers. Cancer, 37, 149–163
31. Kirchner, S. G., Heller, R. M., Kasselberg, A. G. and Greene, H. L. (1981). Infantile hepatic hemangioendothelioma with subsequent malignant degeneration. Pediatr. Radiol., 11, 42–45
32. Baxter, P. J., Anthony, P. P., MacSween, R. N. M. and Scheuer, P. J. (1980). Angiosarcoma of the liver: annual occurrence and aetiology in Great Britain. Br. J. Ind. Med., 37, 213–221
33. Ishak, K. G. (1976). Mesenchymal tumours of the liver. In Okuda, K. and Peters, R. L. (eds). Hepatocellular Carcinoma. pp. 247–307. New York: John Wiley and Sons

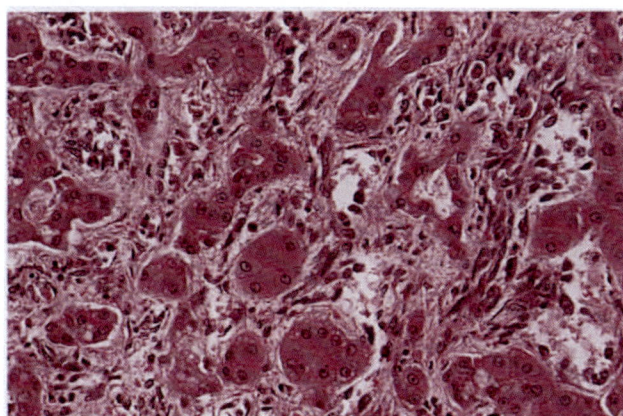

Figure 24.13 Angiosarcoma. Same case as Figure 24.11. This section shows (to left) sinusoidal fibrosis with an occasional atypical elongated cell and (to right) more advanced tumour with multi-layering of atypical cells.

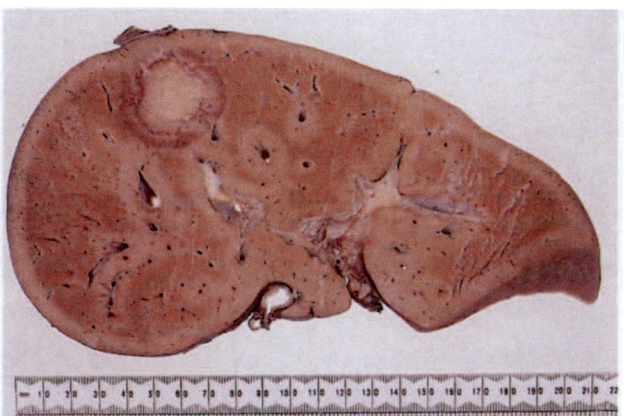

Figure 24.14 Epithelioid haemangioendothelioma. A 29-year-old male presented with multiple tumour nodules, diagnosed on biopsy and treated by liver transplantation. Note the characteristic red blush around the margin of these early lesions.

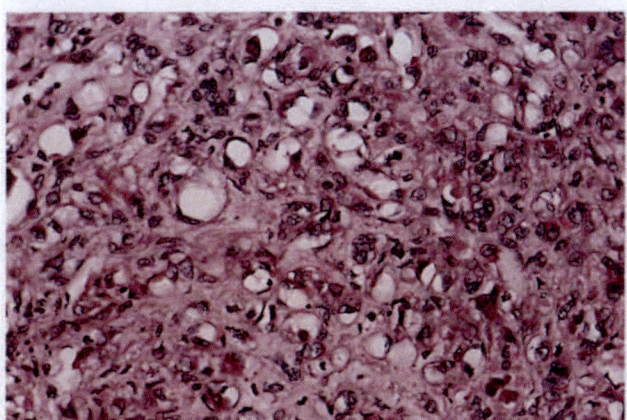

Figure 24.15 Epithelioid haemangioendothelioma. Same case as Figure 24.14. The characteristic tumour cells are embedded in a dense collagenous stroma and can be recognized as endothelial cells by the presence of intracellular lumina.

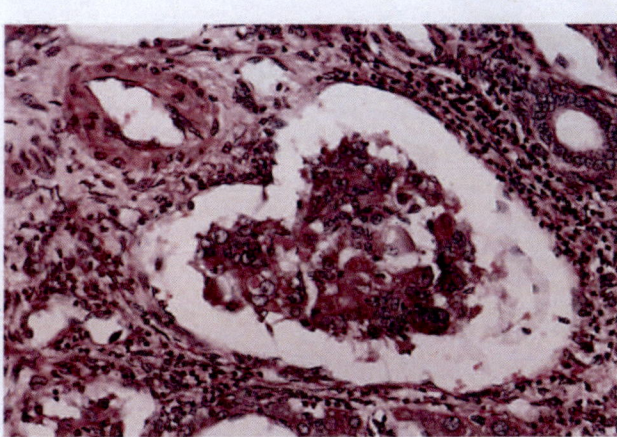

Figure 24.16 Epithelioid haemangioendothelioma. Same case as Figures 24.14 and 24.15, showing epithelioid cells forming a glomerulus-like cluster within a small vein.

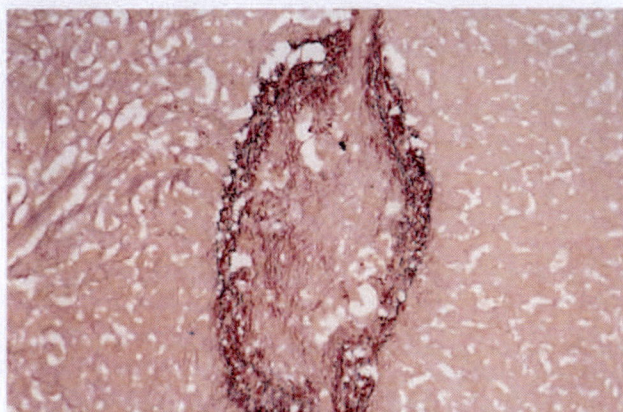

Figure 24.17 Epithelioid haemangioendothelioma. This section shows total obliteration of a terminal hepatic venule by tumour, a widespread change which explains why this patient presented with a Budd-Chiari–like syndrome. Elastic van-Gieson.

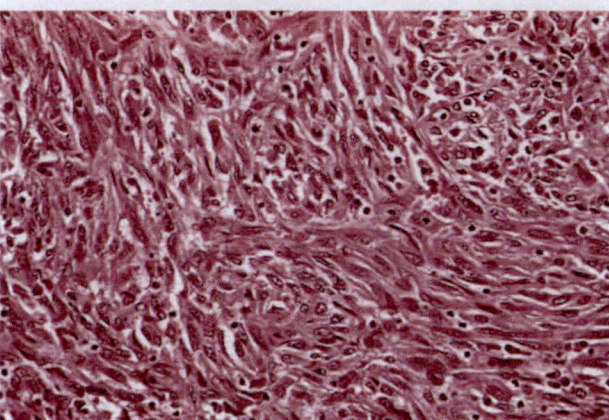

Figure 24.18 Leiomyosarcoma. A 57-year-old male with a liver tumour which at autopsy was found to be confined to the liver. The biopsy shows a typical leiomyosarcoma indistinguishable from one arising in any other site.

34. Guarda, L. A., Ordoñez, N. G., Smith, J. L. and Hanssen, G. (1982). Immunoperoxidase localization of factor VIII in angiosarcoma. Arch. Pathol. Lab. Med., 106, 515–516

35. Thomas, L. B. and Popper, H. (1974). Pathology of angiosarcoma of the liver among vinyl chloride workers - polyvinyl chloride workers. Ann. N. Y. Acad. Sci., 246, 268–277

36. Popper, H. and Thomas, L. B. (1974). Alterations of liver and spleen among workers exposed to vinyl chloride. Ann. N. Y. Acad Sci, 246, 172–193

37. Corrin, B., Manners, B., Millard, M. and Weaver, L. (1979). Histogenesis of the so-called 'intravascular bronchioalveolar tumour'. J. Pathol., 128, 163–167

38. Ishak, K. G., Sesterhenn, I. A., Goodman, M. Z. D., Rabin, L. and Stromeyer, F. W. (1984). Epithelioid haemangioendothelioma of the liver: a clinicopathologic and follow-up study of 32 cases. Hum. Pathol., 15, 839–852

39. Weiss, S. W. and Enziger, F. M. (1982). Epithelioid haemangioendothelioma. A vascular tumour often mistaken for carcinoma. Cancer, 50, 970–981

40. Scoazec, J. Y., Lamy, P., Degott, C., Reynœs, M., Feldmann, G., Bismuth, H. and Benhamou, J.-P. (1988). Epithelioid hamangioendothelioma of the liver. Diagnostic features and the role of liver transplantation. Gastroenterology, 94, 1447–1453

41. Stocker, J. T. and Ishak, K. G. (1978). Undifferentiated (embryonal) sarcoma of the liver. Report of 31 cases. Cancer, 42, 336–348

Lymphoreticular Disease

25

In its physiological state the liver does not contain organized lymphoid tissue. However the liver is probably the most common site for involvement by deposits of lymphoma and infiltrates of leukaemic cells outside the lymphoreticular system. In general, lymphomatous infiltrates are confined to, or centred upon, portal tracts, whilst leukaemic infiltrates are mainly sinusoidal.

MALIGNANT LYMPHOMA

The primary diagnosis of lymphoma is rarely made by liver biopsy alone, but when it is[1] it should always be followed by further investigations, including lymph node biopsy. There are a few reports of lymphoma confined to the liver[2], but in the majority of cases it is merely part of systemic disease.

Lymphomas are generally subdivided into Hodgkin's disease (HD) and non-Hodgkin's lymphoma (NHL). Whilst the Rye classification of HD has been universally accepted, the detailed classification of NHL is less stable[3,4], but most such neoplasms can now be subdivided as B-cell or T-cell neoplasms on the basis of their immunophenotype and genotype.

Cirrhosis accompanying malignant lymphoma is distinctly rare, although some authors believe there is a significant link, possibly through chronic active liver disease[5,6].

Hodgkin's disease

Involvement of the liver in Hodgkin's disease is almost always as part of systemic disease, but its presence has considerable therapeutic implications. It may be suggested by hepatomegaly or jaundice and is more common in those patients with systemic symptoms such as fever. Jaundice is encountered in about 10% of patients and is most often due to either massive hepatic infiltration, to biliary obstruction by tumour deposits or to haemolysis associated with hypersplenism[7]. In a small proportion of cases, however, no cause can be found[8].

In general, clinical and biochemical parameters are poor predictors of liver involvement by HD. In patients with known HD, positive results with at least two imaging techniques can be taken as evidence of hepatic involvement[9]. Open biopsy enables direct sampling of visible lesions and thus doubles the yield of positive biopsies, as compared with blind needle biopsy[10]. However, even in the absence of visible deposits, surgical wedge biopsies are superior to four quadrant needle biopsies[11], perhaps because deposits are commoner in the subcapsular region. The yield of positive cases at staging laparotomy is of the order of 5–10%, whilst at autopsy this figure rises to as much as 60%. Liver involvement has been shown to be distinctly unlikely in the absence of splenic disease[12]. Any type of HD may affect the liver, but lymphocyte predominant HD, now recognized to be a B-cell proliferation quite distinct from the other forms[13], rarely does so. With improved understanding of the disease process, combined with better imaging techniques, the need for staging laparotomies in HD has declined sharply[14] and is now only necessary if the findings would alter the treatment plan.

Macroscopically, tumour deposits may resemble those in the spleen and vary considerably in size, ranging from small discrete pale nodules to large bulky and irregular masses. Other livers may show multiple miliary nodules, or both patterns may be observed.

Microscopically, advanced lesions usually pose no diagnostic problems and resemble the type of deposit seen in the spleen, with Reed-Sternberg cells as the hallmark of HD (Figures 25.1 and 25.2). The absence of visible deposits does not rule out hepatic involvement in HD, but the earlier microscopic lesions may be much harder to identify. These lesions are always located in portal tracts and may be difficult to distinguish from non-specific cellular infiltration of portal tracts-'portal triaditis'-which is seen in up to half of patients in the absence of frank HD of the liver (Figure 25.4)[12,14]. Rappaport stipulated that Reed Sternberg (RS) cells (Figure 25.2) should be found before making a definitive diagnosis[15]. Multiple or serial sections through the liver will often reveal typical RS cells, especially if the infiltrate initially contains atypical mononuclear cells[10,16]. It is for this reason that many authors will accept mononuclear cells alone as evidence of HD of liver provided that they have the nuclear morphology of RS cells and that there is satisfactory biopsy evidence of HD elsewhere in the body (Figure 25.2). Possession of the characteristic RS cell immunophenotype (CD45–, CD15+, CD30+) would add strength to the presumption that such cells are part of HD. In lymphocyte-depleted disease, the infiltrate may be wholly composed of these cells, which are often deeply stained with pleomorphic angular nuclei.

In non-specific portal triaditis the portal tract usually is not expanded and contains a variable mix of non-neoplastic chronic inflammatory cells, occasionally including eosinophils (Figure 25.3). This lesion, too, appears more common in the subcapsular liver and thus is more often seen in wedge biopsies. Epithelioid and giant cell granulomas are another non-specific change found in about 10% of cases (Figure 25.4). These are usually in the portal tract, but may also be parenchymal in distribution. Sometimes they are very numerous, but they do not correlate at all well with Hodgkin's deposits which may or may not be present. Other non-specific changes seen in HD include congestion, sinusoidal dilatation and even peliosis hepatis (Chapter 18). Fatty change of variable degree is common (Figures 25.1 and 25.4). Siderosis and Kupffer cell hyperplasia may also be seen. In common with other lymphoreticular diseases, isolated megakaryocytes may occasionally be seen in sinusoids.

Non-Hodgkin's lymphoma

The presence or absence of liver involvement by non-Hodgkin's lymphoma has much less therapeutic significance than in HD and thus liver biopsy is not regularly part of a staging procedure. However liver infiltration has been found in more than 50% of cases in both biopsy and autopsy material[17]. In common with HD, there is poor correlation of liver involvement with clinical, biochemical and scan data. Most non-Hodgkin's lymphomas involving the liver are of B-cell origin, although T-cell lymphomas have also been described, particularly those encountered as a complication of coeliac disease (Chapter 20)[2]. The liver may also be involved in 40% of cases of Burkitt's

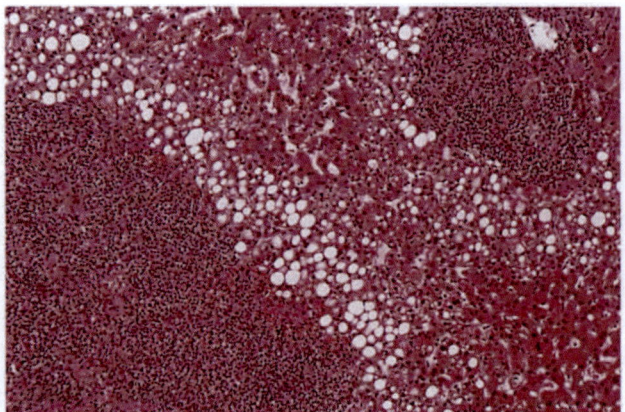

Figure 25.1 Hodgkin's disease. A 60-year-old male patient who presented with pyrexia and general ill-health. Laparotomy revealed enlarged mesenteric nodes (HD mixed cellularity) and obvious hepatic nodules. The biopsy shows large irregular deposits in portal tracts with fatty change in periportal liver cells. The cellular infiltrate is mixed and contained Reed-Sternberg cells as well as lymphocytes and histiocytes.

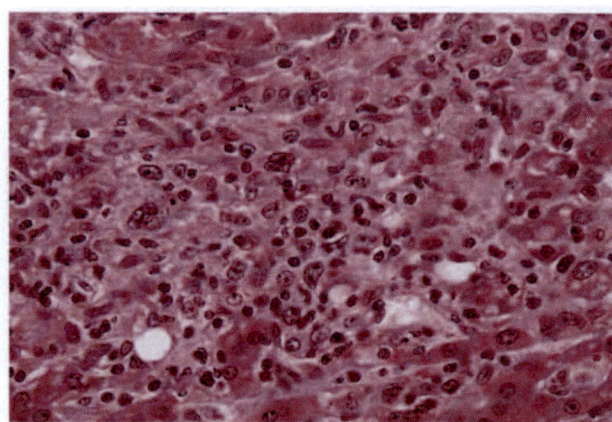

Figure 25.2 Hodgkin's disease. Another patient with known HD. Liver biopsy at staging laparotomy reveals this mixed infiltrate with both mononuclear and typical binucleate Reed-Sternberg cells. Note that lymphocytes are rather sparse and all the deposits in spleen and lymph nodes were similarly lymphocyte-depleted.

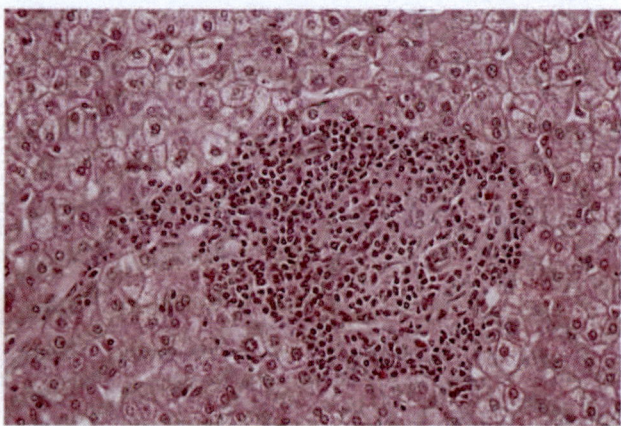

Figure 25.3 Hodgkin's disease. Another patient with known HD. Liver biopsy at staging laparotomy revealed these dense portal tract infiltrates which are composed of lymphocytes and macrophages and a few plasma cells and eosinophils. No atypical cells were seen and thus this is regarded as a non-specific finding, negative for HD. The spleen was also negative in this case.

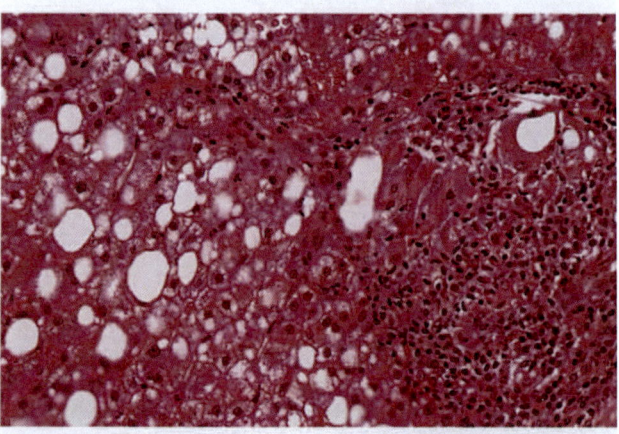

Figure 25.4 Hodgkin's disease. Another patient with known HD. Liver biopsy at staging laparotomy revealed non-specific portal infiltrates and a number of epithelioid and giant cell granulomas. This one is rather ill—defined and contains numerous lymphocytes and macrophages also. Note a large lipid droplet in a giant cell, possibly attributable to lymphangiography performed prior to laparotomy. There is also moderate fatty change in the liver.

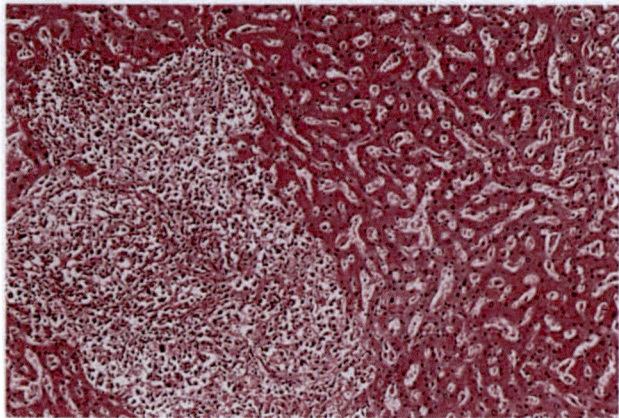

Figure 25.5 Non-Hodgkin's lymphoma. A fatal case of NHL. At autopsy there was extensive nodal disease but no gross deposits in the liver. The section shows an expanded but well-defined portal tract filled with atypical lymphoid cells. Sinusoids are not significantly involved. All portal tracts were abnormal.

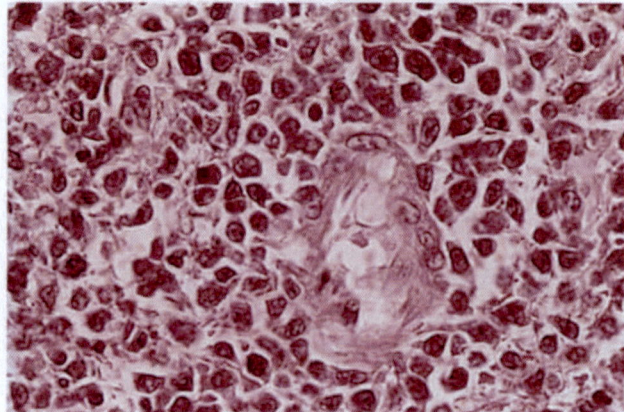

Figure 25.6 Primary hepatic lymphoma. Several deposits of B-cell lymphoma, probably EB-virus related, were an incidental finding at autopsy in this patient who had previously received a liver transplant and was accordingly under immunosuppression. The tumour was confined to the liver.

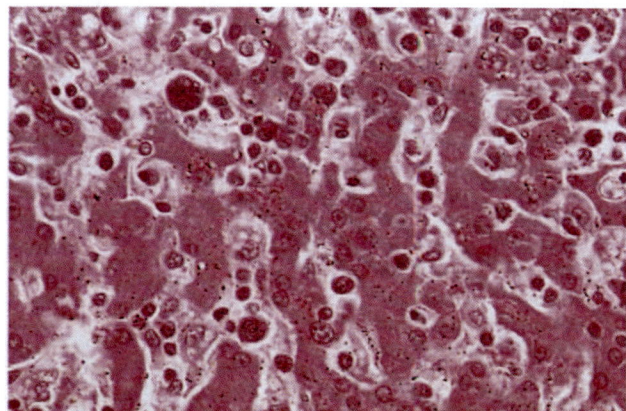

Figure 25.7 Coeliac-associated T-cell lymphoma (previously termed malignant histiocytosis of the intestine). A 59-year-old female with a long history of adult coeliac disease developed a rapidly progressive fatal illness. At autopsy there was a malignant ulcerating lesion in the jejunum; this, together with lymph nodes, spleen and liver, contained the characteristic microscopic lesions of large-cell lymphoma. The liver appeared normal macroscopically, but the section shows sinusoidal infiltration by pleomorphic histiocyte-like malignant cells.

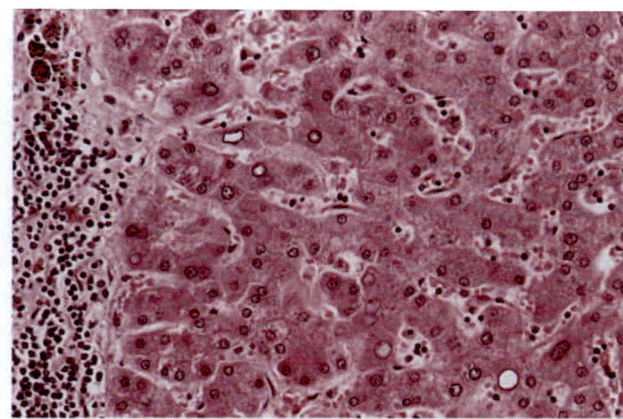

Figure 25.8 Chronic lymphatic leukaemia. An elderly patient died with CLL. The liver appeared normal macroscopically, but the section shows a dense portal tract infiltrate of small lymphocytes. As is usual in CLL, there is little sinusoidal infiltration. Note the haemosiderin-filled macrophages (top left) attributable to haemolysis.

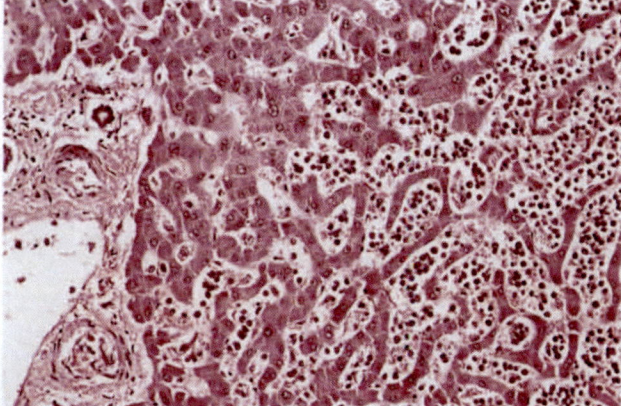

Figure 25.9 Chronic myeloid leukaemia. A fatal case of CML. At autopsy there was no macroscopic evidence of liver involvement, but the section shows large numbers of leukaemic cells in sinusoids, portal and efferent veins.

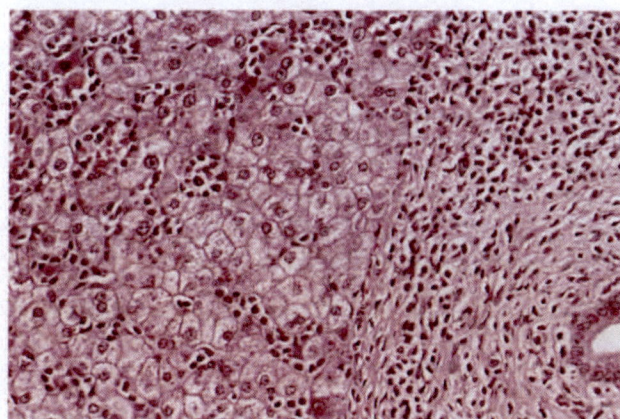

Figure 25.10 Hairy cell leukaemia. A 38-year-old female presented with hepatosplenomegaly and pancytopenia. Liver biopsy shows the very characteristic picture of evenly spaced uniform cells, each with a narrow clear halo, infiltrating both portal tracts and sinusoids.

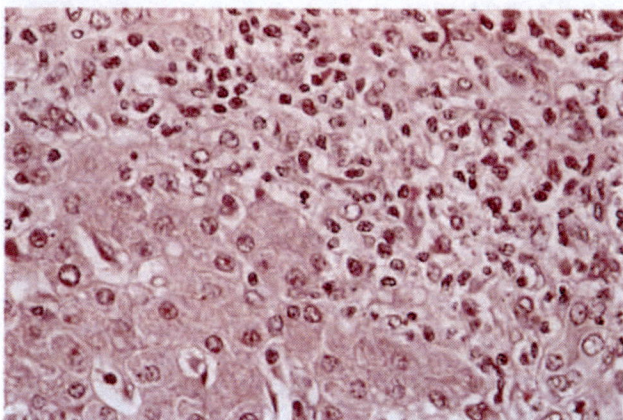

Figure 25.11 Langerhans histiocytosis (Letterer-Siwe syndrome). An 18-month-old infant with progressively febrile systemic disease with characteristic clinical, radiological and bone marrow findings. The post-mortem liver section shows a predominantly portal tract infiltration by large pale histiocytes, which were S 100 protein positive, accompanied by lymphocytes and other mononuclear cells.

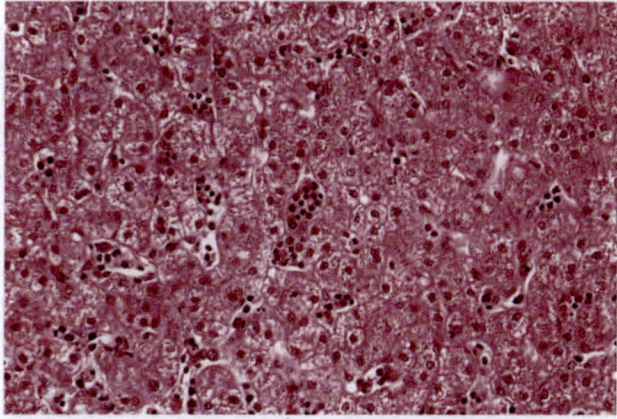

Figure 25.12 Myeloid metaplasia. A 35-year-old male with a chronic myeloproliferative disorder. Liver biopsy shows widespread extra-medullary haemopoiesis. In the absence of megakaryocytes, as here, careful examination is required to determine that these cells include normoblasts.

lymphoma[14], and in AIDS associated lymphoma[18], both of which are also lymphomas of B-cell lineage.

Deposits may be large, irregular masses resembling metastatic carcinoma or may diffusely infiltrate portal tracts where they may scarcely be visible to the naked eye (Figure 25.5). As a rough guide, the high-grade lymphomas are more likely to lead to large deposits and are associated with a poor prognosis. Conversely, low-grade NHL leads to diffuse portal tract involvement and has a favourable prognosis. As in HD, liver involvement in NHL is rare in the absence of splenic disease.

Microscopically, the cytological features of NHL are the same as those in any other organ and diagnosis depends mainly upon recognition of the immunopheno-type, and where appropriate, genotype of the cells in the infiltrates.

Non-specific cellular infiltrates and granulomas are much less common than in HD. Microscopically the deposits are predominantly portal and show the same features as those in other organs with the same problems over classification and nomenclature. Extension into sinusoids usually is an indication of involvement of the bone marrow or the peripheral blood.

Primary hepatic lymphoma

Lymphomas arising in and restricted to the liver are rare[19], although it is not always clear how rigorously disease elsewhere is or can be excluded. The majority of cases are large cell lymphomas of the B-cell lineage (Figure 25.6)[20]. It is possible that such tumours represent high grade lymphomas of the mucosa associated lymphoid tissue (MALT), which might account for their localization in the liver. Rare primary lymphomas of the liver have been reported in AIDS[21]. There is at least one report which describes a predominance of T-cell lymphomas amongst a series of 10 cases[22], although Wright[14] argues that these are more likely to represent T-cell rich B-cell lymphomas, the T-cells being merely benign and reactive rather than neoplastic.

DIFFERENTIAL DIAGNOSIS

As already stated, liver biopsy is not usually the primary means of diagnosis of malignant lymphoma, and wherever possible lymph node biopsy should be undertaken for definitive diagnosis. Problems in distinguishing HD from non-specific portal tract inflammation have already been mentioned. Distinction from conditions such as cholangitis, primary biliary cirrhosis or chronic hepatitis C, may not always be easy. Differentiation depends on the detection of mononuclear or binucleate RS cells in HD or the presence of cytological atypia, together with more intense, diffuse and monotonous infiltrate in NHL. It may also be necessary to distinguish a number of other neoplastic and non-neoplastic conditions:

Malignant histiocytosis

Our understanding of the condition previously called *malignant histiocytosis* (histiocytic medullary reticulosis) has undergone several revolutions. Many cases were probably examples of virus-induced haemophagic syndromes[14], whilst others were true lymphomas in which neoplastic T-cells produced lymphokines that induced activated, but non-neoplastic, macrophages to phagocytose red cells and other particles (Figure 25.7). A recent reexamination of 15 previously reported cases[23] concluded that most were large cell anaplastic lymphomas (eight were CD30 positive), nine of T-cell origin, two were B-cell, but none expressed the macrophage marker CD68.

Angioimmunoblastic lymphadenopathy (AIL)

Angioimmunoblastic lymphadenopathy is another condition which, on the basis of gene rearrangement studies, has now been redefined as a T-cell lymphoma of AIL type[24]. Others may be T-cell rich B-cell lymphomas[14]. Nevertheless, liver involvement occurs in a high proportion of patients with AIL. The portal infiltrates contain, as well as blast cells, variable numbers of lymphocytes, plasma cells, macrophages and eosinophils, and thus may be confused with HD. Distinction may well, in the end, depend on other parameters.

Metastatic carcinoma

Metastatic *oat cell carcinoma* (Chapter 23) of the bronchus may occasionally simulate lymphoma or leukaemia, especially when it permeates sinusoids widely.

Leukaemias

Apart from those cases that began as lymphomas, leukaemic involvement of the liver has little practical significance, usually being observed for the first time at autopsy (Figures 25.8 and 25.9).

Hairy cell leukaemia, however, has a more chronic course and is not infrequently seen in liver biopsy material. The infiltrate is found in both portal tracts and sinusoids. The cells may resemble those of chronic lymphatic leukaemia, although this does not usually involve sinusoids, but the nuclei are usually larger and paler with a narrow clear rim leading to very regular spacing of the cells in the tissues and giving a frog-spawn-like appearance (Figure 25.10). Unusual and distinctive angiomatous lesions, similar to the pseudosinuses found in the spleen, composed of dilated blood spaces lined by hairy cells, may be found in portal tracts or sinusoids[25].

Langerhans histiocytosis

This condition, also known as histiocytosis X, can usually be readily distinguished by its clinical features. Hepatic involvement is usually seen in young children as part of the Letterer-Siwe syndrome and the infiltrates (Figure 25.11) can be distinguished by cells with relatively abundant cytoplasm and the characteristic grooved 'coffee-bean' nucleus, which are stainable with antibody to S100 protein[26]. Ultrastructurally the cells contain Birbeck granules.

Other conditions

Infectious mononucleosis (Chapter 3) may be difficult to distinguish from lymphoreticular neoplasms when taken out of context. Here there are quite intense portal infiltrates of lymphocytes and lymphoblastoid cells, and the same cells are usually also seen in sinusoids, where they may be associated with small focal necroses of liver cells. *Lymphomatoid granulomatosis*[27] and *Felty's syndrome* (Chapter 21) may also produce a similar picture. *Tropical splenomegaly syndrome* (Chapter 6) may also be similar, although generally with fewer cells in portal tracts. The liver may be involved as part of systemic mastocytosis[14]. Benign *inflammatory pseudotumour*[22], which has an excellent prognosis, may also be confused with malignant lymphoma. The main diagnostic features are a high proportion of plasma cells and lack of clonality.

MYELOID METAPLASIA (HEPATIC EXTRAMEDULLARY HAEMOPOIESIS)

This is a normal feature of the fetal liver and is also frequently seen in the first few weeks of life. In adult life it usually occurs as a complication of a myeloproliferative disorder but is also encountered in other marrow replacement syndromes, such as metastatic. carcinoma and multiple myeloma. It is also a regular feature of angiosarcoma (Chapter 24) and hepatoblastoma (Chapter 23). Haemopoietic cells are seen in sinusoids and portal tracts as clumps of rather variable cells. Although the leukocytes may be indistinguishable from those associated with other conditions, such as leukaemias, it is usually possible to recognize either normoblasts or megakaryocytes (Figure 25.12). The former have characteristically dense nuclear chromatin and the latter large multilobed, often distorted, or crushed nuclei. Occasionally megakaryocytes are seen in isolation and there is not always an obvious marrow disorder.

REFERENCES

1. Ludwig, J. and Boon, S. E. (1980). Liver biopsy diagnosis of unsuspected or unconfirmed lymphoproliferative or myeloproliferative disorders. Hepatogastroenterology, 27, 17–19
2. Isaacson, P. G., O'Connor, N. T. J., Spencer, J., Bevan, D. H., Connolly, C. E., Kirkham, N., Pollock, D. J., Wainscoat, J. S., Stein, H. and Wright, D. H. (1985). Malignant histiocytosis of the intestine: a T cell lymphoma. Lancet, 2, 688–690
3. National Cancer Institute. (1982). Sponsored study of classifications of non–Hodgkin's lymphomas. Summary and description of working formulation for clinical usage. Cancer, 49, 2112–2135
4. Stansfeld, A. G., Diebold, J., Kapanci, Y., Rilke, F., Kelényi, G., Sundstrom, C., Lennert, K., van Unnik, J. A. M., Mioduszewski, O. and Wright, D. H. (1988). Updated Kiel classification for lymphomas. Lancet, 1, 292–293
5. Heimann, R., Ray, M. B. and Desmet, V. J. (1977). HBsAg, chronic lymphoproliferative disorders, and cirrhosis of the liver. J. Clin. Pathol, 30, 817–821
6. Naparstek, J. and Eliakim, M. (1978). Malignant lymphoproliferative disorders in chronic liver disease. Am. J. Dig. Dis., 23, 887–892
7. Bouronde, B. A., Old, J. W. and Vazques, A. J. (1962). Pathogenesis of jaundice in Hodgkin's disease. Arch. Intern. Med., 110, 872–883
8. Piken, E. P., Abraham, G. E. and Hepner, G. W. (1980). Investigation of a patient with Hodgkin's disease and cholestasis. Gastroenterology, 77, 145–147
9. Lister, T. A., Crowther, D. and Sutcliffe, S. B. (1989). Report of a committee convened to discuss the evaluation and staging of patients with Hodgkin's disease: Cotswolds meeting. J. Clin. Oncol., 7, 1630–1636
10. Bagley, C. M., Roth, J. A., Thomas, L. B. and De Vita, V. T. (1972). Clinicopathological correlation of liver biopsies in 127 patients with Hodgkin's disease. Ann. Intern. Med., 76, 219–225
11. Glees, J. P., Thomas, N., Redding, W. H., Hefney, M. and Gazet, J.-C. (1978). Liver biopsy at lymphoma laparotomy. Lancet, 1, 210–211
12. Kim, H., Dorfman, R. F. and Rosenberg, S. A. (1976). Pathology of malignant lymphomas in the liver: application in staging. In Popper, H. and Schaffner, F. (eds). Progr. Liver Dis. V. pp. 683–698. New York: Grune and Stratton
13. Hansman, M. L., Stein, H., Dallenbach, F. and Fellbaum, C. (1991). Diffuse lymphocyte-predominant Hodgkin's disease (diffuse paragranuloma). Am. J. Pathol., 138, 29–36
14. Wright, D. H. (1992). Involvement of the liver by lymphoreticular disease. In Millward-Sadler, G. H., Wright, R. and Arthur, M. J. P. (eds). Wright's Liver and Biliary Disease. 3rd edn. pp. 1138–1154. London: W B Saunders
15. Rappaport, H., Bernard, C. W., Butler, J. J., Dorfman, R. F., Lukes, R. J. and Thomas, L. B. (1971). Report of the committee on histopathological criteria contributing to staging of Hodgkin's disease. Cancer Res., 31, 1864–1865
16. Dich, N. H., Goodman, Z. D. and Klein, M. A. (1989). Hepatic involvement in Hodgkin's disease. Clues to histologic diagnosis. Cancer, 64, 2121–2126
17. Paradinas, F. J. (1993). Liver tumours and tumour-like conditions. In Wight, D. G. D. (ed.). Liver, Biliary Tract and Exocrine Pancreas. Vol. 11. Systemic Pathology. Symmers, W. S. C., series ed. 3rd edn. Edinburgh: Churchill Livingstone
18. Hamilton-Dutoit, S. J., Pallesen, G., Franzmann, M. B. et al. (1991). AIDS related lymphoma. Histopathology, immunophenotype and association with Epstein-Barr virus as demonstrated by in situ nucleic acid hybridization. Am. J. Pathol., 138, 149–163
19. Jaffe, E. S. (1987). Malignant lymphomas: pathology of hepatic involvement. Semin. Liver Dis., 7, 257–268
20. Scoazec, J. Y., Degott, C., Brousse, N., Barge, J., Molas, G., Potet, F. and Benhamou, J.-P. (1991). Non-Hodgkin's lymphoma presenting as a primary tumour of the liver: presentation, diagnosis and outcome in 8 patients. Hepatology, 13, 870–875
21. Caccamo, D., Pervez, N. K. and Marchevsky, A. (1986). Primary lymphoma of the liver in acquired immunodeficiency syndrome. Arch. Pathol. Lab. Med., 110, 553–555
22. Anthony, P. P., Sarsfield, P. and Clarke, T. (1990). Primary lymphoma of the liver: clinical and pathological features of 10 patients. J. Clin. Pathol., 43, 1007–1013
23. Wilson, M. S., Weiss, L. M., Gatter, K. C., Mason, D. Y., Dorfman, R. F. and Warnke, R. A. (1990). Malignant histiocytosis. A reassessment of cases previously reported in 1975 based on paraffin section immunophenotyping studies. Cancer, 66, 530–536
24. O'Connor, N. T. J., Crick, J. A., Wainscot, J. S., Gatter, K. C., Falini, B. and Mason, D. Y. (1986). Evidence for monclonal T-lymphocyte proliferation in angioimmunoblastic lymphadenopathy. J. Clin. Pathol., 39, 1229–1232
25. Nanba, K., Soban, E. J., Bowling, M. C. and Berard, C. W. (1977). Splenic pseudosinuses and hepatic angiomatous lesions. Distinctive features of hairy cell leukaemia. Am. J. Clin. Pathol., 67, 415–426
26. Heyn, R. M., Hamoudi, A. and Newton, W. A. (1990). Pre-treatment liver biopsy in 20 children with histiocytosis X: a clinico-pathologic correlation. Med. Pediatr. Oncol., 18, 110–118
27. Schjølseth, S. A. (1978). Lymphomatoid granulomatosis of lung, liver and spleen. Scand. J. Haematol., 21, 104–108

Transplantation

26

LIVER TRANSPLANTATION

Starzl and his colleagues carried out the first human allograft in 1963, and Calne followed in Cambridge in 1968. The procedure remained confined to a small number of centres until the NIH Consensus Development Conference in 1983[1]. The meeting concluded that liver transplantation was by then an acceptable form of treatment which should be offered more widely. Recent figures suggest that the current transplant rate is about 5 per million population in 69 centres in Europe and about 9 per million in 66 centres in the USA[2]. The acceleration in the world transplant rate has been matched in Cambridge where nearly 700 patients had been treated by mid-1992.

Although the early results were discouraging there has been a significant improvement in survival over the last few years, and the one-year figure now exceeds 80% for certain diagnoses such as biliary atresia[3]. The indications for liver grafting include almost any fatal liver disease. In recent years, because of the very high recurrence rate, fewer primary tumours are now treated by transplantation, but the number of children has increased dramatically. More patients with acute hepatic failure, for example following drug-induced hepatic necrosis, are also now being considered for treatment in this way.

Monitoring graft outcome

In clinical practice, both blind core biopsy and fine needle aspiration biopsy (see below) can be used to monitor the progress of the graft. Both have their place. In our series, contrary to our early experience[4], biopsy is now performed routinely at the end of transplantation ('time zero'), and on day 7, and thereafter when clinically indicated, especially before modifying immunosuppressive therapy.

Most post-transplant biopsies need to be processed urgently. If the clinicians are to be persuaded to await the results before initiating treatment, a result will have to be available within a few hours. With modern processing machines a turnaround time for formalin fixed material of $3-3\frac{1}{2}$ hours should be easily achieved[5], without significant loss of quality. Because of the need to provide a rapid answer the interpretation is generally made solely on haematoxylin and eosin sections. Our own current practice is to cut 50 serial sections at 5 μm from the block, placing about five sections per slide. The first, fifth and tenth slides are then stained. The remainder of the mounted sections are subsequently stained or filed for later retrospective studies.

Although conventional histological diagnosis must take precedence over other techniques, with modern Menghini-type disposable biopsy needles there is usually enough tissue to spare for both electron microscopy and for frozen sections. Even if not immediately used samples for the latter should be taken and stored whenever possible.

The interpretation of transplant biopsies is not always straightforward. In contrast to the position with routine biopsy practice, where one expects to find a unifying single disease to explain the patient's illness, more than one diagnosis is extremely common in transplant material[2]. There may often, for example, because it is so common, be evidence of rejection together with some other condition such as bacterial infection. These difficult-

ies often magnify with increasing time after the operation[6]. Also, abnormalities may be very focal and so it is most important to examine all the stained sections.

Fine needle aspiration biopsy (FNAB)

FNAB was developed in Helsinki firstly in the context of renal grafts[7], and then subsequently applied to liver transplants[8]. To eliminate the problem of contamination of the aspirate by blood, white cell differential counts are performed simultaneously on FNAB and blood smears and the latter is then subtracted from the former. The technique has the advantage that it can be frequently repeated, even more than once daily if necessary, because of the low risks associated with the fine calibre of needle used. It is particularly useful for monitoring the quality of the infiltrate in acute cellular rejection, since, especially with the help of monoclonal or polyclonal antibodies, the identification of individual cell types may be easier than in histological preparations. Limited information can also be obtained on parenchymal changes since hepatocytes are also aspirated. Tissue biopsy is, however, essential when an assessment of architectural changes is needed, especially for example when irreversible lesions are suspected. As the chances of finding acute rejection are much lower more than a few weeks after transplantation, so the accuracy of FNAB diagnosis diminishes. Kirby et al.[9] found that in samples taken later than two months after transplantation no less than 40% gave inaccurate information.

The complications of liver transplantation, which can broadly be divided into those which affect the graft and those which affect the host, are shown in Table 26.1

Table 26.1 Complications of liver transplantation

Those which affect the graft	Those which affect the host
Technical	Infection
Rejection	Graft-versus-host disease
Disease recurrence	New tumours
Drug toxicity	

Technical complications

The favoured operation is removal of the diseased liver and insertion of the graft in an orthotopic position in the hepatic fossa. The donor liver, obtained from a patient with an intact circulation who has been declared brainstem dead[10], is cooled by perfusion through the portal vein and hepatic artery and the biliary tree and gallbladder are flushed with perfusate. The liver is then dissected free and can be satisfactorily preserved for up to 20 hours, allowing transportation from another centre if necessary. Technical complications tend to be maximal in the first two weeks after surgery. The recipient operation, technically demanding in any case, is frequently complicated by portal hypertension with often numerous adhesions between the liver and other organs and the parietal peritoneum, each the source of portal-systemic anastomoses. Impaired haemostasis aggravates the situation in many of these cases. Conversely, one of the vascular anastomoses, especially that of the hepatic artery, may thrombose. Problems with the biliary anastomosis, once a major cause of morbidity and mortality, seem to have been largely overcome by careful attention to technique[11].

Post-perfusion injury

This is the term used for damage to the donor organ sustained either during the donor's last illness or during storage prior to transplantation. It may be severe, resulting in a complete failure of function, or it may merely cause minor biochemical and histological abnormalities. The histological abnormalities are seen mainly in the first few days after transplantation and range from extensive necrosis to occasional small foci of ballooning (Figure 26.1) and acidophilic necrosis of hepatocytes[2]. Fine droplet fat is common but variable in extent. Severe forms may prevent any graft function after surgery, a rather heterogeneous group often referred to as *primary non function*.

Rejection

Although rejection was once thought to be of little importance in liver transplantation, it is now clear that this was because of the high rate of other complications. As these have been overcome, rejection of the liver is now the major challenge in terms of patient management. Rejection is defined as graft damage cause by an immunological response by the recipient and in the kidney is traditionally classified into hyperacute, acute and chronic.

Hyperacute rejection

Hyperacute rejection is due to the presence of preformed circulating antibody directed against donor-specific antigens within the graft. It was once thought not to occur in the liver, which is clearly more resistant to this form of damage than the kidney, since grafts across ABO blood group barriers frequently survive. However, it was first clearly demonstrated experimentally in certain hyperimmunized rat models, and now is well documented in clinical transplantation, albeit very rare[12]. The time scale is much longer than is seen in kidney rejection, taking some hours to days (and therefore rendering the term hyperacute inappropriate). The liver is swollen and deeply congested with patent major vessels. Microscopically, the appearances resemble those of ischaemia with eosinophilic necrosis of both parenchyma and portal tracts, with associated haemorrhage and neutrophilic infiltration (Figure 26.2). Fibrinoid necrosis of vessel walls is unusual. Distinction from preservation injury or from ischaemic necrosis due to vascular thrombosis may not be easy on biopsy alone, but immunostaining techniques should detect immunoglobulin, C1q and C3 in vessel walls.

Acute rejection

Acute rejection is the principal form of rejection encountered in clinical transplantation and occurs in 60–80% of all patients, occurring most often in the second or third weeks. Acute rejection causes elevation of serum bilirubin, alkaline phosphatase and transaminases, often coupled with systemic symptoms such as fever and leukocytosis. Although there are now many other investigative techniques available, histology remains the 'gold standard' for the diagnosis of acute rejection against which the other techniques are measured.

Acute rejection has three cardinal features, portal tract inflammation, bile duct damage and vascular inflammation[13,14], which may be quite patchy requiring examination of a number of different levels. The portal infiltrate is dominated by lymphocytes, including blast cells, and eosinophils, which may spill over into the parenchyma at the limiting plate (Figures 26.3–26.5). Bile duct damage consists of infiltration of biliary epithelium by lymphocytes and/or neutrophil polymorphs and associated degenerative changes such as vacuolation or nuclear loss (Figure 26.3). The vascular damage, or *endotheliitis*, consists of attachment of lymphocytes to the endothelium of portal and hepatic venules with infiltration beneath the intima, and, in the case of the latter, extension for a short distance into the adjacent parenchyma (Figure 26.6). More extensive involvement of the parenchyma is extremely unusual, although canalicular cholestasis is common though nonspecific.

Distinction from post-perfusion injury, infection, drug-related disease or biliary obstruction (or more than one, in any combination) is not always easy, but biliary tract disease can usually be confidently excluded by other investigations such as a T-tube cholangiogram. Infection is also best excluded by other means, but it is important to recognize that otherwise uncomplicated acute rejection may be associated with quite striking neutrophil infiltration in and around bile ducts (Figure 26.3).

Acute rejection generally responds to boosted immunosuppression and as the portal inflammation recedes and the proportion of blast cells, and of lymphocytes in general, diminishes. Cholestasis may persist rather longer.

Chronic rejection

Chronic rejection occurs in between 10 and 20% of patients who survive beyond the first month, and generally appears between one month and six months. It has two defining components, bile duct loss (or *Vanishing Bileduct Syndrome*), which affects mainly ducts less than 75 mμ in diameter (Figures 26.7 and 26.8), and foam-cell endovasculitis (or *Transplant Atherosclerosis*), which affects mainly larger first, second and third order branches of the hepatic artery (Figures 26.8–26.10)[2,15]. When fully developed, diagnosis is straightforward since portal tracts of a size normally sampled by a biopsy needle are completely without bile ducts. The vascular lesion is only seen in biopsies in about 10% of cases, but in the removed liver it stands out as bright yellow thickening of the major branches of the hepatic artery. Most patients have two additional features, marked canalicular cholestasis and persistent dropout of centrilobular hepatocytes (Figure 26.11).

Chronic rejection is thought to be irreversible and is thus an absolute indication for retransplantation.

Recurrent disease

All forms of malignancy have a high risk of recurrence[16], ranging from about 70% with HCC to 90% for CCA, although patients with 'small' HCC found incidentally may fare better. Hepatitis B also has a very high chance of recurrence, usually from 4 to 8 weeks after transplantation. The same is probably true of hepatitis C, although the data are still incomplete. Budd-Chiari Syndrome has a small but definite risk of recurrence, probably because the majority of patients have an underlying haematological disorder causing increased thrombotic tendency. Autoimmune chronic active hepatitis has a small risk of recurrence, whilst the true risk of recurrence of primary biliary cirrhosis and of primary sclerosing cholangitis remains a matter for debate[2].

All of these conditions have the same histological characteristics as in non-transplant patients.

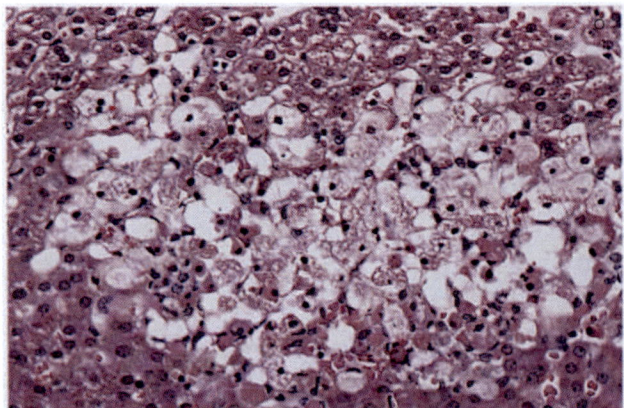

Figure 26.1 Post–perfusion injury. Liver function tests were slow to recover in the days following transplantation. This biopsy was taken at 5 days and shows ballooning of hepatocytes in zone 3, a change which is usually fully reversible.

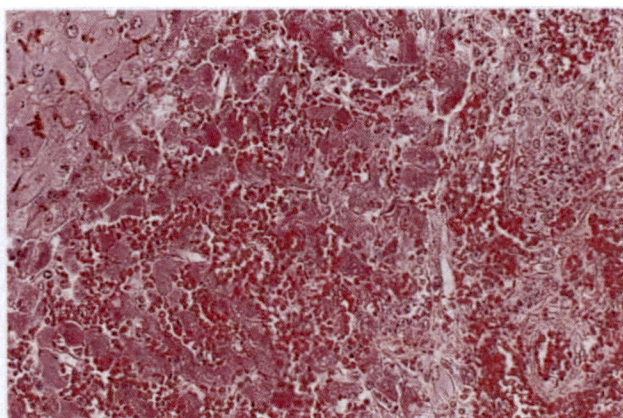

Figure 26.2 Hyperacute rejection. Acute haemorrhagic necrosis of this graft following an ABO blood group mismatch.
The author is deeply indebted to Prof. Michel Reynès who kindly supplied the slide from which this photograph was prepared.

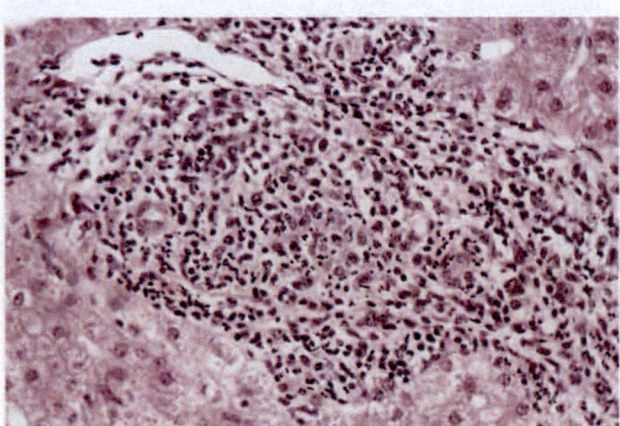

Figure 26.3 Acute rejection. Vigorous acute rejection occurring on the fourth day after transplantation. Note the marked expansion of this portal tract which is filled with inflammatory cells. These are mainly mononuclear, except at the site of the small bile ducts, which have become totally disrupted, and here the cells also include neutrophil polymorphs.

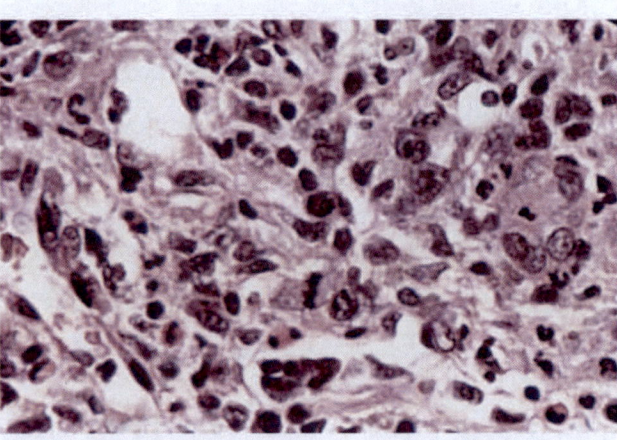

Figure 26.4 Acute rejection. Seventh day after transplantation. High magnification showing that the infiltrate is mainly mononuclear and includes a number of blast cells and other cells in mitosis.

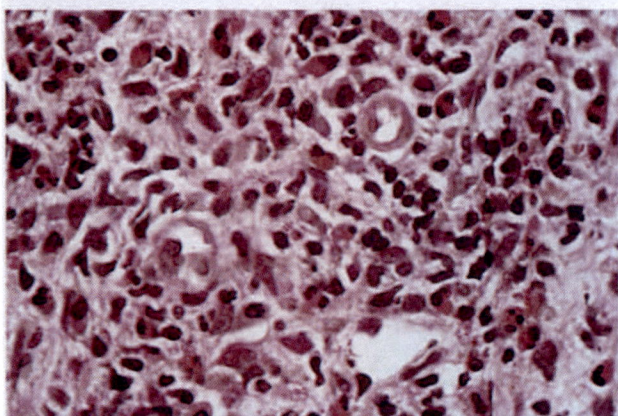

Figure 26.5 Acute rejection. Another example, from the thirteenth day, showing a significant proportion of eosinophils in the infiltrate.

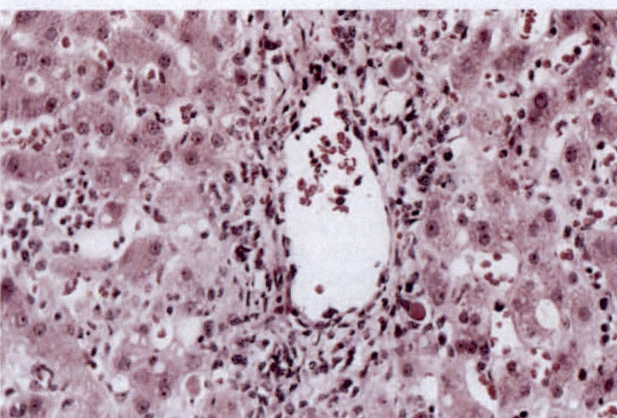

Figure 26.6 Acute rejection. Severe acute rejection on the sixth day after transplantation showing endotheliitis of this terminal hepatic venule, and extension into the adjacent parenchyma along the sinusoids. Hepatocytes are almost entirely unaffected by the process.

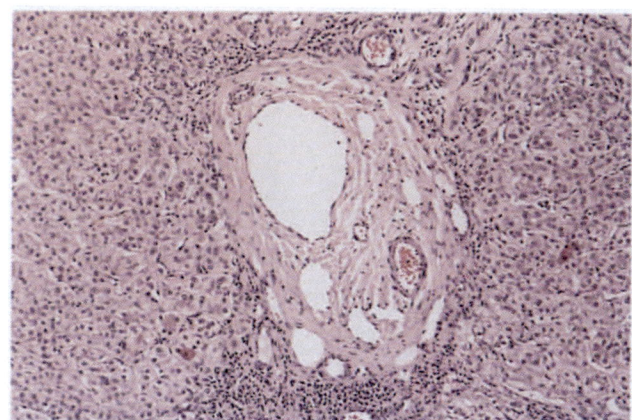

Figure 26.7   Chronic rejection-vanishing bile duct syndrome. A 52-year-old female received a liver graft for hepatocellular carcinoma. Progressive jaundice following surgery. Normal biliary tree. Biopsy at 6 months shows a small portal tract completely devoid of bile ducts. Note also the absence of inflammatory cells.

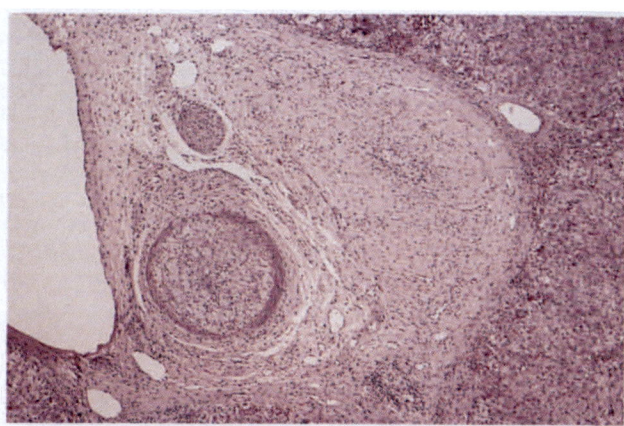

Figure 26.8   Chronic rejection. Another similar case to Figure 26.7, showing a septal portal tract in which the bile duct is represented by a fibrous scar, and the accompanying artery is completely occluded by subintimal foam cells.

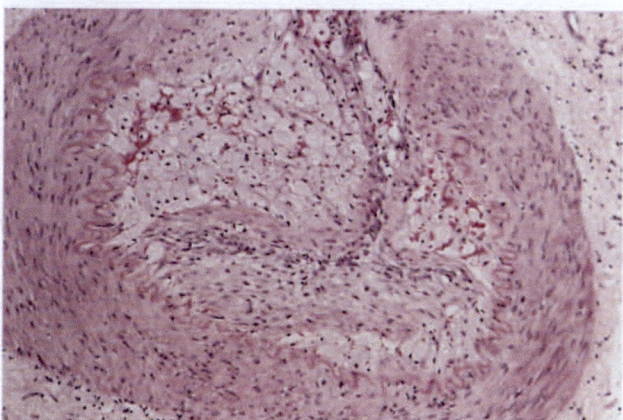

Figure 26.9   Chronic rejection-arteriopathy. Similar case to that shown in Figures 26.7 and 26.8, this specimen from the subsequent hepatectomy. The artery is one of the first order branches at the hilum, and shows complete obliteration of the lumen by subintimal foam cells.

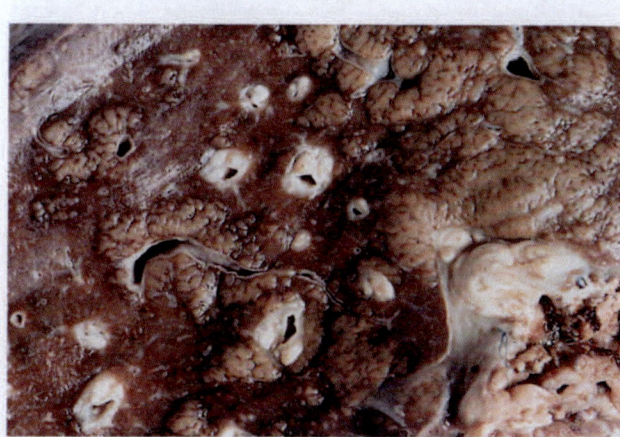

Figure 26.10   Chronic rejection. A 22-year-old female who received a liver transplant eight months previously for subacute viral hepatitis. The macroscopic picture shows the yellow profiles of the hepatic arteries, all of which contained large numbers of foam cells. Note also the extensive ischaemic parenchymal collapse.

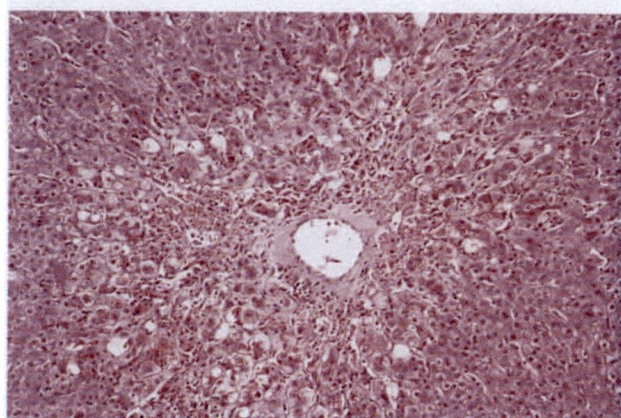

Figure 26.11   Chronic rejection. Same patient as Figure 26.10. Note the zone 3 canalicular cholestasis and liver cell loss, which are common secondary findings in chronic rejection.

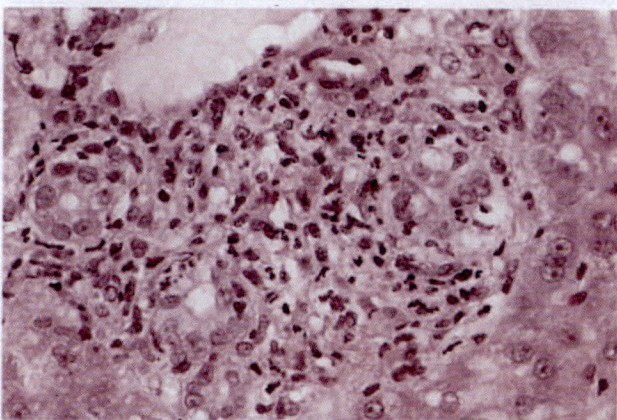

Figure 26.12   Graft-versus-host disease. Progressive jaundice following bone marrow transplantation for chronic myeloid leukaemia. This biopsy, taken on day thirty-seven, shows mononuclear cell infiltration of portal tracts, and especially of bile duct epithelium. Note the resemblance to acute liver transplant rejection.

Drug and toxic injury

Drug and/or toxic injury in the hepatic allograft is difficult to identify with certainty[17]. Whilst all patients receive a variety of potentially toxic drugs, it may be very difficult to distinguish their effect from those of other factors such as infection or rejection. Cyclosporin, FK506, azathioprine, corticosteroids, total parenteral nutrition, and various antibiotic drugs have all been implicated[17], but most have no associated specific morphological features. Azathioprine may be the exception in this respect, and may cause cholestasis and veno-occlusive disease in a small number of patients[18,19].

Complications affecting the host

As with any immunosuppressed patient, there is an increased risk of bacterial, viral, fungal and protozoal infections. These are mostly diagnosed by non-histological means, but are important in differential diagnosis. Viral infections include the opportunist viruses, especially cytomegalovirus and to a lesser extent the other herpesviruses, and the hepatitis viruses especially hepatitis B and hepatitis C (non-A, non-B). The appearances are the same in transplant patients as in non transplant patients.

All transplant patients have a small increased risk of malignant lymphoma, almost exclusively B-cell, probably mostly EB virus related[20]. Graft-versus-host disease has been described in a small number of patients and affects the skin and gastrointestinal tract in the same way as in bone marrow grafts (see below)[21], but the liver, since it is the source of the foreign lymphocytes, is spared.

BONE MARROW TRANSPLANTATION

Bone marrow transplantation is now a common treatment for both aplastic anaemia and acute leukaemias in many centres in Europe and North America. Graft-versus-host disease is one of the principal complications of allogeneic grafts and affects about 70% of patients[22]. The effects of this are felt mainly in the epithelia of the skin, gut and liver, leading to a characteristic erythroderma, diarrhoea and jaundice. As with liver transplants, the interpretation of the liver lesions is often complicated by the uncertain influence of other factors such as opportunistic infections, drugs and irradiation. However, the changes are well documented[22,23]. The primary lesion is bile duct damage. This takes the form of degenerative changes, with cell swelling, nuclear atypia or pyknosis and, in later cases, frank necrosis of the epithelium. These changes are closely similar to those observed in acute rejection of liver grafts (see above, Figure 26.12). The veno-occlusive disease described in a number of reports is probably attributable to non-immunological factors such as prior drug treatment, especially azathioprine, and irradiation[18]. Cholestasis and Kupffer cell hyperplasia are almost invariable seen[24]. Bernau and her colleagues[24] noted close membrane contacts between lymphocytes and both hepatocytes and bile duct epithelium and suggested that the necrosis was a manifestation of direct lymphocyte cytotoxicity, and that all the other findings were secondary to these primary lesions. This view is supported by other authors. although most have found portal lymphocytes to be rather sparse[25], an observation which perhaps can be explained by the long interval between graft and histological examination in many of these cases.

LIVER DISEASE IN RENAL TRANSPLANT RECIPIENTS

Liver disease is a common complication of renal transplantation, but is largely non-specific[26]. Acute viral hepatitis, cytomegalovirus and herpes simplex are all quite common

as opportunistic infections. Chronic hepatitis is a serious problem which affects up to 16% of patients and progresses to cirrhosis in at least half.

REFERENCES

1. NIH. (1984). National Institutes of Health Consensus Development Conference Statement. Hepatology, 4, 107S–110S
2. Wight, D. G. D. (1993). The pathology of liver transplantation. In Wight, D. G. D. (ed.). Liver, Biliary Tract and Exocrine Pancreas. Vol. 11. Systemic Pathology. Symmers, W. S. C., series ed. 3rd edn. Edinburgh: Churchill Livingstone
3. Bismuth, H., Castaing, D., Ericzon, B. G., Otte, J. B., Rolles, K., Ringe, B. and Sloof, M. (1987). Hepatic transplantation in Europe. First report of the European Liver Transplant Registry. Lancet, 2, 674–676
4. Wight, D. G. D. (1984). The morphology of rejection of liver of liver transplants. In Calne, R. Y. (ed.). Transplant Immunology, Clinical and Experimental. pp. 385–435. Oxford: Oxford University Press
5. McCue, P. A. and Santoianni, R. A. (1988). Expedited handling of transplantation biopsies. Am. J. Surg. Pathol., 12, 155–157
6. Nakhleh, R. E., Schwarzenberg, S. J., Bloomer, J., Payne, W. and Snover, D. C. (1990). The pathology of liver allografts surviving longer than one year. Hepatology, 11, 465–470
7. Häyry, P. and von Willebrand, E. (1984). Transplant aspiration cytology. Transplantation., 38, 7–12.
8. Lautenschlager, I., Höckerstedt, K. and Häyry, P. (1991). Fine-needle aspiration biopsy in the monitoring of liver allografts. Transplant Int., 4, 54–61
9. Kirby, R. M., Young, J. A., Hübscher, S. G., Elias, E. and McMaster, P. (1988). The accuracy of aspiration cytology in the diagnosis of rejection following orthotopic liver transplantation. Transplant Internat., 1, 119–126.
10. Conference of Medical Royal Colleges and the Faculties in the United Kingdom. (1976). Diagnosis of brain-stem death. Br. Med. J., 2, 1187–1188.
11. Klein, A. S., Savader, S., Burdick, J. F., Fair, J., Mitchell, M., Colombani, P., Perler, B., Osterman, F. and M, W. G. (1991). Reduction of morbidity and mortality from biliary complications after liver transplantation. Hepatology, 14, 818–823
12. Demetris, A. J., Jaffe, R., Tzakis, A., Ramsey, G., Todo, S., Belle, S., Esquivel, C., Shapiro, R., Markus, B., Mroczek, E., van Thiel, D. H., Sysyn, G., Gordon, R., Makowka, L. and Starzl, T. (1988). Antibody-mediated rejection of human orthotopic liver allografts. A study of liver transplantation across ABO blood group barriers. Am. J. Pathol., 132, 489–502
13. Snover, D. C., Freese, D. K., Sharp, H. L., Bloomer, J. R., Najarian, J. S. and Ascher, N. L. (1987). Liver allograft rejection. An analysis of the use of biopsy in determining the outcome of rejection. Am. J. Surg. Pathol., 11, 1–10
14. Wiesner, R. H. (1992). Hepatic Allograft Rejection. Semin. Liver Dis., 12, No 1 [whole issue]
15. Freese, D. K., Snover, D. C., Sharp, H. L., Gross, C. R., Savick, S. K. and Payne, W. D. (1991). Chronic rejection after liver transplantation: a study of clinical, histological and immunological features. Hepatology, 13, 882–891
16. O'Grady, J. and Williams, R. (1988). Long-term management, complications, and disease recurrence. In Maddrey, W. C. (ed.). Transplantation of the liver. Current Topics in Gastroenterology. pp. 143–165. New York: Elsevier
17. Demetris, A. J., Kakizoe, S. and Oguma, S. (1990). Pathology of liver transplantation. In Williams, J. W. (ed). Hepatic Transplantation. pp. 59–111. Philadelphia: W B Saunders
18. Weitz, H., Gokel, S. M., Loeschke, K., Possinger, K. and Eder, M. (1982). Venoocclusive disease of the liver in patients receiving immunosuppressive therapy. Virch. Arch. [A], 395, 245–256
19. Sterneck, M., Wiesner, R. H., Ascher, N., Roberts, J., Ferrel, L., Ludwig, J. and Lake, J. (1991). Azathioprine toxicity after liver transplantation. Hepatology, 14, 806–810
20. Wilkinson, A. H., Smith, J. L., Hunsicker, L. G., Tobacman, J., Kapelanski, D. P., Johnson, M., and Wright, F. H. (1989). Increased frequence of postransplant lymphomas in patients treated with cyclosporine, azathioprine and prednisolone. Transplantation, 47, 293–296
21. Jamieson, N. V., Joysey, V., Friend, P. J., Marcus, R., Ramsbottom, S., Baglin, T., Johnston, P. S., Williams, R. and Calne, R. Y. (1991). Graft–versus–host disease in solid organ transplantation. Transpl. Int., 4, 67–71
22. Snover, D. C., Weisdorf, S. A., Ramsay, N. K., McGlave, P. and

Kersey, J. H. (1984). Hepatic graft–versus–host disease: a study of the predictive value of liver biopsy in diagnosis. Hepatology, 4, 123–130

23. Knapp, A. B., Crawford, J. M., Rappeport, J. M. and Gollan, J. L. (1987). Cirrhosis as a consequence of graft-versus-host disease. Gastroenterology, 92, 513–519

24. Bernau, D., Gisselbrecht, C., Devergie, A., Feldmann, G., Gluckman, E., Marty, M. and Boiron, M. (1980). Histological and ultrastructural appearance of the liver during GVH disease complicating bone marrow transplantation. Transplantation, 29, 236–244

25. Sloane, J. P., Farthing, M. J. G. and Powles, R. L. (1980). Histopathological changes in the liver after allogeneic bone marrow transplantation. J. Clin. Pathol., 33, 344–350

26. Sopko, J. and Anuras, S. (1978). Liver disease in renal transplant recipients. Am. J. Med., 64, 139–146

Index

Numbers in italic type refer to colour figures

The manufacturer's authorised representative in the EU is Springer
Nature Customer Service Centre GmbH, Europaplatz 3, 69115 Heidelberg,
Germany. If you have any concerns regarding our products, please
contact ProductSafety@springernature.com

Printed and bound by CPI Group (UK) Ltd, Croydon, CR0 4YY

06/05/2026

02100427-0001